Revision Note
MRCP 2 PACES

Revision Notes for
MRCP 2 PACES

Shibley Rahman

MA MB BChir PhD (Cantab) MRCP (UK) LLB (Hons)

British Lung Foundation

London (UK)

Avinash Sharma

MBBS MRCP (UK)

Consultant Physician

Luton and Dunstable NHS Foundation Trust

Luton, UK

JAYPEE BROTHERS MEDICAL PUBLISHERS (P) LTD

London (UK) • St Louis (USA) • Panama City (Panama) • New Delhi • Ahmedabad
Bengaluru • Chennai • Hyderabad • Kochi • Kolkata • Lucknow • Mumbai • Nagpur

Published by
Jitendar P Vij
Jaypee Brothers Medical Publishers (P) Ltd

Corporate Office
4838/24 Ansari Road, Daryaganj, **New Delhi** - 110002, India, Phone: +91-11-43574357, Fax: +91-11-43574314

Registered Office
B-3 EMCA House, 23/23B Ansari Road, Daryaganj, **New Delhi** - 110 002, India
Phones: +91-11-23272143, +91-11-23272703, +91-11-23282021
+91-11-23245672, Rel: +91-11-32558559, Fax: +91-11-23276490, +91-11-23245683
e-mail: jaypee@jaypeebrothers.com, Website: www.jaypeebrothers.com

Offices in India

- **Ahmedabad**, Phone: Rel: +91-79-32988717, e-mail: ahmedabad@jaypeebrothers.com
- **Bengaluru**, Phone: Rel: +91-80-32714073, e-mail: bangalore@jaypeebrothers.com
- **Chennai**, Phone: Rel: +91-44-32972089, e-mail: chennai@jaypeebrothers.com
- **Hyderabad**, Phone: Rel:+91-40-32940929, e-mail: hyderabad@jaypeebrothers.com
- **Kochi**, Phone: +91-484-2395740, e-mail: kochi@jaypeebrothers.com
- **Kolkata**, Phone: +91-33-22276415, e-mail: kolkata@jaypeebrothers.com
- **Lucknow**, Phone: +91-522-3040554, e-mail: lucknow@jaypeebrothers.com
- **Mumbai**, Phone: Rel: +91-22-32926896, e-mail: mumbai@jaypeebrothers.com
- **Nagpur**, Phone: Rel: +91-712-3245220, e-mail: nagpur@jaypeebrothers.com

Overseas Offices

- **North America Office, USA,** Ph: 001-636-6279734
  e-mail: jaypee@jaypeebrothers.com, anjulav@jaypeebrothers.com
- **Central America Office, Panama City, Panama,** Ph: 001-507-317-0160
  e-mail: cservice@jphmedical.com, Website: www.jphmedical.com
- **Europe Office, UK,** Ph: +44 (0) 2031708910, e-mail: dholman@jpmedical.biz

Revision Notes for MRCP 2 PACES

© 2010, Jaypee Brothers Medical Publishers

First Edition: **2010**

ISBN 978-81-8448-893-7

Typeset at JPBMP typesetting unit

Printed at Rajkamal Electric Press, Plot No. 2, Phase-IV, Kundli, Haryana.

PREFACE

The authors had two principal aims in writing this text: namely, (i) to explain the ethos and format of the examination, and (ii) to provide a core body of information useful for the examination. Whilst this examination is demanding, it is still essentially simply an assessment of basic competence required for higher specialist training. The Royal College of Physicians believe that have developed an examination, which they intend to be fair and to be an appropriate test of postgraduate knowledge in Doctors preparing for higher specialist training and since 2001 the examination has been running very successfully. The academic aims of the MRCP(UK) examination are stated clearly:

- To test a wide range of up-to-date medical knowledge so that physicians in training are encouraged to develop their full clinical and professional potential;
- To maintain and improve the practice of clinical medicine;
- To provide a sound basis for continuing medical education.

Much of this book has been derived from authors; own experiences regarding the examination, and where possible sample instructions have been given for individual cases in the real examination. However, the content of the book closely follows the syllabus as published in the **MRCP Clinical Guidelines.** The authors to their knowledge have been aware of all of these cases having appeared in the Membership clinical examination at least once.

Management issues/guidance/protocols are all subject to change with time, and therefore the reader is advised to supplement his/her reading with other sources, for example, from the Royal College of Physicians or the National Institute of Clinical Excellence.

Whilst the delivery of the examination is possibly subject to change with modernisation of the medical curriculum, the content of the higher specialist training is unlikely to change in the imminent future. Please consult the *www.mrcpuk.org* website for current schedules. The marksheets are available in the Clinical Guidelines and on the website.

Much of this book has been derived from a synthesis of teaching and examining for the examination nationally in the UK, although the standards in international centres are exactly the same as in the UK.

The authors wish to emphasise that whilst there is much factual material in this book, this examination is essentially a test of clinical skills, and candidates with much general medical clinical experience pass and those who do not have this experience fail.

As in all good movies, any reference to a real person in the fictitious scenarios contained in this book is purely coincidental. Good luck!

Shibley Rahman
Avinash Sharma

ACKNOWLEDGEMENTS

Dr Rahman would like to acknowledge his parents and relatives for their invaluable inspiration. Dr Sharma would also like to thank Laura for her unending support.

CONTENTS

CONTENTS

PLATE (1)

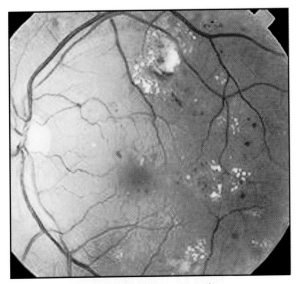

Figure 8.2: Diabetic retinopathy

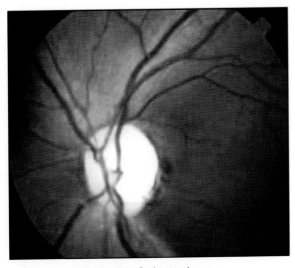

Figure 8.3: Optic atrophy

PLATE (2)

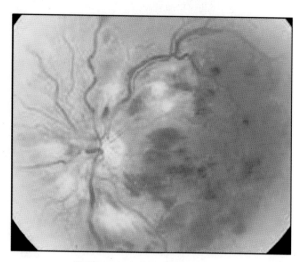

Figure 8.4: Retinal vein occlusion

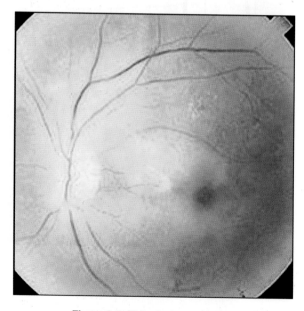

Figure 8.5: Retinal artery occlusion

PLATE (3)

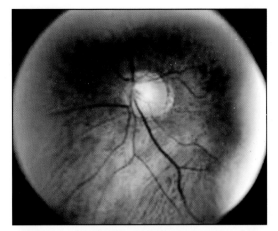

Figure 8.6: Glaucoma

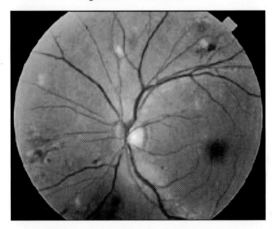

Figure 8.7: Hypertensive retinopathy

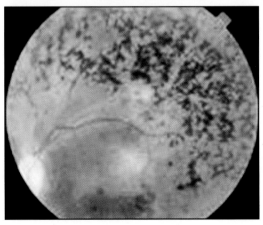

Figure 8.8: Retinitis pigmentosa

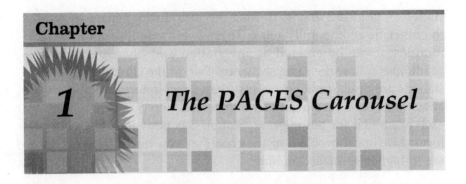

Chapter

1   *The PACES Carousel*

WHY PACES?

PACES is the acronym for 'Practical Assessment of Clinical Examination Skills', the practical component of the MRCP examination. It was first held in June 2001 replacing the previous clinical (long case and short cases) and oral examination. The introduction of a huge revision of the examination involved major changes for candidates, examiners, teachers, local organisers, and central administration throughout the world.

What are the Aims of the PACES Examination?

The aims of the PACES examination have been clearly stated in the curriculum (*MRCP(UK) Part 2 Clinical Examination (PACES) and clinical guidelines 2001/2*). They are to:
- Demonstrate the clinical skills of history taking
- Examine a patient appropriately to detect the presence or absence of physical signs
- Interpret physical signs
- Make appropriate diagnosis
- Develop and discuss emergency, immediate and long-term management plans
- Communicate clinical information to colleagues, patients or their relative
- Discuss ethical issues

How does the PACES Carousel Work?

Five candidates rotate through five 20 minute stations, separated by upto 5 minutes for change-over and waiting (Fig. 1.1). The cycle begins with a five minute wait which enables candidates at the two talking stations (stations 2 and 4) to read the introductory material, whilst the other three hopefully relax. The whole cycle therefore lasts 125 minutes; it can be entered at any station and, thereafter, the five candidates follow the same sequence. Two of the clinical examination stations are double stations; two systems, respiratory and abdominal, at station 1, and cardiovascular and central nervous, at station 3, are each examined for ten minutes. Station 5 is now an assessment of a focussed clinical problem of the type that you might be expected to see in higher specialist training.

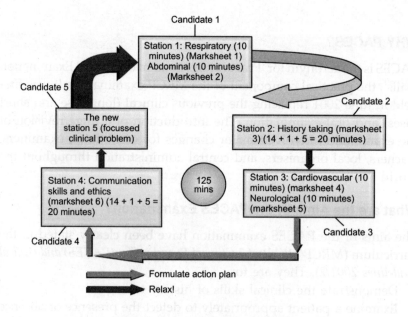

Figure 1.1: Carousel of PACES stations

The talking stations, stations 2 and 4, begin with an al limportant waiting period outside the room, when the candidates read the instructions and introductory material and should devise an action plan for what is to follow. Within the station, they will spend 14 minutes talking to the patient/subject or surrogate, followed by one minute's reflection, during which the subject usually leaves the room and, then, a five minute discussion with one or both examiners.

Time
Time-keeping is a key to success for both the PACES examination and the candidate to succeed. The traditional system of bells and verbal

warnings are used together with additional prompts, for a slow candidate running out of time. Bells are rung at the beginning and end of the five 20 minute stations and, usually, at 10 minutes in the two double stations (1 and 3). The examiner will often draw the candidate's attention to a clock, or, better still, will start a stop clock in the room. In the two talking stations (2 and 4), a verbal 2 minutes warning will be given at 12 minutes. Time management is also increasingly important in every clinician's daily work. Although, it is not explicitly tested in PACES, it is implicit in the strict, but relevant, time limits set to undertake the various tasks.

It may occur to the candidates that if they prolong their time examining a patient, it may shorten the discussion time (and, of course, potential hostile questions). This is not advisable; although examiners will award some marks for the candidate's examination technique they are observing, the majority of marks will go to the candidate's correct clinical findings, the interpretation of them in a diagnosis or differential diagnosis, and discussion of further relevant management. As in all examinations, the way to avoid difficult questions is for the candidate to be pro-active and try, if possible, to control the discussion by talking good sense. Most examiners will not interrupt them if what they are saying is relevant. Examiners get irritated by the slow candidate who, in addition, may go back to repeat their examination, suggesting a lack of confidence in their findings.

The times allocated for the tasks you are given at each station, and substation, are realistic by the standards that apply in everyday practice. On exception to this, which was soon appreciated by PACES examiners, is that candidates would not have time to perform a full neurological examination, in the detail specified in the guidelines, in the time allocated. The solution lay in the introduction to the case where candidates should be directed specifically to which part of the CNS they would be required to examine, e.g. "the arms", "the legs", "the cranial nerves", "speech" etc. Such limitation placed on the examination of a particular system should not preclude the candidate from saying in their presentation that he or she would investigate further. A generous examiner would even supply the missing information!

If you are uncertain about the instructions given relating to the examination, or any other aspect of the case for that matter, **please ask the examiner for clarification.** Examiners will frequently ask the candidates, after they have read the written instructions, *"Do you understand?"*

Marksheets

You must be familiar with the contents of the seven marksheets as they are the cornerpiece of the PACES examination. They are easily accessed, either on the website, or in the Regulations (free), in the references above. More than recording the marks awarded, they contain the necessary demographic information and detailed breakdown and checklist of the component parts of each problem posed at each station. This is essential to the fairness of the marking systems and also enables detailed feedback to be given to candidates, as well as forming the basis of counselling on the rare occasions that this is recommended.

Each marksheet has four sections and, partly, uses boxes to be filled using a 2B pencil, to facilitate computer scanning:

1. Candidate

The candidate prints their NAME and fill in their EXAMINATION NUMBER and the CENTRE NUMBER boxes on each of the seven pairs of sheets handed to them by the organising registrar (the sheet number boxes corresponding to the station is already filled in).

2. Examiner

The examiners write in (a box) a brief description of the CASE followed by PRINTING and SIGNING their name, and, finally, their EXAMINATION NUMBER.

3. Conduct of Case

Except for Station 5 (Marksheet 7), which is appreviated, there are three parts for the four major clinical substations.

At stations 1 and 3, the first part is headed "Physical examination", followed by bullet points relevant to that system; the second part is headed "Identification and interpretation of physical signs" with three bullet points: "Identifies abnormal physical signs correctly", "Interprets signs correctly", and "Makes correct diagnosis". The third part is headed "Discussion related to the case" with two bullet points: "Familiar with appropriate investigation and sequence" and "Famililar with appropriate further therapy and management".

These second and third parts are identified for the four major systems (marksheets 1, 2, 4 and 5) and examiners are expected for each of the three parts to fill ONE of the four boxes: Clear pass, pass, fail, clear fail. Station 5 (marksheet 7) is divided into the four minor systems examined and each, in turn, subdivided into the three parts discussed above (which now become bullet points as there is no room on the sheet to subdivide them further). For each of the four systems overall the examiner is required to fill ONE of the four boxes as above. The crucial part of each marksheet is the bottom line – mirroring life. The box in the bottom right-hand corner requires the examiner to make an "overall judgment" using the same four item scale which is translated into marks: clear fail – 1 mark, fail – 2 marks, pass – 3 marks, clear pass – 4 marks. Adjacent to it is a "Comments" box which every examiner must complete to explain the decision to give a fail or clear fail. If the examiner is particularly concerned about some aspect of the failure which needs to be further explored with the candidate, another adjacent box, "Counselling Recommended", is filled in. This will NOT automatically lead to the candidate being counselled but will be discussed with the other nine examiners, at the completion of the cycle, to decide whether further action is required.

The format of the marksheets for the two talking stations, Station 2 (History Taking) (Marksheet 3) and Station 4 Communication Skills (Marksheet 6) have the same tripartite structure as those for the major clinical systems, appropriately adapted, but requiring each examiner to fill in boxes, as well as, identical to the other sheets, the overall judgement, comments, and counselling boxes. Thus, the first part of Marksheet 3, is "Data gathering in the interview". The second is "Interpretation and use of information gathered", and the third, "Discussion related to the case", all with appropriate bullet points, and the examiner (and candidate). Similarly, in marksheet 6, the three parts are headed "Communication skills – conduct of interview", "Communication skills – exploration and problem negotiation" and "Ethics and law" (The bullet points are described below under the two stations).

The marksheets can be downloaded from the official MRCP website: http://www.mrcpuk.org/Pages/Home.aspx

Marking System

The overall judgement that determines each examiner's mark is not intended to be the numerical mean of the intermediate assessments made in the various sections of marksheets 1 – 6, or, even, of the separate marking of the four minor systems in marksheet 7. This is because each box filled does not carry equal weight. The value of the multiple judgements is primarily in providing feedback to candidates but also enhances broad objective marking by the examiners. It may help to avoid that they be not overimpressed by one thing the candidate has done well, ignoring several things not well done, or *vice versa*. A further aid to the examiners, available to candidates at the same sources as the marksheets, are the anchor statements. Thse try to give substance to the four gradings in assessment, under six headings: "System of examination", "Language and communication skills" (in patient encounters when examining clinical systems as well as the tarking stations", "Confidence and rapport", "Clinical method", "Discussion and appreciation of patient's concerns" and "Clinical thinking". When writing comments on a candidate who is being given an overall fail or clear fail, examiners are encouraged to select appropriate statements that define the mark; evenn if the patient achieves an overall pass or clear pass, it can still be helpful to point out deficiencies (along the way) as an individual examiner will know nothing of the assessment by the other nine examiners until afterwards.

The pass mark for each of the three diets of PACES held annually is agreed by the Clinical Examining Board at end of the examination. The maximum mark attainable by a candidate is to receive a clear pass from each examiner at every station or substation: $14 \times 4 = 56$. The minimum mark would be $14 \times 1 = 14$. An "ideal" cut off would be that the candidate should get a pass from each examiner: $14 \times 3 = 42$. Often the pass mark is simply 41.

Examiners

Examiners are widely recruited. There is no lower age limit but they will usually have been consultant physicians, or equivalent, for atleast 4 years, and have been elected FRCP of one of the UK colleges. They must have some acute general medicine content in their working practice; therefore, superspecialists may not be eligible but can contribute to question-setting. Examiners usually retire within 1 to 2 years after retirement from active clinical practice. Increasing emphasis is placed on examiner training at regular sessions and briefing before each examination. Observation of an examination, before actually examining, is mandatory. Others with an interest in the examination (teachers, course organisers, examiners from other colleges, and disciplines) may also observe and their non-participatory role will be made clear to the candidate.

The performance of examiners is remarkably consistent. Before each carousel, the paired examiners will see the patients or role players (surrogates) together and assess the ease or difficulty of a case. They will agree the criteria they will use in independently awarding the four grades/marks available. When the candidate has left the examination room each examiner completes the marksheet and puts it into a collecting box before finding out the co-examiner's mark. There is exact concurrence within one mark in over 95% of candidate-examiner encounters and exact concurrence in 60%. If necessary, a brief discussion of any discrepancy within a pair takes place before the next candidate enters.

Patients

It is a privilege that patients help with the examination, and it is therefore it is vital that you are as courteous and kind as possible to the patients. Failure to introduce yourself to and respect these patients – a point which will be repeated in this text – is unacceptable. Many patients are nervous about participating, and also are concerned about saying something that we fail you. Please be courteous to them. Many patients ask afterwards how successful you have been and are genuinely concerned you do well!

Aseptic Techniques

It would be a disaster for the Royal Colleges if patients attended the examination and then developed some form of transferred infection such as MRSA which can be tracked back to the examination. Aqueous gel or hand-washing facilities should be available, and should be used between all patients.

REFERENCE

MRCP(UK) Part 2 Clinical Examination (PACES): A review of the first four diets (June 2001 – June 2002). J Dacre, GM Besser and P White on behalf of the MRCP(UK) Clinical Examining Board. J R Coll Edinb 2003;33:285-92.

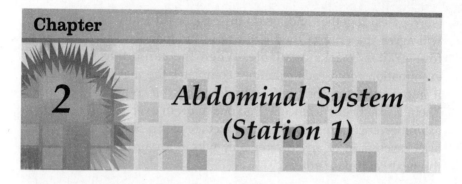

Chapter 2

Abdominal System (Station 1)

INTRODUCTION TO EXAMINATION TECHNIQUE

There are actually probably only a limited number of causes that are suitable for the **PACES** examination!

A good examination technique is critical. Do look carefully and do feel right up to the costal margins. Many candidates use the light palpation to look primarily for areas of tenderness, but if you are careful to use the technique properly it is often possible to feel the liver and spleen at this stage. If you feel an organ during light palpation, you can then check the edge more carefully during deep palpation. You can also check for movement on respiration at this stage.

METHOD OF EXAMINATION TECHNIQUE

Inspection

There are a number of features which are readily found on inspection (Fig. 2.1). The first thing to note is the nutritional status of the patient. However, there are many other signs. Look for any surgical scars.

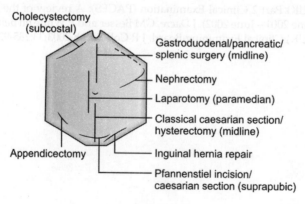

Figure 2.1

It is important to observe the general appearance of the patient, which might be suggestive of particular diagnosis, e.g. α1-antitrypsin deficiency (should be considered if signs of chronic airways disease are evident on inspection – barrel chest, purse lips, respiratory distress), or Wilson's disease: dystonic movements together with Kayser-Fleischer rings on slit-lamp. Other common features are cachexia, icterus, excoriation and bruising. Jaundice is usually detected clinically when the serum bilirubin level is more than 40 μmol/litre. Tattoos can also be seen, and may be relevant to a liver case.

Look at the shape of the abdomen: The candidate should be able to recognise different shapes of abdomen and understand their significance (e.g. symmetry or asymmetry, flatness or distension, hernias). Previous surgery (e.g. laparoscopy, laporotomy), stretch marks, intertrigo, haemorrhage, evidence of superficial veins and direction of flow.

Examine the skin for certain features: colour (anaemia, jaundice, pallor, ashen grey of Addison's disease), the evidence of previous surgery (e.g. herniotomy, laparotomy), monilial infection, bruising and evidence of superficial veins, and evidence of pigmentation (telengectasia, spider naevi, hyperpigmentation of palmar creases). Scratch marks would suggest pruritus (cholestasis). Loss of secondary sexual hair may signify genital hypoplasia. Examine for skin movement: The candidate should be able to recognise abnormal movement with respiration, visible peristalsis, or pulsations.

Examine the hands: Confirm the findings on inspection, feeling in particular for the nodular contracture of Dupuytren or any xanthoma at the elbow, parotid swelling, *fetor hepaticus*. Clubbing (chronic liver disease, inflammatory bowel disease), leukonychia (low protein state), koilonychias, Beau's lines, Dupuytren's contracture, palmar erythema (Causes: Cirrhosis, hyperthyroidism, rheumatoid arthritis, pregnancy, polycythaemia). One can examine for a flapping tremor if one suspects that the patient is encephalopathic: A coarse flap (need to evaluate for 30 s to safely rule out presence).

Examine the eyes: Note any xanthelasma around the eyes. Any arcus (white rim) is often seen around the pupil in those aged 40 and above. Look for conjunctivae pallor (retract lower eyelid) and scleral icterus (retract upper eyelid).

Examine the mouth: There are several clinical signs to be found in the mouth, including angular cheilitis (iron deficiency), glossy red stomatitis (B_{12} deficiency or Kawasaki disease), ulcers within the oral cavity (Crohn's disease), telengectasia (hereditary haemorrhagic), pigmentation at the vermilliform border (Peutz-Jehgers), buccal hyperpigmentation (Addison's disease).

Look for evidence of superficial veins: Look for these determine the direction of flow (away from umbilicus = portal hypertension; upwards from the groin = inferior vena cava obstruction). Common causes of inferior vena cava obstruction are trauma, thrombosis, renal cell carcinoma, retroperitoneal fibrosis, radiation therapy, aortic aneurysm, ascites, surgery, filter replacement, and cancer in the vena cava. Whatever the cause, patients usually develop additional or collateral veins to compensate for the occlusion. As the flow is towards the head, not away from the umbilicus (as in caput medusae of portal hypertension), the two can be delineated.

Examine for lymphadenopathy: Briefly examine from the front for Virchow's node (left supraclavicular fossae). If enlarged nodes are present, a more comprehensive examination may be required. Ideally sit the patient up. This will also enable you to look for nephrectomy scars at the lower back. You can also palpate for inguinal lymphadenopathy. It is not a good idea to miss lymph nodes if you are to perform this examination.

Other Considerations

- Inspect the antecubital fossae for the presence of arteriovenous fistula (polycystic kidney disease).
- Look for scars in the iliac fossae and lumbar regions (nephrectomy and transplanted kidney).
- Different shapes of abdomen (symmetry/asymmetry, flatness or distension). Is the entire abdomen enlarged (ascites) or are there identifiable masses within the abdomen (transplanted kidney). Ask the patient to lift only his or her shoulders off the bed to reduce any hernia that may be present.
- Don't forget to look at the umbilicus, where a superficial carcinomatous nodule may be present (Sister Mary Joseph's nodule).
- Note any gynaecomastia in the male breast. (Causes: Physiological, puberty and senility; Klinefelter's syndrome; cirrhosis; drugs, e.g. spironolactone and digoxin; testicular tumour/orchidectomy; endocrinopathy, e.g. hypo/hyperthyroidism, Addison's disease).
- Are there any pulsatile masses? Look for visible peristalsis.

Palpation

The mark scheme clearly states that organomegaly or masses should be correctly palpated. Candidates need to be able to estimate the size of an organ (e.g. liver, spleen) and to differentiate the organs that are palpable from each other. As well as kidneys, liver and spleen, other swellings may be due to:

- Gallbladder.
- Pelvic masses (e.g. bladder, uterus, ovary). The bladder and bowel may be felt in normal individuals. The bladder rises out of the pelvis in the mid-line and pressure may induce a desire to micturate. Faeces in the bowel can be idented by the examining finger, a unique feature.
- Solid masses (e.g. cancer of the stomach, caecum, abdominal lymph nodes).
- Cystic masses (e.g. pancreatic, mesenteric, ovarian). A pancreatic pseudocyst, if large, can be felt in the epigastric region; they feel fixed and do not extend.
- Pulsatile swelling (e.g. hepatic, aortic); place both hands on either side of the mass. Remember that the abdominal aorta bifurcates at the level of the umbilicus and may be easily palpable in thin patients. Always test for expansile pulsation which is present with aortic aneurysm but not if the pulsation is being transmitted. Auscultate over the swelling, a loud bruit (in the absence of a similar bruit in the heart) *supports* the diagnosis of aneurysm. The normal diameter of the aorta is 3 cm.

Table 2.1: Common causes of abdominal masses

Right iliac fossa	Left iliac fossa
• Carcinoma of the caecum • Crohn's disease • Appendix mass	• Carcinoma of the colon • Diverticular abscess
Less common	*Less common·*
• Ileocaecal TB • Ovarian cyst • Pelvic or transplanted kidney • Iliac lymphadenopathy	• Crohn's disease • Ovarian cyst • Pelvic (or transplanted) kidney • Iliac lymphadenopathy

(Causes of an epigastric mass are discussed later)

Percussion

Percussion to estimate the size of an organ (e.g. liver, spleen). Percussion should also be used to assess ascites, if considered appropriate.

Auscultation

The mark scheme includes that the candidate is expected to auscultate for bowel sounds – increased, normal, absent, and bruits – arterial, venous hum. A succussion splash may also be heard.

Conclusion of the Examination

The candidate should close with other relevant features of the abdominal examination.

One may offer to examine the external genitalia and rectum, but **MRCP Clinical Guidelines** state candidates *must not* perform rectal or vaginal examinations.

Offer to perform a urinary dipstix, especially in the renal case.

Ask for the temperature chart, BP, urinalysis, oxygen saturations.

The candidate should have acquired the ability to recognise: Nasogastric tube, gastrostomy, continuous ambulatory peritoneal dialysis or other dialysis catheter, ileostomy or colostomy, nephrostomy or vesicostomy, indwelling central venous access device for parenteral nutrition.

Common Cases

Once the abnormal signs have been elicited, they need to be presented correctly. The signs should be interpreted correctly within the context of a diagnosis or differential diagnosis. Common abdominal cases are listed below, along with related discussion of investigation and sequence, therapy and management.

CHRONIC LIVER DISEASE

This person who has been abstinent from alcohol for 5 years was found to have some abnormalities on a GP review for a mortgage. Please examine his abdomen to see if you can find any abnormality.

* Look for Dupuytren's contracture, parotid hypertrophy, features of Wernicke's encephalopathy, features of dilated cardiomyopathy. Conditions with which Dupuytren's contracture are associated are: alcoholism, chronic antiepileptic therapy, systemic conditions such as diabetes, cirrhosis, epilepsy and tuberculosis, thickening of the corpora cavernosa of the penis (Peyronie's disease), Garrod's knuckle pads, and retroperitoneal fibrosis.
* Other features (tattoos, track markers).
* Leukonychia, clubbing, palmar erythema.

- Spider naevia (small capillary angiomas found in the distribution of the superior vena cava in chronic liver disease) and caput medusae.
- Pallor/anaemia.
- Paucity of body hair.
- Muscle wasting.
- Purpura and bruising may be seen in patients with thrombocytopaenia and coagulation defects.
- Small testes.
- Ascites and ankle peripheral oedema.
- Autoimmune disease (autoimmune hepatitis)
- Xanthelasma (primary biliary cirrhosis).

Causes of chronic liver disease: Alcohol, viral hepatitis, autoimmune chronic active hepatitis, primary biliary cirrhosis, haemochromatosis, cryptogenic, cardiac failure, constrictive pericarditis, Budd-Chiari syndrome, biliary cholestasis, toxins and drugs (methotrexate, methyldopa, isoniazid, amiodarone), Wilson's disease, α_1-antitrypsin deficiency, other metabolic causes.

Causes of palmar erythema: Cirrhosis, hyperthyroidism, rheumatoid arthritis, pregnancy, polycythaemia.

Causes of cirrhosis: Chronic alcohol abuse (parotid enlargement, multiple fractures), viral hepatitis (HBV or HCV infection, i/v drugs), autoimmune disorders (primary biliary cirrhosis, primary sclerosing cholangitis; ANA and anti-SMA antibodies are positive), genetic disorders (α_1-antitrypsin deficiency, Wilson's disease, haemochromatosis), others (Budd-Chiari syndrome), drugs (e.g. amiodarone, methyldopa and methotrexate).

Complications of cirrhosis: Variceal haemorrhage, hepatic encephalopathy, spontaneous bacterial peritonitis.

Investigations of cirrhosis: Liver screen, coagulation screen (PT, APTT, TT), liver ultrasound, liver biopsy, ANA, dsDNA, anti-smooth muscle and mitochondrial antibodies, 24 hours urinary copper and serum caeruloplasmin, serum ferritin, viral hepatitis serology (hepatitis B and hepatitis C), α_1-antitrypsin levels, immunoglobulins, EEG for encephalopathy.

   Alcohol misuse is characterised by raised γ-GT, MCV, thrombocytopaenia, and low urea; although psychiatrists may make use of urine toxicology and hair samples.

Evidence of decompensation: Altered consciousness, ascites, liver flap.

Evidence of treatment: Ascitic drain, surgical scars.

Treatment of chronic hepatitis C infection is usually reserved for those patients with persistently elevated transaminases, increased hepatitis C viral load and changes on liver biopsy. This treatment is with peg interferon-α and standard dose ribavarin. Assessing a patient with hepatitis C involves FBC, U&E, LFTs, HCV viral load and phenotype, α-FP, abdominal ultrasound and arrangements for an elective liver biopsy to exclude fibrosis.

ASCITES

This 55-year-old lady noticed some swelling of her tummy, and she feels that she has become more itchy because of a longstanding food allergy. Please examine her abdomen and report your possible diagnosis.

In the exam, the most frequent cause reflecting epidemiology of liver disease probably is alcohol, with primary biliary cirrhosis, right heart failure, and intra-abdominal malignancy less so. Rarely untapped – look for needle marks and comment. Prepare to answer questions about the management of ascites/sepsis.

Ascites: Abdominal distension, fluid thrill and shifting dullness, everted umbilicus.

Useful background investigations are: Urinary dipstix (nephrotic syndrome), FBC (infection), LFTs (deranged in liver disease), and u/s abdomen (confirms ascites and presence of intraabdominal masses).

The causes can be listed by virtue of the protein content of ascitic fluid:

Transudate (<25 g/l): Congestive cardiac failure, constrictive pericarditis (elevated JVP, shortness of breath, third heart sound), Meig's syndrome (ovarian fibroma, ascites, pleural effusion), hypoproteinaemic states/nephrotic syndrome (generalized oedema, proteinuria), cirrhosis.

Exudate (>25 g/l): (Cirrhosis (portal hypertension)), peritonitis, malignancy (abdominal, pelvic, peritoneal mesothelioma), myxoedema (hypothyroidism), Budd-Chiari syndrome (hepatic vein obstruction), portal vein thrombosis, tuberculosis, chylous ascites (obstruction of lymphatics, e.g. surgery, lymphoma).

Other measures include serum ascites–Albumin gradient measurement; ascitic leucocyte and neutrophil count or lymphocyte count: Spontaneous bacterial peritonitis is confirmed when ascitic leucocyte count > 500 or neutrophil count > 250 cells/high-power film.

Ascitic fluid should be analysed using cell count and differential, protein, albumin, amylase (pancreatic ascites), glucose (low in bacterial infections), bilirubin (elevated in bile ascites), cholesterol (raised in chylous ascites), cytology (malignant ascites), Gram stain. The macroscopic appearance of ascitic fluid is also important – straw coloured (most causes), turbid (pyogenic causes, TB), bloody (malignancy, TB), chylous (pancreatitis).

Pathophysiology of ascites: It is assumed that the theoretical aspects of ascites are examined in the written parts of the examination. However, candidates should not be made to look embarrassed without a basic mechanism as it underlies potential treatment pharmacologically (and these issues may come up in the discussion). Over 75% of ascites is due to liver disease. The pathogenesis is uncertain, but contributing factors include hypoalbuminaemia and portal hypertension. It is also likely that peripheral vasodilatation promotes sodium and water retention by stimulating the renin-angiotensin-aldosterone system. There is reduced colloid osmotic pressure and decreased renal blood flow as a result of splanchnic vasoconstriction.

Portal hypertension is usually the sequelae of cirrhotic liver disease, whereby the portal pressure in the portal vein is abnormally raised to more than 10 mmHg. The portal vein enters the liver at the porta hepatis and sends a branch to each lobe. When portal flow is obstructed, either from within or outwith the liver, collateral circulation develops to carry blood to the systemic veins. Extrahepatic obstruction is caused by increased resistance to flow, e.g. portal or splenic vein thrombosis. Other causes can include "post-hepatic" obstruction from hepatic vein thrombosis (Budd-Chiari syndrome), or extrinsic compression of the porta hepatis from lymph nodes (prehepatic). Intrahepatic obstruction is usually due to cirrhosis, right heart failure, sarcoidosis and schisosomiasis (worldwide). Varices are commonly oesophageal, derived from the left gastric vein. The clinical consequences of portal hypertension are gastrointestinal bleeding, caput medusae, venous hum, splenomegaly (but the size correlates poorly with portal pressure) and secondary hypersplenism (can cause peripheral blood cytopaenias). The pressure in the tributary veins is raised because of back pressure. Features include gastrointestinal bleeding, caput medusae, venous hum, splenomegaly, and secondary hypersplenism.

Investigations and management of particular significance to the acute presentation of alcohol liver disease: Blood tests include blood cultures and random ethanol level. PT and albumin are important prognostic factors (Maddrey's index- 4.6 × increase in PT over normal + bilirubin; poor prognosis if >32). Ultrasound of the abdomen (confirm portal hypertension). Exclude other causes of an acute hepatitis (hepatitis A IgM, hepatitis B sAg and hepatitis B eAg, liver autoantibodies, immunoglobulins). Give 5% i/v dextrose if not hyponatraemic. Treat for alcohol withdrawal before patient develops signs. Review medications (avoid sedatives). Have a low threshold for giving broad-spectrum antibiotics once cultures taken.

Management of variceal bleeding: It is useful to be aware of the risk of re-bleeding being dependent upon the severity of liver disease, large varices, varices near the oesophagogastric junction, "red sign" on varices, age > 60 years, haemoglobin < 8 g/dl, and renal failure. The management of variceal bleeding consists of resuscitation, catherisation, use of vasoconstrictors (e.g. terlipressin, a vasopressin analogue), balloon tamponade (risk of aspiration), endoscopy with appropriate therapy (sclerotherapy, ligation with rubber bands and combination therapy), and TIPPS/surgery (see below). Spontaneous bacterial peritonitis (SBP) complicates variceal bleeds; the risk is high, therefore use prophylactic antibiotics when indicated.

Management of ascites: This involves identification and treatment of any underlying remediable cause of liver disease, e.g. alcohol, strict sodium and fluid retention, the latter especially if the sodium is very low, bed rest and diuretic therapy, often requiring combination therapy of a loop diuretic such as frusemide, together with a potassium sparing diuretic such as spironolactone. If this fails, bumetanide or metolozone should be considered. <40–60 mmol of salt daily is ideal but difficult to achieve; <80 is more reasonable. Therapeutic paracentesis may be necessary for tense ascites, and occasionally concurrent administration of albumin is indicated. Repeated therapeutic paracentesis should be avoided as the ascites just reaccumulates and only increases the risk of peritonitis which can decompensate the underlying liver disease.

Transjugular intrahepatic portosystemic (TIPPS) shunting creates a side-to-side anastamosis between the portal and hepatic veins in order to relieve the high venous pressures. It decompresses a high pressure portal system, and is very effective at stopping bleeding in around 90%. However, it does not influence mortality – therefore, sometimes used in less severe liver disease. Complications include encephalopathy, infection, bleeding and stent stenosis. Other methods of shunting in diuretic-resistant ascites are peritonoeovenous shunting (Le Veen shunt), where a subcutaneous silastic catheter is used to drain the fluid into the jugular vein, and the Denver shunt (a modification adding a small subcutaneous pump that can be compressed externally).

Complications: Spontaneous bacterial peritonitis, pleural effusion, inguinal, femoral or umbilical hernia, mesenteric venous thrombosis, functional renal failure.

SPLENOMEGALY

This man has felt discomfort in his tummy. Please examine his abdomen and discuss your findings with the examiners.

The functions of the spleen are to produce IgM, capture and process foreign antigen. It filters especially capsulated microorganisms, e.g. pneumococcus. It sequesters and removes old red blood cells and platelets. It recycles iron and pools platelets (30% of total platelets within the spleen).

Usual position of the spleen: 9-11th ribs. A solid organ mass in the left hypochondrium; candidates often feel too close to the midline or miss the spleen because they did not feel it on light palpation then missed the edge on deep palpation. It should be dull to percussion, if it is not a kidney–atleast identify the inconsistency. Splenomegaly is supported by the inability to get above or ballot the mass. It usually moves on respiration. The splenic notch on the superiomedial edge is rarely palpable–do not forge physical signs. The differential diagnosis of a LUQ mass includes large left colon cancers, an enlarged spleen, a pancreatic mass (mainly a carcinoma of the tail), and enlarged left kidney.

Look for signs of anaemia, lymphadenopathy, and enlarged splenic edge to beyond the umbilicus.

Signs of infective endocarditis: Splinter haemorrhages, murmur, etc. Look for rheumatoid hands.

Examine for hepatomegaly.

Enquire about foreign travel and symptoms of possible haematological malignancy.

Causes of Splenomegaly

Mild

a. *Portal hypertension:* Did you see signs of chronic liver disease?
b. *Lymphoproliferative conditions:* Hodgkin's lymphoma, chronic lymphocytic leukaemia or a low grade (follicular) lymphoma are possibilities because the patients often have stable disease with organomegaly. If you are allowed to look for nodes, do so, but do it properly, missing them is not a good idea.
c. *Myeloproliferative syndromes:* Primary proliferative polycythaemia (increased red cell mass with normal *erythropoietin*; predominantly a disease of middle-aged and elderly, with facial plethora, suffusion of conjunctivae and engorgement of retinal vessels; presents with headaches, lethargy, dyspnoea, fluid retention, bleeding, weight loss, night sweats or pruritus which are exacerbated by a hot bath; neutrophil alkaline phosphatase (NAP) score is high) or myelofibrosis, both stable disorders with good signs, chronic myeloid leukaemia—usually treated so that spleen disappears and therefore uncommon in the examination.
d. Infection (EBV, infective endocarditis, infective hepatitis).

Moderate

a. Lympho-/myeloproliferative disorders
b. Infiltration (Gaucher's and amyloidosis).

Massive

a. Myeloproliferative disorders (CML)
b. Myelofibrosis
c. Tropical infections such as visceral leishmaniasis and malaria, rare in the exam – is there a travel history?
d. Hairy cell leukaemia
e. Storage disorders (such as Gaucher's disease).

Other Causes

a. *Storage disorders:* Rare and often treated, so that signs are missing so uncommon in the exam,
b. *Haemoglobinopathies:* Sickle rarely gives splenomegaly in adults, thalassaemia intermedia is ↑ possible—usually a mediterranean person,

c. Hereditary spherocytosis is a possible cause (icteric, splenomegaly and anaemia),
d. Infection – EBV,
e. Felty's syndrome (leg ulcers, neutropenia, rheumatoid arthritis).

A quick summary of important haematological malignancies

Chronic myeloid leukaemia is an abnormal proliferation of mature granulocyte precursors in the bone marrow that arises as a result of genetic aberration in these cells. WCC is high (50–500 $\times$ 10^9/L) and thrombocytosis. NAP score is low. This results in the constitutive activation of tyrosine kinase receptor in those cells that occurs following juxta-position of the *abl* gene with the *bcr* inducer gene. Karyotype analysis reveals the Philadelphia chromosome in 95% of patients. Natural history: Initial chronic phase of chronic myelopoiesis progresses inevitably to an accelerated phase with new cytogenic changes and finally to blast cell crisis). Anaemia and a high platelet count often coexist. Splenomegaly may cause pain and abdominal distension. The condition is treatable with hydroxyurea which lowers the white cell count and reduces the size of spleen, and is now treatable with metabolic receptor blocking agent as well as bone marrow transplantation.

Chronic lymphatic leukaemia is the most common leukaemia and tends to occur in the elderly, with widespread lymphadenopathy and moderate hepatosplenomegaly or splenomegaly. Look under armpits. There may be a petechial rash and pallor. There are mutations in B lymphocyte precursors. CLL is not curable. The long natural history means that patients may remain asymptomatic and die from an unrelated problem. Treatment is for symptomatic disease, aiming to decrease tumour cell load since CLL is not curable.

Polycythaemia rubra vera (PRV) is predominantly a disease of middle age and elderly. There is often facial plethora, suffusion of the conjunctivae and engorgement of retinal vessels. It may present with headaches, lethargy, dyspnoea, fluid retention, bleeding, weight loss, night sweats or pruritus. Polycythaemias are characterised by an increased haemoglobin concentration, packed cell volume and RBC count. Platelet count is also usually elevated. Treatment includes venesection and hydroxyurea. Causes of secondary polycythaemia are arterial hypoxaemia, abnormal release of oxygen from haemoglobin (e.g. carboxyhaemoglobinaemia, interference with tissue oxygen metabolism), and physiologically inappropriate erythropoietin production (e.g. neoplasms such as hepatocellular, renal cell cancer and haemangioblastoma). The diagnosis of PRV has almost been one of exclusion, but there is increasing interest in the JAK2 mutation as it affects the phosphorylation of erythropoietin as a possible genetic test, whilst it is not specific to PRV. One candidate was given an onset of chorea in a 80-year-old patient, and it turned out that he was told that the underlying cause in the patient's case was PRV!

Hodgkin's disease (associated with Reed-Sternberg cells, lymphadenopathy, splenomegaly, and B symptoms (fever, night sweats and weight loss) and Non-Hodgkin's disease (low-grade – indolent course but can transform to high-grade; high-grade – aggressive disease; bone marrow and CNS are sometimes involved). *Myelofibrosis:* Fibrosis in the bone marrow, resulting in extramedullary haemopoiesis in the liver and spleen.

Investigations: Further examination for nodes, full blood count, film with markers on blood for diseases such as CLL, CT chest/abdomen/pelvis for staging of disease, histology, cytogenetics and molecular genetics for classification of haematologial malignancy and are of prognostic significance, biopsy of lymph nodes, Coombs' test (if anaemic), ESR, liver ultrasound, ANA, RhF, C3/C4, dsDNA, ACE, blood cultures, viral serology (hepatitis, HIV), urinalysis – haematuria (endocarditis), proteinuria (myeloma), thick and thin films for Malaria, echocardiogram, brucella antibodies.

Further Notes

Splenectomy: Causes include rupture (trauma), but splenectomy is indicated when splenomegaly results in hypersplenism (destruction of all blood cell types), most often the case in hereditary spherocytosis, Gaucher's disease, autoimmune haemolytic anaemia and thalassaemia. Other indications include symptoms of mass effect from massive splenomegaly. Appearances of the blood film post splenectomy are an increased platelet count and large platelets, increased neutrophils, and nucleated red cells with Howell-Jolly bodies and target cells.

Patients should be informed pre-operatively of the life-long risk of simple infections and the need to take prophylactic antibiotic cover with oral penicillin and the need for immunisation against the common pneumococcal pathogens (pneumovax). Splenectomy work up is 2/52 prior vaccination against pneumoccocus, meningococcus, Hib, prophylactic penicillin and medicalert.

Note causes of generalized lymphadenopathy: Lymphoreticular disorder, chronic lymphatic leukaemia, infectious mononucleosis (likely to be tender), sarcoidosis, tuberculosis, brucellosis, toxoplasmosis, cytomegalovirus, thyrotoxicosis, progressive generalized lymphadenopathy of HIV. Investigations include lymph node biopsy, CT scan and ENT examination.

POLYCYSTIC KIDNEYS/RENAL ENLARGEMENT

This 48-year-old lady, whose only recent medical history includes headaches, noticed occasional discolouration of her urine, but she reports that she loves eating beetroot. Please examine her abdomen and discuss your findings with the examiners, particularly in relation to what you will advise about next.

An Extremely Common Case

It is important to be able to distinguish between a kidney and a liver:

The liver moves down with inspiration, the kidney being a retroperitoneal structure moves very little with respiration.

- The kidney can be bimanually ballotted, the liver cannot.
- The percussion note overlying the liver is usually dull (unless it is cystically enlarged), whereas it is usually resonant over the kidney due to superposition of bowel loops.
- Examining hand can get between enlarged kidney and costal margin.

Evidence of renal replacement therapy – look for arteriovenous fistulae at wrist/forearm.

Bi/unilateral ballottable masses in the loin regions with little or no movement with respiration, and transplanted kidney in the right/left iliac fossa.

Liver cysts causing irregular hepatomegaly.

Kidney transplant: Look for the characteristic J-shaped scar in the iliac fossa. Side effects of immunosuppressive treatment.

Anaemia is uncommon due to overproduction of erythropoietin.

Neurological deficit: Associated Berry aneurysms, resulting in subarachnoid haemorrhage in the minority of patients.

Adult polycystic kidney disease is an autosomal dominant condition affecting 1 in 400 to 1000. It may cause renal impairment, hypertension and haematuria.

Cysts in the liver may also occur (more common in infantile polycystic disease) producing nodular liver enlargement/hepatomegaly. Cysts may develop in the pancreas, spleen and brain. There is a predisposition to mitral valve prolapse. Other associations include berry aneurysms of the cerebral arteries (be attentive for signs of focal neurological defect). PKD1 is on chromosome 16 and encodes for polycystin-1, PKD2 is situated on chromosome 4 and codes for polycystin-2.

Differential diagnosis of a renal mass: Renal cell carcinoma (associated with weight loss, lymphadenopathy and paraneoplastic syndromes), hydronephrosis, adrenal mass–phaeochromocytoma, carcinoma.

Adults generally present with polycystic kidney disease: Pain, haematuria, recurrent urinary tract infections, sensation of a mass/loin pain, polycythaemia, family history.

Complications include loin pain from bleeding into cysts/infected cysts, mitral valve prolapse, anaemia of chronic renal failure, chronic renal failure, polycythaemia, distal renal tubular acidosis, cerebral aneurysms and subarachnoid haemorrhage.

Look for blood pressure, family history and haematuria.

In adults, there is a genetic linkage to chromosome 16 of the PKD locus, and the condition is inherited in an autosomal dominant manner. In children, there is linkage to chromosome 4, and the trait is inherited as an autosomal recessive manner. Children and siblings with established ADPKD should be offrered screening. Poor prognostic factors include male, polycystin-1 mutations, early onset hypertension, episodes of gross haematuria. Incidence 1:1000.

There are bilateral masses in the flanks that are ballotable and the patient may appear uraemic or may have evidence of an arteriovenous fistula, permacath or a Tenckoff catheter for dialysis. Polycystic kidneys are frequently left *in-situ* following transplantation, so also check for a mass with an overlying scar in the right iliac fossa.

Uraemic symptoms are anorexia, nausea and vomiting, cramps and restless legs, peripheral neuropathy, cognitive disturbance and drowsiness, hiccups, itch, pericarditis symptoms, myoclonus. Three things to assess in renal failure are uraemic symptoms, fluid status (fluid overload is indicated by hypertension, elevated JVP and sacral/peripheral oedema), and metabolic/biochemical status.

Factors which cause a progressive decline in renal function are hypertension, poor glycaemic control, persistent proteinuria (reduced with ACEIs and ARBs), dyslipidaemia corrected with statins, smoking, hyperphosphataemia and anaemia. Smoking needs to stop.

Treatment includes bed-rest and analgesia for pain, treatment of acidosis if present, nephrectomy/dialysis/renal transplant (patients require regular renal monitoring as 80% of patients have endstage renal failure by their 8th decade). Hypertension should be carefully controlled as it may result in deterioration of renal function and predispose to an intracranial event. Family members should be counselled and screened with ultrasound – cysts can be identified at about 18 years of age (currently there is no widely available genetic test), a positive family history of subarachnoid haemorrhage requires MRI scanning of the brain, as 20% will have a cerebral aneurysm.

Causes of unilateral enlargement:
a. Simple cysts
b. Renal cell carcinoma
c. Polycystic kidney disease
d. Hydronephrosis.

Causes of bilateral enlargement:
a. Polycystic kidney disease
b. Bilateral renal cell carcinoma (5%)
c. Bilateral hydronephrosis
d. Amyloidosis.

Investigations: U & E, urine cytology, ultrasound abdomen ± biopsy, IVU.
- CT if carcinoma is suspected.
- Genetic studies (ADPKD).

RENAL TRANSPLANT

This man feels tired. Please examine his abdomen and discuss your findings with the examiners, especially in relation to potential important reasons for his tiredness.

An Extremely Common Case

Patients have a scar in the iliac fossa with a smooth ovioid non-mobile swelling underneath, midline laparotomy scar. Ensure that you look for signs that the transplant is still functioning – an arteriovenous fistula, permacath, or a Tenckhoff catheter may indicate a return to dialysis. A good candidate should also pick up on potential causes of the renal impairment such as adult polycystic kidney disease, diabetes (lipohypertrophy/lipoatrophy, insulin injection marks, medic alert/ SOS bracelets), SLE or systemic sclerosis. Look also for gum hypertrophy (ciclosporin), Cushingoid facies, parathyroidectomy scar, hearing aid (Alport's syndrome, Wegener's granulomatosis).

Look for skin signs (malignancy, dysplastic change, SCC, BCC), Infection (viral warts and cellulitis).

Commonest causes of end-stage renal failure: Diabetes mellitus, hypertensive renal disease, IgA nephropathy, polycystic kidney disease, bilateral chronic pyelonephritis.

Aetiology: Lipodystrophy associated with glomerulonephritis, polycystic kidneys in the abdomen, signs of diabetes, e.g. glucometer, glucose stix, foot ulcers and poor vision, other autoimmune conditions, e.g. SLE (rashes), vitiligo.

Differential diagnosis for a mass in the right iliac fossa: Crohn's disease, primary malignancy, iliac TB mass, appendicular abscess, caecal carcinoid. 2,000 transplants take place in the UK every year, with an 80% 5 years success rate for live donors with one matched haplotype. Success rates are lower for cadaver kidneys.

Steps taken to ensure graft survival in transplant patients: Preoperatively, assiduous immunological matching is performed in unrelated donor-recipient pairs including HLA and ABO blood group matching. Blood transfusions are avoided and any comorbidity minimised, e.g. CABG performed for chronic angina prior to renal transplant. Live as opposed to cadaveric donors are preferred, and measures taken to prevent cold ischaemic damage to allograft.

Postoperatively, immunotherapy is started and continued longterm. The standard regimen includes: Prednisolone, azathioprine and ciclosporin, which requires dose monitoring and adjustment. Rejection is most likely to take place in the first three months. Newer agents are used to minimize episodes of acute rejection (tacrolimus, mycophenolate mofetil, monoclonal antibodies directed against the IL-2 receptor, and sirolimus). Reduction in the dose of ciclosporin (in patients already taking mycophenolate mofetil and sirolimus) after 1 year may be associated with improved renal function, blood pressure, lipid and homocysteine levels. There needs to be adequate treatment of hypertension and dyslipidaemia.

Vascular supply of the transplanted kidney: The donor renal artery is anastomosed to either the internal or external iliac cartery. The donor renal vein is reattached to the external iliac vein. The ureter is attached separately to the patient's bladder. The renal pelvis is the most anterior structure, then artery and vein most posterior.

Management of renal transplant patients: Monitor serum creatinine levels, observe for signs of rejection and secondary malignancy, immunosuppressive drugs, address cardiovascular risk factors.

Most patients in the exam will have a transplanted kidney that is functioning well. Symptoms pointing towards graft rejection include declining renal function, tenderness over the graft, hypertension, increased shortness of breath (fluid retention) and decreased urine output.

Types of graft rejection: Hyperacute (preformed antibody mediated ABO mismatch), acute mixed humoral and cellular response which may respond to high dose methylprednisolone and/or anti-lymphocyte antibodies (OKT3), and chronic (cell mediated inflammatory response) resulting in interstitial fibrosis, and tubular obliteration, is irreversible and treatment is therefore supportive for the management of chronic renal failure.

Complications include opportunistic infections (e.g. herpes zoster virus, *Pneumocystis carinii pneumonia*, CMV), premature coronary artery disease, hypertension primarily to ciclosporin, lymphomas and skin cancers, hypersensitivity reaction and bone marrow suppression (azathioprine), complications of steroid therapy such as avascular necrosis of bone.

Increased risk of other pathologies: Seborrhoeic keratosis (increased risk in azathioprine treatment), skin malignancy, lymphoma, hypertension and hyperlipidaemia leading to MI and stroke; immunosuppressant drug side-effects/toxicity: Ciclosporin nephrotoxicity; recurrence of original disease. Focal segmental glomerulonephritis can recur in transplanted kidneys. As this results in graft loss in only 15% of affected patients, it is not a contraindication to transplantation.

Investigations: U&E, FBC (normocytic normochromic anaemia), bone profile, 24-hour creatinine clearance, renal ultrasound, glucose, HBA1c, ESR, urinalysis, ANA, dsDNA, ANCA, anti-GBM, C3/C4, RF, serum protein and urine electrophoresis, antistreptolysin O titre, Hepatitis B and C serology, prostate specific antigen, renal biopsy.

Features of Therapeutic Intervention (Renal Replacement Therapy)

Continuous ambulatory peritoneal dialysis (CAPD): 60% of patients are now treated by this method. The peritoneum acts as a semipermeable membrane; dialysis takes place via a peritoneal catheter. Small abdominal scars remain after removal. Uraemic toxins diffuse into 2-3 litres of dialysate within the peritneum. Excess fluid is removed by osmosis. Dialysis is required up to three times per day and involves attaching bags to the peritoneal catheter. Advantages are that it provides relative freedom from hospital, and is relatively 'gentle'. The main risk is infection (peritonitis). Contra-indications include previous abdominal surgery or diverticular disease.

Haemodialysis: This is performed via a fistula in the forearm and the patient's blood is pumped through a dialyser at 200-500 ml/min; patients often have more than one fistula. Dialysis occurs usually for 3 hours, three times a week in hospital. Satellite dialysis units have improved patient access. An adequate blood pressure and good functioning cardiovascular system are required for haemodialysis as fluid shift is more intense. The advantage is that it is done by others, but there is a risk of sepsis from access.

CAPD vs. haemodialysis: CAPD is more flexible and can be performed at home. However, there is a greater risk of infection and the process needs to be performed three times a day. Haemodialysis requires more time travelling to a dialysis centre and is less flexible, but gives superior electrolyte control. Assessment of dialysis patients includes calculation of their 'dry weight', looking for potassium and ECG changes associated with hyperkalaemia, pulmonary oedema and hypertension.

Complications of dialysis: Acute (peritonitis, bleeding, hypotension, fever, disequilibrium) and chronic (amyloidosis, malnutrition, neuropathy, and acquired cystic disease).

There are four life-threatening indications for emergency dialysis in a known dialysis patient: Serum potassium > 6.5 mmol/l, signs of fluid overload, worsening acidosis, pericardial rub and other signs of severe uraemia.

HAEMOCHROMATOSIS

This 46-year-old man who often spends time abroad as part of his job has asked for advice about skin cancer given his persistent tan. Please examine the abdomen and discuss with the examiners your thoughts on his underlying problem.

Inheritance: Autosomal recessive chromosome 6. HFE gene mutation: regulator of gut iron absorption. Association with HLA-A3.

Homozygous prevalence 1:300, carrier rate 1:10. Males affected at an earlier age due to female protective iron loss by menstruation.

Presentation: Fatigue and arthritis, chronic liver disease, incidental diagnosis onl family screening.

Signs: (will depend on how late the presentation was and how well treated). Skin pigmentation, slate grey (associated with deposition of melanin), sometimes with arthropathy, hepatomegaly, testicular atrophy, splenomegaly, cardiac disease – usually failure. Stigmata of chronic liver disease such as spider naevi, palmar erythema, ascites, jaundice. Diabetes mellitus. Arthropathy. Cardiac involvement (cardiomegaly, congestive cardiac failure). Hepatocellular carcinoma develops in 33% of cirrhotic patients.

Scars: Venesection weekly until the haemoglobin concentration falls below 11g/dl and the patient is marginally iron deficient, liver biopsy, joint replacement, abdominal rooftop incision (this incision is otherwise known as the "double Kocher" incision, which allows good access to the liver and spleen, and is particularly useful for intrahepatic surgery, radical pancreatic and gastric surgery and bilateral adrenalectomy).

Evidence of advanced liver disease: Loss of body hair, ascites and gynaecomastia.

Evidence of complications: Endocrine "bronze diabetes", congestive cardiac failure, joints (arthropathy).

Investigations: Fasting serum transferrin saturation > 50% is the best screening test (remember to suggest checking relatives). Serum ferritin is markedly raised if there is advanced disease – may be normal in early disease and is not a good screening test. C282Y H63D gene tests are useful for family studies. It serves as a useful screening tool as studies have shown that 83-100% of patients exhibit this mutation. Remember the usual Part 1 catch that ferritin is an acute phase reactant, and therefore can be raised in an inflammatory process. Liver biopsy is only required to confirm cirrhosis, usually done if ferritin > 1000 mcg/L.

Management: Aim to have normal transferring saturation and serum ferritin at around 50. Phlebotomy, most patients tolerate weekly 450 ml maintaining Hb of 12 g/dl. During treatment the serum ferritin concentration decreases. As iron depletion approaches, serum iron and Hb concentration falls. The frequency of phlebotomy should be reduced and a maintenance of 2-6 units removed each year for the rest of the patient's life. Desferroximine as a continuous infusion; a poor and expensive alternative to phlebotomy. Possibly, avoid alcohol, Indian Balti curries, and shellfish. Surveillance for HCC.

Family screening: Iron studies. If positive, liver biopsy and genotype analysis.

Prognosis: 200 X increased risk of HCC if cirrhotic; reduced life expectancy if cirrhotic; normal life expectancy without cirrhosis and effective treatment.

Liver transplantation in haemochromatosis: Over 50% 1 year survival, high mortality: Cardiac + infectious complications.

   Consider also blood glucose (diabetes), ECG, CXR and echo (cardiac failure), liver ultrasound and α-fetoprotein (hepatocellular carcinoma).

CARCINOID SYNDROME

This lady has frequent episodes of diarrhoea. Please examine her abdomen and discuss your findings with the examiners.

   Gut primary with liver metastasis secreting 5 HT into the systemic circulation.

   Symptoms include diarrhoea, wheeze and flushing.

   Secreted mediators scar and thicken the right-sided heart valves resulting in tricuspid regurgitation and/or pulmonary stenosis.

   Rarely, a bronchogenic primary tumour can release 5-HT into the systemic circulation and cause left-sided valve scarring.

HEPATOMEGALY

This 40-year-old man originally from Pakistan has received abnormal liver function tests, and yet he has never drunk alcohol. He once received a blood transfusion after a car accident. Please examine his abdomen and discuss your findings with the examiners.

   Start by palpation in the right iliac fossa and move upward with the fingers of the right hand perpendicular to the costal margin. Determine the nature of that enlargement (smooth, hard, craggy).

   Establish that the mass is truly hepatic by attempting to get above it.

   Establish that the mass, if hepatic, is not just a downwardly displaced liver (COPD) by percussing downward from the ipsilateral nipple until dullness is detected.

Look for signs of chronic liver disease, lymphadenopathy, no visually obvious hyperinflated lungs, enlarged liver margin 3-4 breadths below costal margins, smooth and uniformly enlarged or hard and craggy with irregular edge, gynaecomastia, supraclavicular nodes, Dupuytren's contracture, raised JVP, jaundice, testicular atrophy, pedal oedema, absence of secondary sexual hair.

Look for evidence of an underlying cause of hepatomegaly: Tattoos and needle marks (infectious hepatitis/alcohol), pigmentation (haemochromatosis), cachexia (malignancy), midline sternotomy scar (CCF).

If the liver is felt, ascertain the following:

- Soft (normal), firm (inflamed or infiltrated) or hard (advanced cirrhosis or metastases)?
- Smooth or nodular – if nodular, micronodular or macronodular?
- Pulsatile? – tricuspid regurgitation (TR)
- Tender? – TR, Budd-Chiari syndrome, hepatitis, hepatocellular cancer, abscess
- Reidel's lobe (a tongue-like projection from the inferior surface of the right lobe, it can extend to the right iliac fossa).

The differential diagnosis for a RUQ mass includes hepatomegaly, enlarged gallbladder and colonic carcinoma of hepatic flexure.

Evidence of treatment: Ascitic drain/tap sites and peritonovenous shunts, surgical scars.

Causes of Hepatomegaly

- Physiological (Reidel's lobe, hyperexpanded chest)
- Infection – bacterial (TB, liver abscess), viral hepatitis (EBV, CMV, hepatitis A, B, and C), protozoal (malaria, histoplasmosis, amoebiasis, hydatid, schistosomiasis)
- Alcoholic liver disease (fatty disease, liver cirrhosis)
- Malignant disease (lymphoma, carcinoma or metastatic deposits, leukaemia, hepatocellular carcinoma, myeloproliferative disorders)
- Metabolic/genetic disease (Wilson's disease, AA amyloidosis, Gaucher's disease, haemochromatosis, sarcoidosis, primary biliary cirrhosis, polycystic disease)
- Cardiovascular (right heart failure, hepatic vein thrombosis (expect, however, ascites and splenomegaly)).

Initial investigations: FBC (for example, raised WCC in infection), ESR, U&Es, LFTs including albumin and gamma-glutamyl transferase, PT,

APTT, TT, abdominal ultrasound (the first line investigation used to define the liver architecture, size and clues to the pathology), CXR, cirrhosis screen, ECG and echocardiography, malignant disease – abdominal CT/MRI scanning (useful to further investigate solid lesions), α-fetoprotein (hepatocellular carcinoma), serum iron and ferritin levels, serum caeruloplasmin levels and urinary copper levels, serum blood glucose, Hepatitis viral serology (including hepatitis A, B, C, EBV, CMV, toxoplasma), autoimmune screen (ANA, dsDNA, rheumatoid factor, antimitochondrial antibody, antiphospholipid antibodies), α_1-antitrypsin level, serum ACE.

Evidence of decompensation: Ascites, asterixis, altered consciousness.

Differential diagnosis: Enlarged gallbladder, nephromegaly, enlarged lymph nodes, collection in the Pouch of Rutherford-Morrison, adrenal tumour, colonic tumour of the hepatic flexure, dilated bowel loops.

It can be difficult to define the edge, if so:

Is percussion helpful?

Does the person look like someone with metastasis?

Are there signs of chronic liver disease, look for hair loss, feel for gynaecomastia. Prepare to debate what is or is not a spider naevus.

Is there jaundice, tell the examiner that you would like to examine the testicles in males.

Remember that the patient with cirrhosis may not have a palpable liver.

Complications of cirrhosis: Variceal haemorrhage due to portal hypertension, hepatic encephalopathy, spontaneous bacterial peritonitis.

INFLAMMATORY BOWEL DISEASE

This 27-year-old lady has frequent diarrhoea. Please examine her abdomen and discuss your findings with the examiners.

Aspects of history: Nature and frequency of blood passed, onset of symptoms, patient's definition of diarrhoea, associated nocturnal diarrhoea (ulcerative colitis), number of bloody stools per day, abdominal pain/urgency/tenesmus, straining, constipation and pain (fissure), rectal lumps/masses, previous GI history (haemorrhoids, bleeding disorders, food poisoning), drug history (NSAIDs, anticoagulants, iron and bismuth), alcohol history, FH of GI neoplasia and polyps, concerns of patient particularly cancer. Systemic features such as anorexia and malaria.

Differential: Colonic cancer, ulcerative colitis, Crohn's disease.

Clinical signs: Pallor, anaemia, slim build, oral ulceration, surgical scars, tenderness, palpable masses (right iliac fossa mass in Crohn's disease, colonic tumour in UC), perianal disease.

Acute severe UC: Usually total disease with severe rectal bleeding and profuse diarrhoea (> 6 stools/day), abdominal pain, systemic disturbance (i.e. tachycardia, pyrexia, pallor, wasting). Moderately active UC: moderate rectal bleeding with some signs of systemic disturbance, failing to respond to treatment. Mild UC: Little or no rectal bleeding, no systemic disturbance.

Active Crohn's disease: Frank bleeding less common.

Investigation: Stool microscopy and culture to exclude infective cause of diarrhoea, FBC, inflammatory markers, AXR to exclude toxic dilatation in UC and small bowel obstruction, sigmoidoscopy and colonoscopy for histological confirmation, and bowel contrast studies: Strictures, fistulae in Crohn's disease.

Treatment

- Medical treatment (including non-pharmacological treatment)
  Crohn's disease: Smoking cessation. Steroids are the mainstay of treatment in patients with acute Crohn's disease. Tapering steroids are required to induce remission. A new agent budesonide has a rapid first-pass metabolism and is poorly absorbed. Maintenance therapy: Azathioprine, methotrexate, infliximab (particularly useful for some patients who do not respond to steroids or immunsuppressive therapy). Metronidazole and ciprofloxacin are useful as well.
  Ulcerative colitis. Oral or topical 5-ASA, i/v steroid and i/v ciclosporin. Colonoscopic colorectal surveillance is needed and usually begins no later than 10 yeas after diagnosis.
  Maintenance therapy: Oral steroid and 5-ASA.
- *Nutritional support:* High fibre, elemental and low residue diets
- Psychological support
- Surgical treatment.

Aims of surgery: To restore health in patients with chronic disease, e.g. nutritional failure. To eliminate the risks of side-effects of steroids in long-term.

Crohn's disease: Obstruction from strictures, complications from fistulae and perianal disease and failure to respond to medical therapy.

Ulcerative colitis: Chronic symptomatic relief, emergency surgery for severe refractory colitis and colonic dysplasia following premalignant change on colonoscopic surveillance or carcinoma.

Emergency surgery is required in perforation, severe haemorrhage, toxic dilatation > 6 cm (megacolon) as there is a high risk of perforation and faecal peritonitis, stricture causing obstruction, fistulae or abscess formation, sepsis.

Complications

Crohn's disease: Malabsorption, anaemia, abscess, fistulae, intestinal obstruction.

Ulcerative colitis: Anaemia, toxic dilatation, perforation, colonic carcinoma (higher risk in patients with pancolitis 5-10% at 15-20 years), surveillance (2 yearly colonoscopy for patients with pancolitis > 10 years is usually recommended), colectomy if dysplasia is detected. Some key extra-intestinal manifestations are shown in Table 2.2.

Table 2.2: Extra-intestinal manifestations

Mouth	Aphtous ulcers
Skin	Erythema nodosum, Pyoderma gangrenosum
Joint	Large joint arthritis, Seronegative arthritides
Eye	Uveitis, episcleritis, conjunctivitis
Liver	Primary sclerosing cholangitis

PRIMARY BILIARY CIRRHOSIS

This 56-year-old lady noticed some changes in the appearance of her face. Please examine the abdomen to suggest why.

Consider this in a pigmented patient with prominent excoriations due to marked pruritus and icterus. Look carefully for xanthelasma and xanthomata over joint, skin folds, and sites of trauma (including venepuncture). Other xanthomata frequently occur over joints, skin folds and at sites of trauma. Finger clubbing is common and should be looked for. The spleen is palpable (50% of cases).

Remember that steatorrhoea in the condition can lead to easy bruising, osteoporosis and osteomalacia (test for tenderness over the spine).

Complications: Oesophageal varices, steatorrhoea and malabsorption, osteomalacia.

Important associations: Rheumatoid arthritis, dermatomyositis, autoimmune thyroiditis, the CREST syndrome, Sjogren's syndrome and renal tubular acidosis.

Serum antimitochondrial antibody is positive in 95-99%, smooth muscle antibody positive in 50% and ANF positive in 20%. There is impaired biliary excretion of copper with excessive copper deposition in the liver.

Treatment: Ursodeoxycholic acid improves serum biochemistry, decreases the rate of referral for liver transplantation and decreases pruritus, but has no effect on histology or long term survival.

HEPATOSPLENOMEGALY

This 50-year-old man has noticed for a long time some lumps in his neck. Please examine his abdomen and discuss your findings with the examiners.

No other signs: Myeloproliferative disorders, lymphoproliferative disorders, cirrhosis of the liver with portal hypertension.

Hepatosplenomegaly with palpable lymph nodes: Chronic lymphatic leukaemia, lymphoma.

Other causes of hepatosplenomegaly: Malaria (on a world-wide basis), hepatitis B or C, brucellosis, Weil's disease, toxoplasmosis, cytomegalovirus, pernicious anaemia and other megaloblastic anaemia, storage disorders, amyloidosis, other signs of portal hypertension (e.g. Budd-Chiari syndrome).

EPIGASTRIC MASS

The differential diagnosis for this includes gastric carcinoma, pancreatic pseudocyst, pancreatic carcinoma, and abdominal aortic aneurysm. Two 'catches' are: (i) Liver (either left lobe or a post-necrotic nodule of a cirrhotic liver), and (ii) Large recti (these appear to enlarge when the patient sits forward). You should always suspect gastric or pancreatic carcinoma in a cachectic patient complaining of pain, dyspepsia, anorexia and significant weight loss. You may not always feel a mass.

Characteristics of a gastric carcinoma: Hard, irregular mass, cannot get above it, and moves with respiration. Think immediately of checking for a left supraclavicular node (Virchow's or Troisier's node).

Characteristics of a pancreatic pseudocyst: Cannot get above it, indistinct lower border, resonant to percussion, and moves slightly with respiration.

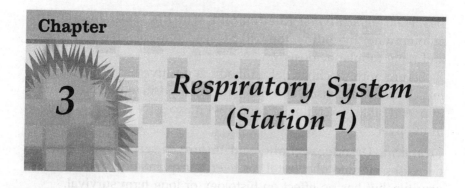

Chapter

3

Respiratory System (Station 1)

INTRODUCTION TO EXAMINATION TECHNIQUE

Inspection

The mark scheme makes clear that general inspection is an important component of the respiratory system examination.

Look for scars: Thoracotomy scar (lobectomy and other thoracic operations including for treatment of foreign body aspiration, bronchiectasis, old TB, bronchial carcinoma; note that whereas right thoracotomy scars are for respiratory procedures left thoracotomy scars can be used for cardiovascular procedures), aspiration sites for pleural effusions (often posterior or lateral), and old chest-drains (2nd intercostals spaces in the mid-clavicular line or 5th intercostals space).

On general inspection, assess the nutritional status (e.g. cachexia). Look for obvious features of systemic disease, such as:

- *Pickwickian syndrome:* Obese, somnolent, malar facies, audible wheeze.
- *Systemic sclerosis:* Beaked nose, shiny tight skin over face, telengectasiae (associated apical fibrosis)
- *Ankylosing spondylitis:* Kyphotic spine (associated apical fibrosis)
- *Rheumatoid arthritis:* Symmetrical destructive arthropathy of the hands
- *Horner's syndrome:* Ptosis, meiosis, enophthalmos, anhydrosis.

Examine for finger clubbing (suppurative lung disease – abscess, bronchiectasis or empyema; fibrosing alveolitis absent in upto 60%, bronchial carcinoma, mesothelioma) and cyanosis; demonstration of the flap of carbon dioxide in the hands.

Examine for cyanosis: Are there any additional features of superior vena caval obstruction (facial and upper limb oedema, dilated superficial thoracic veins and fixed dilatation of the neck veins), lip pursing, subcutaneous emphysema?

Assess for respiratory distress: Use of accessory muscles, tachypnoea, grunting, intercostal/subcostal recession

Listen carefully during your inspection for the sounds of polyphonic (multiple) or monophonic (large single) wheeze that results from airways obstruction, particularly in expiration. Is the respiratory cycle of normal duration (inspiration longer than expiration)? Sounds of upper airway obstruction may also be evident (grunting, gurgling, noisy/heavy breathing).

CHEST WALL SHAPES

The *Clinical Guidelines* report that candidates are expected to be aware of different types of chest wall shapes. Not only is this important for the general examination anyway, but the authors are aware of various instances where this has specifically be enquired about in the actual MRCP examination (Fig. 3.1).

- *Kyphoscoliosis:* Kyphosis is exaggerated antero-posterior curvature of the spin. Scoliosis is lateral curvature of the spine. This may be apparent only as a 'S' shape of the thoracic spine but as the condition progresses the vertebral bodies are rotated so that the ribs protrude backwards using a "hunch" back. This may be idiopathic (80%), or secondary to polio.
- *Barrel chest:* This is seen in patients with longstanding hyperinflation of the lungs, as in emphysema and sometimes in kyphosis. This appearance is due to an increase in AP diameter.
- *Pectus carinatum:* Is protruberant sternum. It may be congenital or secondary to *severe childhood asthma*, rickets or congenital heart disease. It consists of a localised prominence of the sternum and adjacent costal cartilages, often accompanied by indrawing of the ribs to form symmetrical grooves (*Harrison's sulci*).
- *Pectus excavatum:* Is a depressed sternum. This is congenital and not secondary to lung disease. It may be a forme fruste of Marfan's syndrome and is associated with mitral valve prolapse. The distance between the spine and sternum is reduced resulting in an apparent enlargement of the heart on chest radiograph and functional systolic murmur. The lower end of the sternum is depressed, though when severe the whole sternum and costal cartilages are sunken. It may cause a displaced apex beat, cardiac murmur, apparent cardiomegaly and abnormal lung function if very severe.
- *Harrison's sulci:* These are horizontal grooves at the bottom of the rib cage in children caused by persistent indrawing of the ribs.

- *Thoracoplasty*: Note any *scars* from previous surgery or trauma. Before chemotherapy for tuberculosis was available, a *thoracoplasty* consisting of pushing in part of the ribcage to collapse the underlying lung was sometimes performed.
- *Chest wall shapes:*

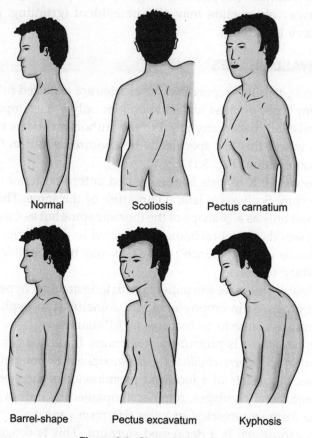

Figure 3.1: Chest wall shapes

Purse-lip breathing: Seen in chronic obstructive airways obstruction (especially emphysema). Not necessarily a sign of distress, as is a means of increasing the intra-thoracic pressure to collapsed bronchioles.

Rate of respiration: Use of accessory muscles of respiration; symmetry of expansion (asymmetrical chest wall movement is suggestive of a reduction in lung volume – collapse, pneumothorax, fibrosis or reduction surgery).

Evidence of previous surgery (e.g. thoracotomy, thoracoplasty, thorascopic biopsy, plombage) or radiotherapy (e.g. telengectasia, burns, limb lymphoedema, Indian ink marks for field identification), evidence of engorged superficial veins (e.g. SVC obstruction) or subcutaneous nodules

Look for a Horner's syndrome and wasting of small muscles of the hand wasting.

Look for signs relating to the skin: the candidate should be able to recognise associated disease (e.g. eczema), the evidence of previous surgery (e.g. thoracotomy, chest drain, Portacath), and engorged superficial veins (e.g. SVC obstruction), subcutaneous emphysema. Superior vena cava obstruction is most often due to bronchial carcinoma and/or associated mediastinal glands, lymphoma, and mediastinal fibrosis and other rare causes. The resulting signs may vary in severity: dilated veins on the anterior chest wall, engorged fixed non-pulsatile jugular veins, swollen face, neck and sometimes arms, and conjunctival oedema.

Surface anatomy: The right lung is divided into three lobes (upper, middle and lower) while the left lung is divided into two lobes while the lingula divides the two (Fig. 3.2).

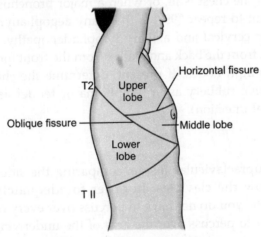

Figure 3.2: Surface anatomy of lungs

Palpation

Examine the hands: Feel pulse (bounding) and examine for the presence of a flapping tremor (carbon dioxide retention). Confirm correct position of the trachea with appropriate warning; check for tracheal deviation by placing the index and ring fingers of the trachea at the sternal angle and using the middle finger to feel the tracheal rings.

Demonstrate appropriate techniques for assessing the position of the upper and lower mediastinum. If you attempt to do this from both sides of the chest, be prepared to give a sensible justification (e.g. confirmation of findings). Assess both the extent and symmetry of movement of two sides of chest wall. Ask the patient *"Could you please take a deep breath in?"*. The thumbs should separate by atleast 5 cm. Confirm the findings from inspection by placing a hand either side of the sternum, and observe any loss of chest wall expansion during inspiration. Ensure that you have assessed the expansion of both the upper and lower lobes bilaterally (this requires this manoeuvre being performed twice; above and below the breast).

Confirm the position of the apex beat, as displacement will signify mediastinal shift. The impulse may be difficult to feel in the hyper-inflated chest.

Assess tactile vocal fremitus or vocal resonance. It is adequate to do one or the other (some examiners are thought to prefer only vocal resonance). It may be more fluent to assess vocal resonance, as this can be done at the end of auscultation. Use the ulnar border of the hand for tactile vocal fremitus. This is increased over consolidated lung and diminished when air, fluid or thickened pleura separates the lung from the chest wall, or when a major bronchus is occluded. Ask the patient to repeat "99". Is there any aegophany?

Palpate for cervical and axillary lymphadenopathy. Examine the patient's neck from the back and axillae from the front for the presence of enlarged lymph nodes. If present, determine the character (hard as in carcinoma, rubbery as in lymphoma or tender as is often the case as in viral infection).

Percussion

Start in the supraclavicular fossae, comparing the sides then move down to below the clavicles. In order to adequately assess the percussion note, you do not have to percuss over every rib space. It is only necessary to percuss over the area of the underlying lobes. This means that the same information can be got by percussing in three places as thirty (remember to percuss in the axillary region to assess the middle lobe).

Auscultation

Both sides of the chest need to be auscultated for bronchial (lobar pneumonia) and vesicular breath sounds, the intensity of breath sounds. Localised decreased breath sounds are found in a pneumothorax, pleural effusion, tumour, pleural thickening and collapse. Generalised decreased breath sounds occur in emphysema, asthma, muscular chest wall, obesity and fibrotic lung disease. Bronchial breathing is heard in consolidation, abscess near a chest wall, bronchial neoplasm, dense fibrosis and the top of a pleural effusion. It can also be heard if one is listening too close to the midline. The chest especially should be examined for added sounds (e.g. crackles, wheeze – inspiratory crepitations/crackles should be timed for when they occur in the respiratory cycle, as this may be a pointer to underlying pathology – early to mid : bronchiectasis, mid to late lung fibrosis (fine) or pulmonary oedema; wheeze = the air passing through an airway that is narrowed and on the point of closure); click and noises from the chest wall in synchrony with cardiac systole. Don't forget the lung apices. Is expiration longer than inspiration (asthma)?

Examine for whispering pectoriloquy or vocal resonance (when appropriate): Voice sounds conducted through consolidated lung tissue, extensive fibrosis and pulmonary collapse associated with a patent bronchus resemble more closely those produced at the larynx than those heard over normal lungs, in that they are louder and more distinct.

The presence of a pleural rub (crunching sound during inspiration) signifies pleural inflammation (usually infection/uraemia).

OTHER POINTS OF THE RESPIRATORY EXAMINATION

The candidate should close with other relevant features of the respiratory examination, viz:
- *Sputum pot:* Significance of copious mucopurulent secretions suggesting bronchiectasis.
- Presence of oxygen cylinder or nebuliser.
- *Oxygen saturation monitor:* Offer to ask for the oxygen saturation.
- *Peak flow:* Measurement of peak flow measurement using an appropriate meter.
- Bedside spirometry
- Arterial blood gas measurement
- *Tracheostomy:* An inference for why the tracheostomy scar is present.
- *Inhaler technique:* The technique of standard inhaler devices and their appropriate application.

Inhaler Technique

This has been known to be assessed in PACES within Station 1, Station 2 or Station 4.

- *Explain the way in which the bronchodilator works:* By relaxing the air passages in your lungs.
- *Explain the need for the bronchodilator solution:* To reach as deep down into your lungs as possible and to stay in your lungs long enough to be absorbed.
- Remove the mouthpiece cover.
- Shake the cannister.
- Hold the inhaler vertically in your dominant hand. Dexterity is important.
- Breathe right out.
- Put the mouthpiece in your mouth with your lips tightly around it.
- Press firmly down on the body of the inhaler as you *start* to breath in. This timing is important.
- Take in a deep breath slowly so that the spray goes deeply into your lungs.
- Hold the breath for 10 sec.
- Breathe out and go through the whole process again.

Common Respiratory Cases

Once the abnormal signs have been elicited, they need to be presented correctly. The signs should be interpreted correctly within the context of a diagnosis or differential diagnoses. Common respiratory cases are listed below, along with related discussion of investigation and sequence, therapy and management.

LUNG MALIGNANCY

This 42-year-old man has been short of breath. Please examine his respiratory system and discuss with the examiners.

Commonest Malignancy in the Western World

Key Signs

Systemic features: Cachexia, anaemia, clubbing, tar-stained fingers, tracheal deviation towards collapse or away (effusion) from the lesion, reduced expansion, percussion note dull (collapse/consolidation) or stony dull (effusion), auscultation (crackles and bronchial breathing) and reduced breath sounds and vocal resonance (effusion), HPOA, lymphadenopathy.

    Chest: None, consolidation, collapse, pleural effusion.

    Metastasis: Bone tenderness, hepatomegaly.

Paraneoplastic: Gynaecomastia, Lambert-Eaton syndrome, SLCL, squamous cell carcinoma, dermatomyositis and acanthosis nigricans.

Endocrine: Ectopic ACTH production (Cushing's syndrome), PTHrp production (squamous cell carcinoma), SIADH.

Dermatological/rheumatological: Dermatomyositis, clubbing, hypertrophic pulmonary osteoparthropathy.

Neurological: Confusion, fits, focal CNS deficits, cerebellar syndrome, proximal myopathy, peripheral neuropathy.

Other features: Superior vena cava obstruction due to mediastinal lymph nodes compressing the superior vena cava impeding venous return (suffused and oedematous face and upper limbs, dilated superficial chest veins and stridor, non-pulsatile elevation of the jugular venous pressure) (Causes: Bronchial carcinoma, enlargement of the thyroid or thymus glands, TB, recurrent laryngeal nerve palsy). Symptoms include painless swelling of the face, headache, visual disturbance with the sensation of fullness in the ears. Investigations for SVCO obstruction are chest X-ray, thoracic CT scan, a venogram. To confirm carcinoma, carry out investigations below. Therapeutic modalities are radiotherapy or chemotherapy, and corticosteroids are useful in reducing laryngeal and/or cerebral oedema.

Aetiology: This is predominantly:

1. Cigarette smoking (this causes the vast majority of adenocarcinoma of the lung),
2. Manufacturing – Asbestosis, chromate, nickel, arsenic, radioactivity – uranium mining.

Investigations

These include:

- Cytology: Sputum and pleural fluid,
- CXR: Opacities, hilar enlargement, consolidation, lung collapse, pleural effusion, bony secondaries,
- FNAC,
- Bronchoscopy ± washings/brushings/transbronchial biopsy, (if the tumour is located centrally),
- Open/VATS biopsy,
- CT, lung function tests,
- Radionuclide scans for bony metastasis,
- PET of the lung (for certain cases).

The purpose of the investigations is to allow the following:

1. Diagnosis of the mass (CXR: collapse, mass, hilar lymphadenopathy) and spiral CT (so small tumours are not lost between slices during a breath).

2. Determine cell type (induced sputum cytology, biopsy by bronchoscopy or percutaneous needle).
3. Stage (CT/bronchoscopy/mediastinoscopy/thoracoscopy). Non-small cell carcinoma: TNM staging to assess operability. Small cell carcinoma: Limited or extensive disease.
4. Lung function tests for operability assessment. Pneumonectomy contraindicated if $FEV_1 < 1.2L$.
5. Complications of the tumour. Metastasis: Increased LFTs, increased calcium, anaemia. NSCLC: PTHrP hypercalcaemia, and SCLC: increased ACTH, SIADH to hyponatraemia.

Treatment

An important aspect, of course, is for the patient to stop smoking if he/she is still smoking.

In the UK, NICE recommends professional guidance on the management of lung cancer: This guidance was published in 2005 in the form of the leaflet CG24, available on their website http://www.nice.org.uk/nicemedia/pdf/CG024niceguideline.pdf

Surgery for fit patients with early disease (IA, IB, II), involving lobectomy or pneumonectomy, excision of peripheral tumours, contraindications to surgery in non-small cell lung cancer: Metastatic carcinoma, transfer factor < 50%, severe pulmonary hypertension, uncontrolled cardiac arrhythmias, poor lung function, left laryngeal nerve palsy, malignant effusion, dysphagia, mediastinal lymph node involvement, superior vena cava obstruction, phrenic nerve palsy, rib or distant metastasis.

Curative radical radiotherapy for those who are unfit for surgery or patients with mediastinal node involvement, neoadjuvant chemotherapy for small cell tumours before radiotherapy, palliative radiotherapy for bronchial obstruction, SVC obstruction, haemoptysis, bone pain, cerebral metastasis, radiotherapy/stenting for SVC obstruction, endobronchial therapy, pleural drainage/pleurodesis, drug therapy (symptomatic)

Small cell lung cancer: Chemotherapy – benefit with six courses.

Palliative care: Dexamethasone and radiotherapy for brain metastasis and SVCO, radiotherapy for haemoptysis, bone pain and cough, chemical pleurodesis for effusion, opiates for cough and pain.

According to the aforementioned NICE guideline, If a chest X-ray or chest computed tomography (CT) scan suggests lung cancer (including pleural effusion and slowly resolving consolidation), patients should be offered an urgent referral to a member of the lung cancer multidisciplinary team (MDT), usually a chest physician.

Finally, an important aspect of advice is access to charities and support groups, such as those offered by the British Lung Foundation, the Roy Castle Foundation, and Macmillan Cancer Support.

CHRONIC OBSTRUCTIVE AIRWAYS DISEASE

This 42-year-old man has been short of breath. Please examine his respiratory system and discuss with the examiners.

An Extremely Common Case

Causes: Environmental (smoking and industrial dust exposure) and genetic (α-antitrypsin deficiency).

Key signs: Nebulizers/inhalers/nasal speculums/sputum pot and its contents, signs of hyperinflation, barrel-shaped chest, tracheal tug, nicotine-stained fingers, low position of the laryngeal prominence, loss of cardiac dullness, and lowering of hepatic dullness, bounding pulse, face and conjunctivae for plethora. Tachypnoea, use of accessory muscles, loss of normal outward movement of the abdomen during inspiration and expiratory wheeze. *Advanced stage:* Pursed lip breathing, cyanosis on the underside of the tongue and vermilion border of the lip, and in-drawing of the lateral rib cage (Hoover's sign) on inspiration. Advancing respiratory failure, cyanosis, restlessness, confusion, coarse tremor and warm peripheries. Percussion note resonant.

Note COPD does not cause clubbing: Therefore, if present, consider bronchial carcinoma or bronchiectasis.

Look carefully for evidence of hyperinflation of the chest:
- Symmetrical diminution of chest expansion
- Increased A-P diameter of the chest (but this may also occur in disorders of the thoracic spine)
- Use of accessory muscles of respiration, especially sternomastoids
- Indrawing of intercostals spaces, supraclavicular fossae and costal margins on inspiration
- Shortening of the distance between the cricoid cartilage and suprasternal notch to less than three finger breadths
- Loss of cardiac and hepatic dullness
- Hyper resonance of the chest to percussion

Blue bloater: Bronchitis (minimal inflation, dyspnoea, cor pulmonale, i.e. raised JVP, ankle oedema, RV heave and loud P2, coarse crepitations): Pink puffer – emphysema (hyperinflated barrel shaped chest, tachypnoea, purse-lip breathing, no pulmonary hypertension/cor pulmonale). Chronic bronchitis is a clinical diagnosis: Cough productive of sputum on most days for >3/12 on >2 consecutive years. *Emphysema:* Pathological diagnosis: Destruction of alveolar walls. Degree of overlap with chronic asthma (main differential diagnosis), although in COPD there tends to be reversibility (<15%).

Cor pulmonale: Cyanosis, respiratory distress, systolic waves in JVP, malar flush, ankle and sacral oedema, parasternal heave, loud P2 with a pansystolic murmur heard best in inspiration at the sternal edge. Cor pulmonale is the enlargement of the right ventricle that occurs as a consequence to raised pulmonary artery pressure (pulmonary hypertension) that occurs secondary to chronic lung disorders (e.g. COAD, bronchiectasis) or disorders of the pulmonary circulation (recurrent pulmonary emboli, pulmonary hypertension). *ECG features:* P pulmonale, right axis deviation, right ventricular hypertrophy.

Investigations: FBC–raised WCC (infection), low albumin (severity); CXR–hyperinflation, flat hemidiaphragms, large central pulmonary arteries, reduced peripheral lung markings, bullae, ABG–type II respiratory failure, ECG–right atrial and ventricular hypertrophy (cor pulmonale), respiratory function tests–low transfer factor and obstructive (obstructive + air trapping).

Management

[Please note that, in the UK, NICE offers authoritative guideline for the management of COPD (please refer to the link http://www.nice.org.uk/guidance/CG12) and the British Thoracic Society offers guideline for pulmonary rehabilitation (http://www.brit-thoracic.org.uk/ClinicalInformation/PulmonaryRehabilitation/tabid/108/Default.aspx).]

Aspects of Management

- Weight reduction, if overweight/obese (support for nutritionists may be sensible here);
- Stop smoking through willpower, literature, advice, clinics (such as stop smoking programmes), psychological intervention, anti-smoking medication; exercise;

- Pulmonary rehabilitation empowering patients to take interest and control of their condition [Please note that the current NICE guideline recommends that all patients with COPD who are unable to go about their day-to-day business should be offered a course of pulmonary rehabilitation classes (The BTS guidelines emphasize that anyone with chronic dyspnoea whose lifestyle is affected should have pulmonary rehabilitation – this applies mainly to patients with COPD, but not exclusively)].
- Bronchodilators such as β_2 receptor agonists (salbutamol) or anticholinergic inhalers such as ipatropium bromide should be offered in patients who are breathless. A trial of oral theophylline should be considered. A trial of corticosteroids may be instituted using oral prednisolone 30 mg daily for 2 weeks, if there is failure to respond to increased bronchodilator therapy. Lung function is measured before and after and an improvement of >15% in airflow limitation indicates the need for inhaled steroids. If no improvement occurs then inhaled steroid is unlikely to be beneficial [The airway defect is largely fixed but may be partially reversible with the use of bronchodilators. A positive test is one in which there is $\geq$ 200 ml increase in FEV_1 from baseline response to bronchodilator or steroid (a more brisk response of $\geq$ 500 mls may indicate asthma rather than COPD)].
- Antibiotics when symptomatic of infection. This is particularly useful (and steroid tablets) for early intervention in an acute exacerbation of COPD [Also see later; please note that reducing the amount of re-hospitalizations for patients with COPD is a key target in the UK National Service Framework for COPD].
- Treatment of heart failure, if present.
- Surgery is indicated in selected patients only (pleurodesis procedures for recurrent pneumothraces, bullectomy for isolated bullous disease and lung volume reduction surgery in emphysema).
- Annual influenza vaccination (if no contra-indication).
- *Long term oxygen therapy:* If PO_2 < 7.3 and FEV_1 < 1.5 litres, evidence of cor pulmonale. 2-4L via nasal prongs for atleast 15 hrs a day is effective. Improves average survival by 9 months. The patient must not smoke and use long-term oxygen therapy because of the obvious risk of flammability.
- *Non-invasive ventilation:* This is now being used more and more frequently as a means of avoiding endotracheal assisted ventilation, from which it is often very difficult to wean patients with COAD off. It provides pressure support through a face mask and has

been shown to be of benefit in those with hypercapnic hypoxia. It is sometimes not well tolerated as the mask needs to be tightly applied to the face. Consider BIPAP when pH < 7.35, hypercapnia, and respiratory rare > 30. C/I to NIPPV include imminent arrest, bulbar palsy, coma, and upper airway obstruction.

[Please note that NICE does not recommend α_1-antitrypsin replacement in patients with proven deficiency and severe symptoms].

Acute Exacerbation

Usual precipitants of an exacerbation – smoking (triggering bronchospasm), infection (most commonly *H. influenzae*, *S. pneumoniae* or *M. catarrhalis*), bronchoconstricting drugs, exercise. Treatment of an acute exacerbation: Controlled oxygen via Venturi mask 24%, nebulised bronchodilators, antibiotics, steroids 7-14 days, i/v aminophylline. Even if the CXR shows no radiological evidence of pneumonia, antibiotics such as Ofloxacin can still be used in patients with severe exacerbations (Lancet 2001;358:2913), where the primary end-point was death in hospital or need for repeat courses of antibiotics. Follow-up involves assessing the patient's ability to cope, measuring FEV_1, checking inhaler technique and the patient's understanding of disease and treatment, and assessment of home nebulizers and LTOT if severe COPD.

Guidelines for specialist referral: Rapid decline in FEV_1, COPD in patients less than 40 years and in patients with less than 10 pack years smoking, bullous lung disease, severe COPD, assessment for LTOT/ trial of steroids/home nebulizers, frequent infections (exclude bronchiectasis), symptoms out of proportion to lung deficit, uncertain diagnosis.

Consolidation

This patient has been acutely unwell for 3 days, with shortness of breath and a productive cough. Please examine his chest.

Community-acquired pneumonia. Common organisms: *Strep. Pneumoniae* 50%, *Mycoplasma pneumoniae* 6%, *Haemophilus influenzae*, *Chlamydia pneumoniae*.

Antibiotics: 1st line: penicillin or cephalosporin and macrolide.

Hospital-acquired pneumonia. Common organisms above plus *Pseudomonas, Staph. aureus, Gram-negative bacilli.* Antibiotics: 1st line: Anti-pseudomonal penicillin or broad-spectrum Cephalosporin ± gentamicin.

Causes of consolidation: Pneumonia, tumour, pulmonary embolus, vasculitis, e.g. Churg-Strauss.

Clinical signs: Tachypnoea (count respiratory rate), oxygen mark, sputum pot (rusty sputum indicates pneumococcus), reduced expansion and increased tactile focal fremitus, dull percussion note, focal coarse crackles, increased vocal resonance and bronchial breathing, ask for the temperature chart. Extra points include: Confusion and hypotension and markers of severity, complications, e.g. parapneumonic effusion, clubbing may indicate an abscess, erythema multiforme (target lesions due to *Mycoplasma*).

Severity score for pneumonia: CURB 65 (urea > 7; respiratory rate > 30; BP systolic < 90 mmHg or diastolic <60 mmHg), WCC <4 or >12, T > 38 or <32, age > 65, PaO_2 <8 kPa, multiple lobes affected.

Prevention: Pneumovax II® to high-risk groups, e.g. chronic disease (especially nephrotic and asplenic atients) and the elderly.

Investigation: CXR consolidation (air bronchogram), abscess and effusion; bloods (WCC, CRP, urea, atypical serology, immuno-globulins), blood (25% positive) and sputum cultures, urine (Legionella antigen, Pneumococcal antigen, haemoglobulinuria: Mycoplasma causes cold agglutinins causing haemodialysis).

Management: Oxygen and antibiotics.

Complications: Lung abscess (*Staph. aureus, Klebsiella,* anaerobes), para-pneumonic effusion/empyema, pneumothorax, haemoptysis, septic shock and multi-organ failure.

PULMONARY FIBROSIS/CRYPTOGENIC FIBROSING ALVEOLITIS

This 42-year-old man has been short of breath. Please examine his respiratory system and discuss with the examiners.

An Extremely Common Case

Key signs: Chest wall movement reduced on side of lesion, tracheal displacement towards side of lesion, percussion note is dull, widespread inspiratory crepitations, tactile vocal fremitus increased, clubbing, rheumatoid hands (bibasal fine crackles end-inspiratory if cryptogenic fibrosing alveolitis). No sputum.

Signs of associated autoimmune diseases: E.g. rheumatoid arthritis (hands), SLE and systemic sclerosis (face and hands) and Crohn's (mouth ulcers). Signs of treatment: E.g. Cushingoid from steroids. 65-85% of patients with fibrosing alveolitis have clubbing.

Underlying diagnoses: Connective tissue diseases, SLE, rheumatoid disease, radiotherapy, drugs, e.g. methotrexate, amiodarone, sulphalasize, gold, sulphonamides, nitrofurantoin, inorganic dust related interstitial lung disease, e.g. asbestosis, granulomatous disease (e.g. sarcoidosis, tuberculosis, beryllosis), offending agents known to cause hypersensitivity pneumonitis (e.g. mushrooms).

Causes of basal fibrosis: Cryptogenic fibrosing alveolitis, asbestosis, amiodarone, connective tissue diseases, aspiration.

Causes of upper lobe fibrosis: Pneumoconioses (excluding asbestosis), EAA, TB, ABPA, ankylosing spondylitis.

Idiopathic cryptogenic fibrosing alveolitis: A histopathological spectrum from inflammatory dequasamative interstitial pneumonitis to fibrosis usual interstitial pneumonitis (UIP). UIP is more common. Overall prognosis is poor, though DIP responds better to steroids. Desquamative interstitial pneumonitis (DIP) is inflammatory in nature, whereas UIP is more advanced inflammation with fibrosis. The overall prognosis in cryptogenic fibrosing alveolitis is poor. The importance of tests supporting an inflammatory picture is that there is likely to be a beter response to steroids and immunosuppression.

Complications: 60% of patients die as a direct consequence of fibrosing alveolitis, pulmonary hypertension and right heart failure, lung cancer.

Investigations: Bloods (ESR, rheumatoid factor, ANA), drug history, spirometry, autoantibodies, CXR (bilateral basal reticulonodular changes), ABG for type I respiratory failure, HRCT (groundglass opacification), bronchoalveolar lavage (lymphocytes predominate in inflammatory and neutrophils do not), pulmonary function tests including diffusion capacity, tests for underlying causes. DTPA scan can be used to assess the probability of deterioration. Serum precipitins for EAA.

HRCT may obviate need for the biopsy. Open lung biopsy (transbronchial or percutaneous biopsy may be required for histology).

Management: Depends on the underlying cause. High dose steroids should be commenced following diagnosis (often involving a high-resolution, thin slice CT of thorax) and then continued for 4 to 6 weeks. If this does not achieve remission, then immunosuppressant drugs such as azathioprine or cyclophosphamide should be considered. Lung transplantation is an option in younger patients with rapidly progressive disease: there is a 60% 1 year survival rate.

Prognosis: 50% mortality at 2 years. There is an increased risk of bronchogenic carcinoma.

Other Points to Note

Apical fibrosis: Possible ipsilateral tracheal deviation, reduced upper zone expansion, dull percussion note, fine inspiratory crepitations in upper zone. *Causes:* Old tuberculosis, radiotherapy, ankylosing spondylitis, connective tissue disorders (anti-Jo-1 dermatomyositis), extrinsic allergic alveolitis, massive pulmonary fibrosis from pneumoconiosis, histoplasmosis.

Other features of old TB: Chest deformity, tracheal deviation towards the side of the lesion (fibrosis), reduced expansion, dull percussion, crackles and bronchial breathing, scars from previous plombage therapy (pingpong balls/sponges used to collapse the infected lobe to prevent aeration and spread of bacilli), previous lobectomy/ pneumonectomy scars (look at back and under axillae), and scars from phrenic nerve crush for diaphragm analysis, kyphosis (Pott's fracture). Streptomycin was introduced in the 1950's. It was the first drug shown to be beneficial in a randomized controlled trial.

Primary TB: Asymptomatic, persistent cough, significant CMI, compression of a bronchus leading to collapse. TB may progress or re-activate: Postprimary TB causes endobronchial symptoms (cough, sputum, haemoptysis), compression of a bronchus by lymph nodes leading to collapse of a lobe or segment, spread via the lymphatics to the pleura, aspergilloma formation within a cavitated lesion. *Tests:* Tuberculin and Mantoux (strongly positive may imply active infection), and Heaf. False –ves, when CMI response is impaired. CXR (patchy upper lobe opacification) and microbiological identification (AFB, early morning urines).

Postprimary TB: This involves necrosis in the centre of the lesion, with discharge of its contents and cavitation. Discharge into the bronchus with endobronchial symptoms can occur, compression of a bronchus by lymph nodes leading to collapse of a segment, spread via the lymphatics to the pleura or pericardium, and aspergilloma formation within a cavitated lesions.

Asbestos-related lung disease: Usually occurs > 20 years after exposure, proportional to the intensity of exposure. Characterized by exertional dyspnoea, dry cough, inspiratory crackles in lower zones. Chest X-ray may show irregular opacities, and with more advanced disease honeycombing. Pulmonary function tests reveal restrictive lung disease with a reduced transfer factor. Lung cancer is increased synergistically with smoking, and the risk of mesothelioma is markedly increased. Patients are eligible for industrial injury benefit. Benign pleural disease involves plaques, diffuse pleural thickening, effusion and calcification. Benign pleural disease is usually asymptomatic and detected on CXR. Patients are usually not eligible for industrial injury benefit. Mesothelioma normally occurs > 30 years, and almost always caused by asbestosis. High risk asbestosis is crocidolite (blue asbestos). Diagnosis is confirmed by pleural biopsy.

Pneumoconioses: Silicosis–upper zone fibrosis with eggshell hilar calcification that predisposes to TB infection; berylliosis – granulomatous lesions resulting in fibrosis, similar to sarcoid; asbestosis–predominantly affects lung bases, pleural plaques and associated mesothelioma; simple coal-worker's lung does not cause pulmonary fibrosis.

Extrinsic allergic alveolitis: Bird fancier's lung (pigeons), Farmer's lung (mouldy hay), Byssinosis–cotton dust. Following exposure there is inflammation of the bronchioles resulting in cough, pyrexia and malaise. If exposure becomes chronic it may result in increasing shortness of breath and non-caseating granulomatous disease. Treatment is with steroids in acute disease and long-term avoidance of precipitating factors.

BRONCHIECTASIS

This 60 or 21-year-old woman presents to your clinic with a chronic cough. Please examine her chest and discuss your finding.

An Extremely Common Case

Bronchiectasis is a term used to describe abnormal and permanently dilated airways.

Points in the examination: Clubbing, central cyanosis, dyspnoeic and tachypnoeic, cachexia and short stature, cough with copious purulent sputum (often bloody) and halitosis, coarse inspiratory crepitations, often cover one or more areas of lung. Look for cystic fibrosis (CF), post infective (pneumonia, TB, measles, whooping cough), ABPA, hypogammaglobulinaemia, primary ciliary dyskinesia/Kartagener's syndrome.

CF: Examine the precordium, Portex reservoir under the skin or Hickman line/scars for long-term antibiotics. CF features: Respiratory, intestinal (obstruction, rectal prolapse, pancreatic failure and malabsorption/failure to thrive, diabetes develops in 20% of adults due to destruction of the islets of Langerhans by mucoid plugging of the pancreatic ducts, biliary cirrhosis, gallstones, meconium ileus), infertility, arthropathy.

Cor-pulmonale: Cyanosis, ankle oedema, RVH, loud P2.

Part of the differential of clubbing and crackles includes interstitial lung fibrosis and malignancy.

Potential complications include anaemia, brain abscess, empyema, cor pulmonae and secondary amyloidosis, chest pain, haemoptysis, metastatic spread of infection, arthropathy.

Investigation: Sputum culture and sensitivity and cytology, CXR shows tramline shadows and high resolution CT scan (thickened bronchial walls), sinus radiography (mucosal thickening and fluid levels), aspergillus precipitins. Look for a specific cause: Bronchoscopy for malignancy, serum immunoglobulins for hypogammaglobulinaemia, aspergillus precipitins and skin prick testing, and saccharine ciliary motility tests (nares to taste buds in 30 min): Kartagener's syndrome.

CF investigations: Screened at birth by low immunoreactive trypsin. Sweat test Na^+ >60 μmol/l (false positive in hypothyroidism and Addison's disease). Genetic screening.

CF genetics: Incidence 1/2500 live births, autosomal recessive chromosome 7q, CFTR, commonest mutation is a deletion Df508. Pathophysiology: Secretions are thickened and the lumens of various structures are blocked (bronchioles leading to bronchiectasis; pancreatic ducts leading to chronic pancreatitis, gut leading to meconium ileus equivalent in adults; seminal vesicles leading to male infertility).

General principles of treatment: Postural drainage, physiotherapy, antibiotic therapy for exacerbations particularly to cover *Pseudomonas*, mucolytics (nebulised rhDNase is effective in patients with viscid sputum), longer-term rotating antibiotics, bronchodilators, if there is any airflow obstruction, surgery is occasionally used for localised disease, gene therapy for cystic fibrosis, replacement of immunoglobulins. Specific treatment of CF; daily chest percussion and physiotherapy, early institution of broad spectrum antibiotics for minimisation of lung damage from infective exacerbations, pancreatic enzyme replacement therapy (e.g. pancrease®), immunization, bronchodilators, aerosol dornase alpha which interferes with sputum neutrophil DNA, immunisation, heart-lung transplantation for poor pulmonary function and purulent bronchiectasis, palliative care, gene therapy.

Causes

1. *Congenital:* Cystic fibrosis Kartagener's syndrome (features are dextrocardia, bronchiectasis, situs inversus, infertility, dysplasia of the frontal sinuses, sinusitis, otitis media; patients have ciliary motility).
2. *Mechanical:* Bronchial carcinoma (suspect if localized bronchiectasis).
3. *Childhood infections:* Whooping cough, measles and TB.
4. *Immune overactivity:* Allergic bronchopulmonary aspergillosis.
5. *Immune underactivity:* Hypogammaglobulinaemia.
6. *Aspiration:* Chronic alcoholics.
7. *Yellow nail syndrome:* The nails are thick, excessively curved from side to side and slow growing, leaving bulbous fingertips uncovered and pale yellow. The cuticles are lost, the lunulae are absent and there is oncholysis. The yellow nail syndrome is usually associated with lymphatic hypoplasia, ankle oedema and a number of pulmonary conditions such as bronchiectasis, pleural effusion, COPD and malignant neoplasms. Other associations include D-penicillamine therapy, nephrotic syndrome, hypothyroidism and AIDS.

Complications: Cor pulmonale, secondary amyloidosis, massive haemoptysis, metastatic infection, e.g. cerebral abscess.

ASTHMA

This 22-year-old man has been short of breath. Please examine his respiratory system and discuss with the examiners.

Look initially for pectus carinatum (see **chest wall shapes** above). Examination reveals a bilateral scattered wheeze, and costal recession. Examine the sputum cup, and comment on accessory muscles of respiration, tachycardia, pulsus paradoxus and whether the patient can utter sentences without stopping to take a breath. The diagnosis is bronchial asthma and comment on the functional status.

Asthma is an inflammatory disorder characterized by hyper-responsiveness of the airway to various stimuli, resulting in widespread narrowing of the airway.

Indications for steroids in chronic asthma: Sleep is disturbed by the wheeze, morning tightness persists until midday, symptoms and peak expiratory flows progressively deteriorate each day, maximum treatment is with bronchodilators, emergency nebulizers are needed.

Investigations: Dynamic spirometry, serial peak flow measurement, skin tests to assess the role of allergens, steroid response test, airways hyperrespnsiveness test (increased sensitivity to histamine ot metacholine bronchial provocation test). For acute episodes, peak flow measurement, arterial blood gases, chest X-ray (to exclude pneumothora or pneumonia), ECG if the cause of breathlessness unclear, and sputum culture.

Complications: Retarded growth rate, pneumothorax, thoracic cage abnormality, recurrent bronchial infection, respiratory arrest, fixed airway obstruction.

Non-pharmacological management of chronic asthma: Avoidance of cold air, diet (high intake of fresh fruit and vegetables), clean mattresses (avoidance of bed mites), removal of other exacerbating factors (e.g. family pets).

Pharmacological management of a patient with acute asthma: Nebulised β-agonists, e.g. salbutamol, oxygen, high-dose steroids (intravenous hydrocortisone or oral prednisolone), blood gases, CXR to rule out pneumothorax.

Table 3.1: Asthma guidelines

BTS guidelines (please refer to the BTS website for the current guidelines)
Step 1 — Inhaled short-acting β-agonists used as required for symptom relief.
Step 2 — Step 1 + regular inhaled anti-inflammatory agents (such as beclomethasone, budesonide, chromoglycate)
Step 3 — Step 1 + high-dose inhaled steroids or low dose inhaled steroids plus a long-acting beta-agonist bronchodilator
Step 4 — Step 1 + high-dose inhaled steroids and regular bronchodilators (long-acting inhaled or oral beta-agonists, sustained-release theophylline, inhaled ipatropium)
Step 5 — Step 4 + oral steroids

LUNG COLLAPSE

This man is stable, but has had a previous procedure. What was that procedure, and why might he have done this? Confine your examination to the respiratory system.

Ipsilateral tracheal deviation, decreased ipsilateral expansion, dull ipsilateral percussion note, reduced ipsilateral breath sounds.

Common causes of lung collapse: Iatrogenic for TB, bronchial carcinoma, bronchial adenoma, lymphadenopathy, mucus plugs (asthma, allergic bronchopulmonary aspergillosis), foreign bodies. Tell the examiner that you would like to look for tar staining (tobacco smoking), clubbing and cachexia.

A Note on Pneumothorax

Unlikely to be in the examination, but the author has experience of some candidates feeling they were given a small apical pneumothorax. The classification of a pneumothorax is given in *Table 3.2*.

Contralateral tracheal deviation, reduced ipsilateral expansion, hyper-resonant ipsilateral percussion note, reduced/absent ipsilateral breath sounds.

Causes of pneumothorax: Spontaneous (usually in thin males), trauma, bronchial asthma, COPD, carcinoma of the lung, cystic fibrosis, TB.

Table 3.2: BTS grading of pneumothorax (see BTS guidelines for current guidelines)

Small	Small rim of air around the lung (those less than 20% in size usually resolve within weeks)
Moderate	Lung is collapsed towards the heart border
Complete	Airless lung, separate from the diaphragm (aspiration which is less painful than intercostals drainage, leads to a shorter admission time and reduces the need for pleurectomy with no increase in recurrence rate at 1 year)
Tension	Any pneumothorax with cardiorespiratory distress (rare and requires immediate drainage)

PLEURAL EFFUSION

This 42-year-old man has been short of breath. Please examine his respiratory system and discuss with the examiners.

An Extremely Common Case

Key signs: Tachypnoea, fullness of intercostal spaces, diminished chest movements on inspection and palpation, apical impulse not visualised, trachea shifted to the opposite side, vocal fremitus and vocal resonance reduced on affected size, stony dullness on percussion, diminished breath sounds. 'Bleating aegophany' may be heard above the level of the effusion.

Extra points: Cancer (clubbing and lymphadenopathy), mastectomy, colostomy or laporomy, radiation scars and tattoos, chemotherapy –

alopecia, mucositis, Cushing's syndrome, radiation scars, tuberculosis/ lymphoma (lymphadenopathy and fever), congestive cardiac failure (raised JVP, third heart sound, peripheral oedema), nephrotic syndrome (generalised oedema and ascites), chronic liver disease/ cirrhosis (leuconychia, spider naevi and gynaecomastia), autoimmune disease (characteristic rash or arthritis), pulmonary emboli (raised JVP, right ventricular heave, loud P2, deep vein thrombosis), hypothyroidism (dry skin, bradycardia, characteristic facies, slow-relaxing reflexes), chronic renal failure (arteriovenous fistula), connective tissue disease (rheumatoid hands), signs of DVT.

Differential diagnosis: Consolidation (bronchial breath sounds), collapse, raised hemidiaphragm, pleural thickening. Dyspnoea on immersion in water is suggestive of diaphragmatic palsy and therefore perhaps the most useful diagnostic investigation are dynamic diaphragm studies.

Causes: Exudate (>30 g/dl protein): Bronchial cancer, pneumonia, mesothelioma, drugs (methotrexate, nitrofurantoin), TB, rheumatoid disease, SLE, sarcoidosis, Dressler's syndrome, PE, pulmonary infarction, metastasis.

Transudate (<30 g/dl protein): Nephrotic syndrome, cirrhosis, cardiac failure, hypothyroidism, yellow-nail syndrome, peritoneal dialysis, Meig's syndrome.

Investigations

- Blood tests (FBC, ESR, U&Es, LFTs, full biochemical profile,).
- CXR (AP and lateral: earliest sign is blunting of the costophrenic angle which may require the presence of at least 300 ml of fluid).
- Aspiration of the pleural fluid (confirm diagnosis, appearance of fluid? chylous suggests malignancy or trauma to the thoracic duct and? bloody suggests malignancy, infarction or trauma, type of fluid – exudates or transudate; exudates favoured by protein concentration pleural fluid: Serum > 0.5, LDH pleural fluid: Serum > 0.6, highly cellular fluid), smear (Gram stain, Ziehl-Nielsen, malignant cells), further tests on aspirate (e.g. amylase > 200 units/ dl is indicative of pancreatitis or occasionally malignancy).
- Sputum examination (AFB, pneumonia, malignant cells).
- Serological tests (RA factor, ANF).
- Pleural biopsy (essential for TB and malignancy).
- Mantoux test.

- Ultrasound of abdomen for hepatic cause.
- Bronchoscopy ± CT-guided biopsy for tissue diagnosis (biopsy is useful for diagnosis of tuberculosis and malignancy)/thoracoscopy.
- CT or MRI chest depending on underlying cause (looking particularly for localized effusions and pleural and parenchymal disease) possibly a bone scan.

Investigations: Pleural fluid cytology (60%) plus pleural biopsy (70%) plus thoracoscopy (90+%), CT of thorax may also be useful.

Complications: Constrictive fibrosis of pleural and restricted lung function, iatrogenic secondary infection, iatrogenic pneumothorax, unilateral pulmonary oedema, and haemorrhage (especially after pleural biopsy).

Management: The principal aim is to treat the aetiology, aspiration if causing respiratory distress, pleurodeses, surgery (persistent collections and for progressive pleural thickening). For infective causes, systemic antibiotics are indicated and intercostal drainage is essential. For tuberculosis, standard oral antituberculosis chemotherapy is indicated. For malignant effusions, pleural effusion indicates inoperability; treatment is guided by symptoms. Agents (tetracycline, talc or bleomycin) are introduced via intercostals drains to cause adhesion of the two layers of pleura and prevent re-accumulation (pleurodesis).

A Note on Empyema

Empyema is a collection of pus within the pleural space. Most frequent organisms are anaerobes, *staphylococci* and Gram-negative organisms. Associated with bronchial obstruction, e.g. carcinoma. *Treatment:* Pleural drainage and IV antibiotics. Intrapleural streptokinase. Surgery.

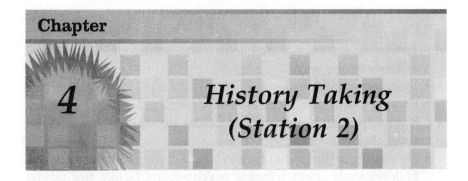

Chapter

4

History Taking (Station 2)

INTRODUCTION TO THE GENERAL APPROACH TO THE HISTORYTAKING STATION

[The MRCP Clinical Examining Board have kindly made available sample scenarios for this Station: these may be viewed and downloaded using the following link: http://www.mrcpuk.org/PACES/Pages/PACESscenarios.aspx]

The timing of the station starts when you enter the station having read the letter. Make sure you take note of the detail in it, and the particular questions that need to be answered. You will probably be asked how you will respond to the GP's request for advice, so focus your history on addressing the problems of relevance, as well as leaving time for more general enquiry. When starting the conversation with the patient remember to take time to introduce yourself, put the patient at ease, and check that the patient's understanding of why he/she is there corresponds to yours – as you would in real life. If the information given by your patient differs from that in the GP letter, try not to panic. As you know, this happens in real life, and you should simply clarify the position with the patient, as you would normally.

Be alert to clues that the patient may give regarding particular concerns, or emotional state – part of the test is to see how good you are picking these up. Is the patient concerned about cancer; are there distressing social circumstances behind the presenting complaint? Towards the end of your time, remember to summarise with the patient the salient points of the history (this allows you to fill in any detail that may have escaped you earlier), to share with the patient your thoughts about the possible nature of the problems, and to explain briefly how you will take matters forward. This also helps you to formulate your problem list. The patient is at liberty to ask for an explanation of any tests you suggest.

1. The key points in the first part of the markscheme, "data gathering in the interview", are:
    *   Presenting complaints are elicited, and documented in a logical and systematic way.
    *   Inclusion of systems review.
    *   Enquiry about past medical history/family/smoking/treatment history (past and present). Candidates surprisingly often omit a drug allergy history.
    *   Do not forget the social history and follow psychosocial clues. Follows leads about relevant psycho-social factors (including: Activities of daily living, work life, home life, tobacco, alcohol, recreational drugs, sexual history, impact of problems on the job).
    *   Appropriate verbal and non-verbal (eye contact, posture etc.) responsiveness, good balance of open and closed questions.
2   The second part of the markscheme deals with "identification and use of the information gathered". This involves:
    *   Checking information is correct with patient. This is in terminology appropriate to the patient.
    *   An ability to interpret history with the patient. You should offer a diagnosis, and then regarding the management go onto explaining the process, risks and benefits of various options, and perhaps explaining some uncertainties regarding diagnosis, outcome or prognosis if relevant. Check for understanding and summarising at appropriate intervals.
    *   A good candidate would also give the patient the opportunity to ask any further questions before closure.
    *   An ability to create a problem list including diagnosis, social problems, concerns or complaints about treatment, and disease complications, is inherent.
3   The third part of the markscheme deals with "discussion related to the case". In the semi-structured oral interview, the candidate is expected to:
    *   Be able to discuss the implications of the patient's problems, both medical and referral to surgery and other specialists including alternative/complementary medicine.
    *   Be able to discuss strategy for solving the problem. This is terminology appropriate to senior examiners!

    In discussing with the examiners, you will be expected to consider how the patient's problems affect lifestyle, social interactions and employment prospects, as well as the purely medical aspects. You will probably be asked for a reasonable differential diagnosis on the basis of what you have accrued, possibly be asked what signs you might look for on clinical examination, and be asked for your strategy for solving the problems – so again this may be a series of tests or may be much broader, and involve other health professionals. Finally, if there have been any specific questions asked by the referral letter, you must address them. The examiners will mark your performance on your handling of the conversation and also the accuracy of information that you have given. Whilst the emphasis will be on history taking and communication skills, if you give a patient or relative seriously misleading or dangerous information you willl be failed. You will also be failed if you do not ask the key questions that would materially affect the treatment of the patient, e.g. other medications.

COMMON SYMPTOMS COMPRISING THE HISTORY

Each history and scenario will be different, but the principles above can still apply. We have included here some common "complaints", both in real life and in examinations both at undergraduate and postgraduate level. These are broadly divided into subject group, although some symptoms may cross more than one group.

CARDIOVASCULAR SYSTEM

Hypertensive

Points in the history Has the hypertension been found before? Relevant symptoms such as cardiac failure, headaches, palpitations, dyspnoea, ankle oedema, blurred vision, tremors, weight change, renal disease, anxiety disorder.

Elicit cardiac risk factors (e.g. ethnic origin, cholesterol, smoking, a relevant family history including relevant disorders renal disease and neurofibromatosis) and previous medical history (previous MI/ CVA, renal infarction, renovascular disease, diabetes); obtain a drug history including previous drug history and side-effects (steroids, NSAIDs, OCP, MAOIs), and some details of lifestyle issues (e.g. smoking, caffeine and alcohol history, domestic situation and its accompanying stresses).

Enquire specifically about certain features suggestive of a cause: For example, weakness in patients with hyperaldosteronism may suggest hypokalaemia; paroxysmal symptoms, palpitations, sweating, pallor flushing suggest phaeochromocytoma; features to suggest Cushing's disease (e.g. weight gain, muscle weakness, hair growth) or acromegaly (headaches, galactorrhoea); pulsation in the neck may be suggestive of an adult-type coarctation of the aorta.

Causes

The causes of hypertension are generally a white-coat effect, primary (essential) or secondary. Important secondary causes include intrinsic renal disease (polyarteritis nodosa, systemic sclerosis, chromic pyelonephritis, polycystic kidneys, renal artery stenosis either due to fibromuscular dysplasia or artheromatous disease, Cushing's syndrome, Conn's syndrome, acromegaly, hyperparathyroidism, coarctation of the aorta, pregnancy and pre-eclampsia, steroid therapy.

Investigations

U&Es, cholesterol, glucose, ECG, urine analysis (for protein, blood), renal ultrasound of the kidneys (e.g. polcystic kidneys, renal artery stenosis), renal arteriogram, 24-hr urinary VMA, 24-hr urinary free cortisol, urinary free cortisol, renin, aldosterone, OGTT (acromegaly), echocardiogram, 24-hour ambulatory blood pressure monitoring for white coat or borderline hypertension.

Management

This includes measurement of the blood pressure (two subsequent clinics are needed where their blood pressure is assessed from two readings using the best conditions available; routine use of automated blood pressure monitoring or home-monitoring devices in primary care is not currently recommended because their value has not been adequately monitored); lifestyle changes initially and then periodically, drug treatment to patients with persistently high blood pressure and monitoring of side-effects. Anti-hypertensive drug treatment initiated in systolic BP > 160 or sustained diastolic > 100 mmHg (<140/90 diabetics). Consider other drugs for cardiovascular risk, e.g. aspirin, statin therapy. A sustained drop in BP is needed, and modifiable risk factors should be addressed before pharmacological treatment is instituted.

Chest Pain

Points in the History

An accurate history of the chest pain is vital: This includes where (ischaemic pain is poorly localised retrosternal discomfort often described as tightness, pressure or burning), nature (ischaemic pain is heavy or tight, often patients deny the symptom of pain and refer to it as discomfort), radiation (may radiate to the arms, neck, jaw, gums or abdomen, and sometimes this may be the only sites), exacerbating factors (including exertion effects, posture, meals), cardiac risk factors. Cardiac pain tends to be heaviness, band, gripping and dull ache. Precipitants are exertion, cold weather, or stress. Non-cardiac pain tends to be a dull ache, sharp, shooting, and precipitated by specific body motion. Enquire about rest and nocturnal pain. A history of hot and shivery symptoms, central chest pain comfortable when sitting upright, inability to sleep lying down, no effect of exertion and eating is suggestive of pericarditis? may be on the background of autoimmune disease. Pericarditis is pleuritic chest pain, varying with posture, classically relieved by sitting forward. Consider predisposing factors to angina: Including obesity, hyperlipidaemia, hypertension, hyperthyroidism, anaemia.

Enquire about previous medical history: Cardiovascular or cerebrovascular disease, cholesterol, diabetes, hypertension, risk factors for PE/DVT, pericarditis risk factors (pyogenic, TB, malignant, uraemia, hypothyroid, autoimmune disorders). Include a drug history, family history of peripheral vascular disease, thrombophilia, familial hypercholesterolaemia, and social history (smoking, occupational lifestyle, recent travel).

Differential Diagnosis

(1) Chronic stable angina, predictable on exercise and may be relieved by rest; worse in cold or windy weather, induced by stress, rapidly improved by GTN, (2) Unstable angina, at rest, (3) Pericarditis: Localized anterior central pain, worse on breathing and lying flat, (4) Aortic dissection, sudden onset radiating to the back, (5) Pleural pain, lateralized and worse on breathing and associated with cough, (6) Oesophageal pain (may be worse on eating and associated with vomiting; oesophagitis may be pain after meals particularly citrus juices or spirits, with relief on sitting or standing up), (7) Spinal pain, mainly in the back but may radiate round to front in a nerve root distribution, (8) Skin pain, usually due to shingles, (9) Musculoskeletal pain, usually tender to palpation, (10) Pulmonary embolism which may cause sudden chest pain, hypotension, dyspnoea, collapse and right heart strain.

Investigations

FBC (neutrophil leukocytosis and thrombocytosis in MI), ECG (resting rhythm, evidence of previous MI, LVH, right-heart strain), glucose, lipids, CK/troponin I, exercuse testing, CXR (focal lung disease, masses, pruning of pulmonary vessels as in pulmonary hypertension), Hb/TFTs (thyroid function can exacerbate pain as can anaemia), V/Q scan (if PE suspected), echocardiogram (structural heart disease), *H. pylori* if suspicion of oesophageal pain (also consider upper GI endoscopy and oesophageal manometry).

Cardiac Failure

Points in the History

Try to confirm that symptoms are consistent with heart failure in the first place, for example traditionally with LVF: Dyspnoea, orthopnoea, paroxysmal nocturnal dyspnoea, nocturnal cough, fatigue. Symptoms are usually worse when lying flat, but this is not specific: For example, consider GORD, postnasal drip and bronchial secretions. RVF: Ankle swelling. Assess symptom severity: The NHYA scale is I–no limitations, II – slight limitation of physical activity, III–marked limitation of physical activity; IV – symptoms at rest.

Consider the patient's thoughts about the causes of the symptoms and expectations of treatment. What can your patient no longer do that he/she would like to do? Does he/she live alone? What family, friends and other supports are there?

Enquire about the possible causes of heart failure: Coronary artery disease, pressure overload (hypertension or aortic stenosis), volume overload (aortic or mitral regurgitation), arrhythmias (including atrial fibrillation), and cor pulmonale (often due to COPD but sometimes parenchymal lung disease or pulmonary emboli).

Investigations

Ask about investigations so far: Assessment of renal function and albumin should be included since fluid overload leading to pulmonary oedema can be due to renal failure or hypoalbuminaemia.

Management

ACE inhibitors improve outcome, and should be used in all patients, apart from where contraindicated. β-blockers have been shown to improve outcome in selected patients with NYHA I-III classes. Everyday experience shows that loop and thiazide diuretics improve symptoms but do not improve outcome. Low dose spironolactone is useful for NYHA III and IV in those already being treated with ACEI and diuretics. Digoxin should be considered for all patients with heart failure and atrial fibrillation.

A NEW MURMUR/ENDOCARDITIS

Points in the History

Murmurs are often asymptomatic and discovered during routine medical examination. New murmurs associated with fever or signs of infection are indicative of endocarditis. Check for points that suggest an underlying aetiology or associated structural disease, e.g. history of rheumatic fever, history of thyroid disease/shunts/chronic liver disease/pregnancy (associated with flow murmurs), previous MI, history of congenital disease/syndrome (valve stenosis and endocardial cushion defects), dizziness/syncope (LV outflow obstruction), angina (associated with aortic stenosis).

Investigations

A transthoracic echocardiogram is clearly the single most important investigation, but other investigations are useful, e.g. ECG for cardiac rhythm (e.g. atrial fibrillation associated with mitral disease; LVH associated with aortic stenosis), and CXR (heart size and aortic contour).

Palpitations

Points in the History

Ask how well tolerated the palpitations are, as this factor will be very important to the patient. Other useful points in the history:
- Ask for the nature of the palpitation (pauses and thumbs suggest extra-systoles with compensatory pauses), irregular or regular (irregular palpitation suggests atrial fibrillation or frequent extrasystoles).
- Ask the patient to tap out the rhythm on the desk (a slow forceful rhythm suggests bradycardia or bigeminy rhythm with compensatory pauses.
- Does the patient experience palpitations as fast or slow? Simple ectopics are usually easy to determine from the history alone: Patients refer to "missed" or "extra" beats. Sudden bursts of fluttering may indicate paroxysmal atrial fibrillation. A clear onset and offset to rapid regular palpitations is characteristic of re-entrant tachycardias.
- Ask about associated symptoms especially chest pain, dyspnoea, faintness (this strengthens the argument for pacemaker implantation with bradycardias), anxiety, tremor, increased

appetite. Palpitations accompanied by diarrhoea, wheezing and flushing may be indicative of carcinoid syndrome.

- Ask also about psychiatric syndromes, e.g. panic attacks, generalised anxiety disorder, depression, somatization.
- How long ago did the palpitations start? How frequent are they?
- Triggering factors (e.g. exertion in VT, posture for vasovagal syndrome, emotional stress, often sinus tachycardia, effect of exercise i.e. patient may notice that extrasystoles disappear during exercise, alcohol for atrial fibrillation, and caffeine which has a questionable relationship to extrasystoles).

Previous medical history: Fever, anaemia, previous history of heart disease (risk factors, previous events), hypertension (most recent blood pressure), mitral valve disease (previous rheumatic fever) or thyroid disorders, phaeochromocytoma, hypoglycaemia, mastocytosis.

Elicit a full drug history, consider beliefs concerns and expectations, and a social and occupational history.

Investigations

ECG, 24-HT, CXR, echocardiogram, bloods, Respiratory System.

Asthma

Points in the History

Questions relating to current symptoms: Onset and duration of symptoms, nature of symptoms (cough, sputum, haemoptysis, worsening wheeze, fever, chest pain, disturbance of sleep, presence of nocturnal cough); any diurnal variation; precipitating factors– infection, contact with known allergens, stress, exercise, poor compliance with medication; how the PEFR has changed.

Questions relating to where the diagnosis was made, underlying stability/severity of disease, reversibility associated with therapy; usual treatment – home nebulisers, steroids; previous exacerbations and their management (?whether in hospital); days taken off work; previous admissions to ITU and whether he was ventilated in the past; primary or secondary care of management.

Previous medical history: Eczema, atopy, nasal polyps, recent surgery.

Drug history: NSAIDs, β-blockers, common allergies (including drug allergies).

Travel history: Recent air travel (?are the symptoms actually suggestive of a pulmonary embolus).

Social history: Anxiety and stress, smoking. Family history: Asthma, clotting disorders.

Investigations

PEFR, pulse oximeter, arterial blood gases, CXR, FBC, U&E, CRP and ESR, sputum MC+S, spiral CT scan, lung funtion tests, serum precipitins.

Management

As well as medication for asthma, the patient should ideally stop smoking and avoid any relevant allergens. Admit if: Hypoxic, PEFR < 50% of patient's normal value; patients with severe attacks requiring urgent reatment and early liaison with ITU, patients with a history of brittle asthma should be admitted even if the symptoms are mild. Follow the BTS guidelines (see **Station 1** section).

Breathlessness/Dyspnoea

Points in the history Assessment of the premorbid state.

Account of symptoms (acute or chronic/progressive; sudden or insidious; episodic, stepwise or continuous?).

- Could the breathlessness be due to a cardiac complaint as well as a respiratory one? (Is the patient on a medication for chronic heart failure?)
- Is the breathlessness progressive as in lung fibrosis, COPD or does it follow a daily rhythm such as in asthma?
- Is the breathlessness of rapid onset (e.g. foreign body, anaphylaxis, anxiety, pneumothorax or pulmonary embolism, where the pain can be localised and worse on inspiration)?
- Does the breathlessness come on over a few minutes or hours? (if the onset lasts a few hours, consider asthma, COPD, chest infection, metabolic acidosis, or left heart failure; asthma is distinguished by the absence of a history of chest pain, the absence of murmurs, and a previous history of asthma);
- Is there a history of antecedent illness? (e.g. pericardial tamponade);
- Is there breathlessness sufficient to wake the patient at night time, for example, paroxysmal nocturnal dyspnoea, or noctural asthma?;
- Does the breathlessness come on over several weeks? (diffuse pulmonary fibrosis, chronic heart failure, recurrent pulmonary embolism, anaemia);

- Is there dyspnoea at rest or exertion?
- Any difficulty sleeping because of symptoms? Usual symptoms during the day? Effects on daily activities? Effects of daily activities on symptoms? Concerns about illness?
- What is the impact of the disease, **both** physical **and** psychosocial?

Enquire about risk factors – Past respiratory disease (recurrent pneumonias, TB), family history, smoking, hypertension, lipid profile, diabetes, atopy; number of exacerbations per year.

Enquire abour relevant triggers, including exercise, cold, smoking, occupational exposure (e.g. asbestos, compost), allergens (house dust mite, dog allergen, cat allergen, birds including parrots, pollen and moulds). Ask about any evidence of winter exacerbations (e.g. COPD).

Take a decent drug history (especially NSAIDs for wheeze, ACE for cough, drug-induced fibrosis, e.g. nitrofurantoin, busulphan), and occupational history including asbestos and compost), social history (passive, pipe and cigarette smoking), travel history (atypical pneumonias and TB).

Differential Diagnosis

Cardiovascular (LV systolic/diastolic failure), LVH, myocardial ischaemia, pericardial disease; respiratory (COPD, asthma, upper respiratory tract obstruction, interstitial lung disease, respiratory infection, pleural effusion), other (anaemia, diabetic ketoacidosis, salicylate poisoning, hyperventilation syndrome). Features of a hyperventilation syndrome include headaches, dizziness, palpitations and peioral paraesthesia.

Investigations

These might include:
- Chest X-ray (emphysema, asthma, consolidation, cardiac failure, pulmonary oedema, pneumothorax, bronchial carcinoma),
- FBC (to exclude anaemia, or polycythaemia),
- ECG (arrhythmias),
- PEFR,
- Full lung function tests including spirometry, reversibility of forced expiratory volume in 1s, arteral blood gases (severity of disease and type of respiratory failure),
- Sputum and blood cultures should be taken if an infective aetiology is suspected. Blood immunological investigations (if relevant),
- Bronchoscopy can be performed if a foreign body is aspirated. CT of thorax can evaluate masses of unknown aetiology,

- An echocardiogram is useful if cardiac failure or a valvular lesion is suspected. A V/Q scan or CTPA is useful if pulmonary emboli are suspected.

Treatment

Consider the following approaches:
- Withdrawal of offending agent (e.g. fungus in hypersensitivity pneumonitis, drug in drug-induced lung fibrosis).
- Symptomatic treatment with bronchodilators and anticholinergics, antibiotics.
- Home oxygen therapy and inhaler technique (depends on degree of hypoxia and blood gases).
- Consider also non-pharmacological treatments (e.g. postural adjustments and breathing exercises to relieve anxiety, fan cooling).

Cough

Points in the History

Features of a good 'cough' history would include the following:
- Ask about the duration of symptoms: Patients often put up with a cough for many years; a morning cough present for many years productive of white sputum is characteristic of chronic bronchitis; a longstanding, highly productive cough is suggestive of bronchiectasis. Is there any diurnal variation?
- Ask about the type of cough. For example, with vocal cord paralysis the cough sounds bovine. Laryngitis, especially in children, leads to a harsh 'croupy' cough.
- Enquire about other respiratory symptoms such as haemoptysis, postnasal drip (symptoms of sputum running down the back of the throat, unpleasant, other ENT symptoms).
- Enquire about features suggestive of specific diagnosis: E.g. tuberculosis, asthma, sarcoid – rashes, eye symptoms, glandular enlargement or shortness of breath, allergy.
- Is the cough related to meals or lying down? This may be due to to gastro-oesophageal reflux.
- Is the cough related to starting medication? Common examples include ACE inhibitor, NSAIDs, or amiodarone (which can cause a pneumonitis).
- What is the impact of cough on the patient? You could ask about the effect on urinary continence and sleep.

- Is there a history of smoking? (Itself can cause a chronic cough, bronchogenic carcinoma and chronic bronchitis) Ask about history of passive smoking.

Enquire about previous medical history: Childhood asthma, atopy, nasal polyps, peptic ulcers, ENT surgery or sinus problems.

Ask about family history (asthma/atopy, lung cancer): Living conditions (overcrowding, damp housing), exposure to pollution. Travel to endemic areas.

Differential Diagnosis

Asthma, cough variant asthma, gastrooesophageal reflux, postnasal drip, postviral infection, allergy, GORD, ACE inhibitor, bronchitis, tuberculosis, inhaled foreign body, lung neoplasm, sarcoid, drugs, psychogenic.

Investigations

FBC (including eosinophilia), CXR (to exclude lung caner, sarcoid and TB), respiratory function tests, U&E, LFTs, bone profile, allergen testing, serum ACE, CT sinuses (postnasal drip), PEFR chart, oesophageal pH monitoring, trial of therapy (particularly important for cough variant asthma or asthma). Bronchoscopy is not required unless CXR is abnormal or RFTs show a restrictive defect (will also require HRCT).

Haemoptysis

Points in the History

Confirm haemoptysis is not a fleck of blood, and is not haematemesis.

Ask therefore about the nature of the haemoptysis fresh-red blood or mixed in with sputum. If from the mouth, a nasopharyngeal source is likely. Blood from the chest is usually red, not brown. Any history of recent trauma such as a sports injury?

When did the haemoptysis develop? How often? What is the approximate volume eggcup or spoonful (any cause),

Ask about related symptoms suggestive of an underlying disorder:

- Pleuritic chest pain, dyspnoea, fever, and recent leg swelling (i.e. DVT) may suggest a PE. If so, elicit relevant risk factors for PE.
- A long history of dyspnoea may be associated with chronic lung disease or mitral stenosis.

- Progressive weight loss is suggestive of TB or bronchial carcinoma.
- Cough and purulent sputum imply infection; tuberculosis can present with fever, night sweats, and haemoptysis.
- Lung cancer is suggested by lethargy, weight loss, lymphadenopathy, bone pain and paraneoplastic syndromes.
- Vasculitis is suggested by fevers, joint pains, haematuria, rash. Epistaxis and haemoptysis occur together with Wegener's granulomatosis and hereditary haemorrhagic telengectasia.

Past history of cardiac or pulmonary (e.g. COPD, pneumonia, tuberculosis, recurrent infections suggesting bronchiectasis), history of vasculitis, and specifically any history of rheumatic fever as a child which may have caused mitral stenosis. Recurrent haemoptysis over several years is common in bronchiectasis, but consider also TB, aspergilloma and lung malignancy.

Drug history (anticoagulants), contact history (areas endemic with TB, air travel), family history (e.g. haemorrhagic telengectasia or a disorder of coagulation/thrombophilia), smoking history, occupational history (exposure to asbestosis).

Differential Diagnosis

Pneumonia, lung cancer, bronchiectasis, pulmonary emboli, TB, overanticoagulation, rare causes (arteriovenous malformation, amyloidosis, sarcoidosis, foreign body, benign tumour, vasculitides, aspergilloma, mitral stenosis).

Investigations

These should be targetted at what is most likely. Possibilities include:
- CXR (lung cancer, COPD, bronchiectasis, TB, pneumonia),
- Sputum (cytology if there is a suggestion of bronchial carcinoma, AFBs in the sputum for TB),
- Blood tests (FBC, U/Es, anti-GBM antibodies, LFTs, clotting screen, cANCA, D-dimers, calcium),
- ECG (right heart strain, atrial fibrillation, urinary microscopy for red cell casts),
- Spirometry,
- Oxygen saturation,
- CT scan of thorax (useful especially for bronchiectasis),
- Bronchoscopy (lung cancer; useful also for other sources of bleeding such as arteriovenous malformations),

- Aspirate of pleural effusion, biopsy of any tumour or relevant organ (e.g. kidney),
- Radioisotope scan (e.g. V/Q for pulmonary embolus),
- Previous investigations and treatment (e.g. surgical, radiotherapy, chemotherapy, palliative care),
- Echocardiogram (useful for both left and right ventricular failure, as well as mitral stenosis).

Tuberculosis

Points in the History

Ask first of all about the duration of symptoms and enquire about specific features is the cough productive, sputum – quantity and colour Is there haemoptysis (see above)?, Is there chest pain often related to pleurisy?, Is there shortness of breath?, Is there a temperature, Is there loss of weight

Pulmonary TB: Typically causes a slow onset of symptoms including productive cough, haemoptysis, weight loss and night sweats.

Neurological TB: Cranial nerve palsies, meningitis, spinal cord involvement. Rashes, e.g. lupus vulgaris, erythema nodosum. Adrenals – lethargy, anorexia and dizziness. Atypical pneumonias. Sarcoidosis.

Previous medical history: BCG vaccination or recent Mantoux/Heaf test; immunosuppression – HIV, immunosuppressive drugs; other recent infections, e.g. shingles.

Drug history: Previous treatment for TB. Family history: TB and contacts with them. Travel history: Especially to areas endemic of TB. Social history: Occupational, crowded accommodation, contacts, alcohol dependence syndrome, living rough. Sexual history: HIV/AIDS.

Investigations

Repeat CXR, sputum smear and microscopy, Gram's stain, Ziehl-Nielsen stain, blood cultures, FBC, film – haemolysis. LFTs prior to anti-TB therapy, hepatitis, U&E – hyponatraemia, complement fixation test; HIV test; Mantoux test; serum ACE; sputum culture for TB, pulmonary function tests; consider pleural biopsy; CT and biopsy.

Management

Triple therapy, side-effects (rifampicin–red urine, tears; isoniazid – impaired LFTs, peripheral neuropathy; pyrazinamide–arthralgia and sideroblastic anaemia; ethambutol–optic neuritis and peripheral neuropathy). TB is a notifiable disease. Regular f/u. Rifampicin results in less effective oral contraception. Treatment plan is triple therapy with rifampicin, isoniazid, pyrazinamide for 2 months followed by rifampicin and isoniazid for another 4 months.

Wheeze

Points in the History

Do not forget an elementary history of recent asthma symptoms including wheeze, cough, dyspnoea, haemoptysis, occupationally-related. Do the symptoms improve on holiday (suggestive of occupational asthma: ask about nature of job)? Ask about exacerbating factors. You will also need to establish any relationship between trigger and onset of symptoms (if on first exposure, irritant, if later, sensitization). Is there a past history of allergy and atopy? Ask about peak flow meter and readings. Ask about social factors (as for asthma) and the concerns of patient.

Differential Diagnosis

Narrowing of airways (asthma, bronchitis, bronchiectasis, foreign body, tumour), left ventricular failure, carcinoid syndrome, pulmonary eosinophilia (e.g. tropical eosinophilia, allergic bronchopulmonary aspergillosis, polyarteritis nodosa).

Investigations

PEFR diaries and lung function.

Management

Asthma is described above and a complete understanding of the management of this is expected. Consider an occupational physician referral, if appropriate. The only effective treatment is avoidance of the precipitant. Financial problems and difficulty finding work may be relevant. Finally, consider that employees with occupational asthma are eligible for industrial injury benefit abdominal system.

Abdominal Swelling

Differential Diagnosis

Gaseous distension (malabsorption syndrome), fat (for example, Cushing's syndrome causing fat deposition in the abdominal wall, or obesity), solid (hepatomegaly, splenomegaly, nephromegaly; if cystic, consider bladder, pancreatic cyst, ovarian cyst), pregnancy (amenorrhoea), ascites. Consider specifically cause of ascites: Non-liver causes including generalised fluid retention, e.g. heart failure, hypoalbuminaemia, constrictive pericarditis, portal or hepatic vein thrombosis; intraabdominal disorders, hypothyroidism, patients on haemodialysis, liver failure. If exudative, consider malignancy, and infection including TB. Drug history: Steroids. Social history: Alcohol intake.

Investigations

Diagnostic tap of ascites is necessary for cytology, microscopy, AFBs and amylase. Neutrophil count is useful for diagnosis of bacterial pericarditis. CT of abdomen is the investigation of choice for an abdominal malignancy. Abdominal X-ray to confirm gas and fluid levels, and to examine for abdominal obstruction.

Abnormal Liver Function Tests

Points in the History

Enquire about any constitutional symptoms or episodes of jaundice (especially with fasting), colour and change of stools and urine, weight loss, new lumps, and features of haemochromatosis (e.g. appearance, arthralgia).

Past medical history of liver disease, abdominal surgery, abdominal pain or gallstones, autoimmune diseases, diarrhoea (associated with Crohn's, ulcerative colitis), previous malignancy (and related investigations, e.g. smear/mammogram).

Drug history: IV drugs (relevant to hepatitis B and C), herbal remedies, regular prescriptions, over-the-counter medications, recent blood transfusions.

Family history: Liver disease, malignancies, autoimmune disease, Gilbert's syndrome.

Social history: Detailed smoking and alcohol history (if there is suggestive of heavy alcohol abuse, this should be taken further), travel abroad, unusual foods (shellfish associated with Hepatitis A). Sexual history: Contraception and Hepatitis B, C, D and HIV risk.

Investigations

LFTs, FBC, viral hepatitis serology, autoimmune profile, serum electrophoresis, liver ultrasound.

Management

Abstention from alcohol (if relevant), treatment aimed at symptoms and underlying cause (e.g. ursodeoxycholic acid for PBC, steroids for autoimmune liver disease; venesection and desferrioxamine for haemochromatosis).

Diarrhoea

In simplest terms, diarrhoea can mean an increase in stool frequency or stool volume.

Points in the History

There needs to be a detailed description of the diarrhoea itself: This should ideally include:
- The frequency of bowel action and timing,
- The volume and consistency (watery/clear/frothy, fluid/brown, semi-formed, solid),
- The presence of blood and slime (melaena is tarry), features of steatorrhoea (implied by pale and difficult-to-flush stools),
- The relationship of bowel actions to eating, and particular foods (e.g. bread, cakes, oats, etc.)
- Any feelings of incomplete evacuation, any accompanying pain, and 'tenesmus' (the feeling of a need to evacuate when the rectum is empty),
- "Alarm" symptoms including anaemia, loss of weight, anorexia, recent onset of progressive symptoms, melaena or haematemesis, dysphagia, abdominal mass.
- If the patient is diabetic, and suffers from nocturnal diarrhoea, especially consider autonomic neuropathy, and consider antibiotic prophylaxis and loperamide in the management; but first of all consider in the history the person's occupation, and also whether there are associated features of autonomic disturbance such as impotence or incontinence.

Obtain a chronological description of its onset and events related to it (the time course, precipitant, exacerbating/relieving factors, other symptoms), an enquiry into the background factors that might explain the cause of the diarrhoea or have resulted from it, and finally an enquiry into related symptoms (particularly if the patent is 'ill' with weight loss, fever, or symptoms affecting other symptoms).

Enquire about symptoms suggestive of an underlying condition.

- Overall, organic pathology is suggested by certain features, for example, symptoms at night, mouth ulcers and unintentional.
- Irritable bowel syndrome is characterized by a flurry of bowel actions in the early morning but nothing later in the day. There may be bloating and colicky pain with IBS. The diarrhoea never occurs at night.
- Abrupt onset implies infections or toxins.
- There may be features of thyroid disease.
- A colonic pathology is suggestive of watery stool often with blood and mucus, possibly with urgency of defaecation). If symptoms suggest large bowel disease, look for other features of clinical syndromes, such as inflammatory bowel disease (eye, mouth ulcers, abdominal pain, skin and eye involvement, arthritis), colorectal carcinoma (per rectum bleeding), diverticular disease and superior/inferior mesenteric ischaemia.
- Small intestine diarrhoea is suggested by features of steatorrhoea, i.e. offensive grossly fatty and difficult to flush stools, often associated with severe back and abdominal pain or weight loss) and exocrine pancreatic insufficiency (steatorrhoea and weight loss). If symptoms suggest small bowel disease, ask about relevant past medical history – thyroid disease, diabetes, surgery; alcohol intake, medications, e.g. recent medications, and the four commonest causes of malabsorption in the UK – coeliac disease (dermatitis herpetiformis), cystic fibrosis, posteneritis enteropathy and giardiasis.

Enquire about features of overflow (for example, constipation or partial bowel obstruction).

Enquire about bleeding through the rectum (spotting and fresh blood on toilet tissue during or following bowel action is found in haemorrhoids or fissure; fresh and profuse bleeding is found in diverticular disease, inflammatory bowel disease, arteriovenous malformation or carcinoma; dark/altered blood usually from lesions in the proximal colon; red-current stool is found in intussusception; mucoid bloody diarrhoea is found in typhoid and amoebiasis).

Previous surgical history: E.g. post-gastrectomy, gut resection.

Previous medical history: Abdominal surgery (bacterial overgrowth), autoimmune disorders. Social history: Stress and depression, smoking and alcohol consumption (alcohol is a potent laxative).

Drug history: E.g. chemotherapy, alcohol, laxatives/purgatives, antibiotics, SSRIs, NSAIDs, excessive laxatives or purgatives. Also enquire about non-prescription medications.

Travel history: Tropical sprue can occur years after travel abroad (Caribbean and Asia). Other lifestyle issues (e.g. high fibre diet, stress, living conditions, sexual orientation if AIDS is a concern).

Family history: A family tree should be drawn with details of age of diagnosis of cancer, age of death, type of malignancy.

Questions Specific to Crohn's Disease

Where was the diagnosis made? Any previous investigations performed (colonoscopy, barium meal/follow through)? Progression of disease remitting-relapsing, previous surgery. Previous response to medical treatment. Features of the disease: Associated abnormal urinary symptoms and change in abdominal size, fevers (disease or abscess), lethargy (malabsorption or anaemia associated with Crohn's disease), any abdominal masses (abscess or Crohn's mass), the ability of the patient to eat/drink, non-GI manifestations (eyes, arthropathy, skin lesions, liver disease). Is there a family history? Social history is especially important: How does the disease affect her home and occupational life and is there good family support? Enquire about smoking as this is thought to exacerbate Crohn's disease.

Differential Diagnosis

As above. In summary, these include: Irritable bowel syndrome, inflammatory bowel disease, GI malignancy, infective diarrhoea, drugs: Laxatives, alcohol history, malabsorption, diverticular disease, thyrotoxicosis.

Investigations

- FBC, ESR, CRP, U&E, LFTs, serum amylase.
- Stool faecal fat – If very high, consider pancreatic cause and monitor a response to pancreatic enzyme replacement (there may be pancreatic insufficiency or inactivation of pancreatic enzymes due to chronic pancreatitis or gastric acid hypersecretion); if high, perform endomysial antibodies (if positive, follow response to gluten-free diet), if these antibodies are negative consider low duodenal biopsy (e.g. giardia, Whipple's disease, amyloid disease, secondary coeliac syndrome, tropical sprue).
- Stool microscopy for infection.

- Sigmoidoscopy/colonoscopy.
- Ultrasound scan if considered to be a collection.
- Further investigations include barium studies for blind-loop syndrome.

Management

This may include some of the following:
- Resuscitate (rehydration and correction of electrolyte imbalances may be necessary) Correct the underlying cause (e.g. pancreatic enzyme replacement). Antidiarrhoeal medication (e.g. opioids).
- For optimisation of Crohn's disease, treat acute pain with analgesia. Chronic pain relief with opiates can be counterproductive (constipation). Optimise medical management: Glucocorticosteroids, aminosalicylates, azathioprine, metronidazole (for severe perianal involvement), infliximab.

Dysphagia

Points in the History

A good "dysphagia" history could comprise:
- Are symptoms getting progressively worse? Chronic and/or intermittent pain is more likely due to a benign stricture or achalasia of the stomach.
- Is there pain on swallowing? Usually this is due to oesophagitis; achalasia where swallowing can provoke pain radiating to the neck; oesophageal cancer (difficulty in swallowing solids occurs at the beginning of the meal, but after a few pain-producing mouthfuls, the rest of the meal passes with relative ease),
- Is the dysphagia for solid food (obstructive) or liquids (motility)?
- Where does the food get stuck? High dysphagia may suggest a compression web, pharyngeal pouch, thyroid swelling.
- What are the associated symptoms? You might ask about episodes of vomiting, choking, splutting, past history of regurgitation or aspiration, haematemesis, heartburn, weight loss, loss of appetite.

Look for features suggestive of an underlying diagnosis:
- Anxiety in a young female, for example, suggests a psychogenic aetiology or globus hystericus.
- Food and liquid regurgitated easily on turning the head is suggestive of a pharyngeal pouch.
- Abnormal skin texture and circulatrion in the hands and fingers is suggestive of systemic sclerosis.

- Parotid gland enlargement, dry eyes and mouth are associated with Sjogren's syndrome.
- Neurological features such as ptosis or fasciculations may prompt enquiry about myaesthenia or motor neurone disease.
- A history of mechanical causes may be elicited such as fish-bones in the piriform fossa or foreign body).
- There may be an inflammatory condition of the mouth (e.g. leukoplakia, carcinoma of the tongue; there may be a history of heartburn suggestive of reflux oesophagitis).

A good drug history may give you useful clues (e.g. NSAIDs, K^+ or aspirin causing infective oesophagitis by Candida, Herpes, CMV).

Other conditions: Carcinoma of the bronchus, benign oesophageal stricture. Ask specifically about risk factors for oesophageal carcinoma (smoking, alcohol excess, possible dietary factors, achalasia of the cardia, Plummer-Winson syndrome, tylosis).

Differential diagnosis: As above.

Investigations

Relevant blood tests, CXR (for aspiration, foreign body, achalasia, bronchial Ca), ECG (left atrium hypertrophy), barium swallow (pharyngeal pouch, achalasia, external compression), upper GI endoscopy (useful for foreign body, candidiasis, stricture, Plummer-Vinson syndrome), CT chest (mediastinal nodes, malignancy).

Management

Treat the underlying cause. Management options therefore vary (e.g. oesophageal dilatation of stricture, surgical excision of tumour and pouch, palliation with stent, remove foreign body).

Epigastric Pain and Dyspepsia

Points in the History

Site of pain, duration, character/nature, whether the symptoms are of new onset, progressive, recurrent, episodic or recurrent, constant or intermittent, radiation to the back or shoulder, precipitating factors such as movement, effect of food or inspiration, other gastrointestinal symptoms (e.g. heartburn, vomiting, dysphagia, haematemesis, change in bowel habit, rectal bleeding, jaundice, pale stools, dark urine, loss of weight and appetitite, bloating), whether previously treated including previous GI investigations, haematemesis – almost always needs further investigation, drug history (NSAIDs, codeine, coproxamol, corticosteroids, aspirin), response to treatment.

Alarm symptoms (anaemia, loss of weight, anorexia, recent onset of progressive symptoms, melaena or haemaemesis, dysphagia, abdominal mass), consider the history also of a Mallory-Weiss tear where the tear results after a bout of severe vomiting.

Take, as usual, a full conventional history. Points to include:

Previous medical history: Cardiac disease, depression, known history of peptic ulcer diseasse or varisces, chronic liver disease, familial blood dyscrasia.

Drug history: Precipiting drugs–NSAIDs, steroids, anticoagulants, alcohol; medication to alleviate symptoms.

Family history: Malignancy. Smoking history and alcohol history. Psychiatric features.

Enquire about occupational history, stress and psychosocial aspects, alcohol and smoking history, and importantly the patient's own concerns.

Investigations

< 45 years, dyspepsia, lack of alarm symptoms, assess H pylori status and eradication therapy, otherwise consider endoscopy. British Society of Gastroenterology guidelines suggest that for first presentation of dyspepsia that patients < 45 years without alarm symptoms should have H. pylori serology checked and receive antisecretory treatment, and patients 44 (or 55 years) or over or patients with alarm symptoms should be referred for UGI endoscopy. For gastric carcinoma, consider gastroscopy and biopsy.

Differential Diagnosis

There are certain features of ulcers well known to medical students and rapidly forgotten by junior Physicians. Duodenal ulcer (epigastric pain occurring before meals, waking them at night, and relieved by food, milk, alkalis and belching), gastric ulcer (pain usually occurs after meals, often making the patient afraid to eat and resulting in a loss of weight; vomiting can relieve the pain), oesophageal reflux, depression, cardiac pain, gallstones, pancreatitis, carcinoma of the stomach (acute haemorrhage, epigastric pain, weight loss, important in the over 60s).

Investigations

FBC, LFTs, calcium and glucose; *Helicobacter* antibodies; endoscopy and CLO testing; ECG if cardiac cause; liver ultrasound. Management: Stop precipitating factors – smoking, stress, alcohol, NSAIDs. If the patient is depressed, professional follow-up.

Jaundice

Points in the History

Ask first of all where the patient first noticed prodromal illness of anxiety, fever, or malaise, whether there was any unwellness before the jaundice, duration, previous episodes, features of cholestasis such as pruritus (primary biliary cirrhosis), upper abdominal pain (gallstones), the colour of stools (pale if obstruction is complete), back pain and fatty stools if pancreatitic involvement, painful jaundice (alcohol, infection, drug-induced, Wilson's disease, hepatitis, biliary colic, pancreatitis, cholecystitis, metastatic and Budd-Chiari) or painless (e.g. hyperbilirubinaemia, Gilbert's, pancreatic or biliary malignancy, haemochromatosis, primary biliary cirrhosis), features of liver failure (reduced attention span, daytime somnolence), respiratory or cardiac symptoms.

Full alcohol history and related social factors (including CAGE questionnaire). Ask also about any recreational drug use or sports-related drug use (e.g. anabolic steroids).

Travel history (schisotosomiasis, viral hepatitis, clonorchiasis, amoebiasis).

Occupational history (hepatitis B or C in health care workers, leptospirosis, alcoholic liver disease, toxins).

Previous medical history (liver, gallstone history, recent blood transfusions, other autoimmune disorders in relation to PBC and CAH), previous surgical history (biliary stricture, retained stones, hepatic metastases, halothane hepatitis), previous episodes of jaundice (viral hepatitis, gallstone).

Risk factors for viral hepatitis (recent travel abroad, shellfish consumption, i/v drug abuse, tattoos, sexual).

Family history (inherited haemolytic anaemias, isolated hyperbilirubinaemia, haemochromatosis, Wilson's disease, α_1-antitrypsin deficiency, contact with hepatitis B or C), drug hepatitis (paracetamol, antibiotics).

Investigations

This essentially involves a blood hepatitic screen.

If unconjugated hyperbilirubinaemia, look for reticulocytosis suggestive of a haemolytic anaemia (stools are normal or dark; urine darkens on standing).

If there is a conjugated hyperbilirubinaemia, and the stools are normal, then consider possibility of hepatocellular carcinoma. If conjugated hyperbilirubinaemia, but the stools are pale and urine dark, it is advisable to perform abdominal ultrasound. If the ultrasound shows normal intrahepatic bile ducts, consider intrahepatic cholestasis. If the ultrasound shows dilated intrahepatic ducts, consider extrahepatic cholestasis.

For rarer causes, consider genetic studies (e.g. haemochromatosis and Wilson's disease), and also for cause in general a liver biopsy.

Management

This may involve discussion of pathology of alcoholic liver disease, consequences of alcohol dependence syndrome.

Lower GI Haemorrhage and Melaena

Points in the History

Nature and frequency of blood passed, onset of symptoms, patient's definition of diarrhoea, associated nocturnal diarrhoea (ulcerative colitis), number of bloody stools per day, abdominal pain/urgency/tenesmus, straining, constipation and pain (fissure), rectal lumps/masses, previous GI history (haemorrhoids, bleeding disorders, food poisoning), drug history (NSAIDs, anticoagulants, iron and bismuth), alcohol history, FH of GI neoplasia and polyps, concerns of patient particularly cancer. Systemic features such as anorexia and malaria.

Differential Diagnosis

Colonic cancer, ulcerative colitis.

Investigations

FBC, routine biochemistry, stool microscopy, flexible sigmoidoscopy, double contrast barium enema, colonoscopy.

Vomiting

Points in the History

Ask about the following:

- Frequency of vomiting.
- Relation to any medication (a full drug history is required).
- Separate evaluation of the nausea, including whether present before and after the vomiting, triggering and relieving factor.
- Time of day of vomiting (mornings suggest raised intracranial pressure).
- Is there any acid brought up?

Enquire about associated clinical features:

- Chemical causes (e.g. digoxin, opioids, uraemia) where nausea tends to be severe and persistent and vomiting produces little or short-lived relief from the vomiting.
- Toxins (e.g. alcohol excess).
- Other GI symptoms present, but where vomiting predominates (e.g. constipation, acid regurgitation, dysphagia, abdominal pain, dyspepsia, bloating, fullness, intestinal obstruction, diarrhoea, haematemesis and melaena), features of hepatitis (abdominal pain, biliary pain, itching and dark urine).
- Past history of gastrointestinal disorders, e.g. reflux oesophagitis, pancreatitis or endocrine disorders, psychiatric disorder (e.g. eating disorders, anxiety).
- Neurological features (raised intracranial pressure, visual field loss – optic chiasm compression, acute labyrinthitis).
- Ophthalmological features (acute angle closure glaucoma).
- Endocrine disorders should be considered, for example, hypothyroidism (constipation, poor memory, depression, headache typically with diurnal variation – intracranial causes), features of adrenal insufficiency (e.g. weight loss, depression, nausea/vomiting, abdominal pain, syncope from postural hypotension), diabetic ketoacidosis, hyperglycaemia, uraemia.
- Pregnancy.

Differential Diagnosis: These are suggested above.

Investigations: Again, as above.

Management: First, correct reversible causes (e.g. remove iatrogenic drug causes, treat hypercalcaemia). Secondly, consider drug treatments (e.g. metoclopramide, side effects: Gastric stasis and bowel disorder; cyclizine: Mechanical bowel obstruction, dystonia). Principles are start with a first-line drug, re-evaluate regularly.

NEUROLOGICAL SYSTEM

Back Pain

Points in the History

Back pain can be due to a problem in the back or any other predisposing conditions that impact upon the back, i.e. prostate, carcinoma of the lung, infection, etc.

Important aspects of the history concerning the back pain include: Nature, onset (sudden implies trauma-related or disc lesions) or gradual (degenerative disease), radiation, frequency, precipitating and relieving factors (e.g. symptoms worse on movement suggests a mechanical cause), other pains (claudication or neck pain), severe and unrelenting symptoms suggestive of neoplasia, pathological fractures (consider myeloma), trauma, impact of pain on life, any involvement of bladder or bowel function, drug history, smoking history, any history of a primary neoplasm. Ask about other symptoms (e.g. infection may be elucidated through a history of night sweats and fever; osteomyelitis may occur in diabetes and the immunocompromised).

Red flags for sinister back pain include:
- Age > 55,
- Non-mechanical back pain with no clear aggravation by movement or change in posture,
- Thoracic pain,
- Past history of carcinoma esp. colorectal, breast, renal, thyroid,
- Past drug history including repeat prescriptions for corticosteroids and neurological symptoms or signs.

Other important points include:
- Violent trauma,
- Alternating/bilateral sciatic,
- Weak legs,
- Weight loss,
- Progressive continuous non-mechanical pain,
- Systemically unwell,
- Localized bony tenderness,

- Spine movement in all directions painful,
- CNS deficit at more than one root level, bilateral signs of nerve root tension.

Features of a osteoporosis history: (1) Past family history of osteoporosis, (2) Psychosocial factors, (3) Risk factors for osteoporosis (e.g. heavy alcohol consumption, early menopause, hypogonadism, endocrine disease such as thyrotoxicosis, prolonged steroid use, immobility, severe chronic illness or malnutrition).

Differential diagnosis: Causes vary across age groups.
- For all age groups, consider trauma/fractures, strenuous activity.
- Younger patients (<40 years): Prolapsed disc, ankylosing spondylitis, spondylolisthesis
- Older patients (>40 years): Osteoarthritis, spinal stenosis and spinal claudication, osteoporosis, Paget's disease of bone, herpes zoster. Other causes include vertebral fractures, TB, metastases, Cushing's disease, psychosomatic, peptic ulcer, pancreatitis, pancreatic Ca, rectal Ca, abdominal aneurysm, renal Ca. Consider also gynaecological causes (e.g. uterine tumours, PID, endometriosis).

Investigations: These are targeted at investigating the underlying cause, and include:
- Bloods (including full blood count, liver function tests, serum immunoglobulins, serum calcium (raised in malignancy, myeloma and bony metastases), bone profile, parathyroid hormone level, PSA, Bence Jones protein),
- Imaging (X-rays). Spine X-ray is useful for trauma (fractures), osteoarthritis (narrowed disc spaces and osteophytes), chronic osteomyelitis (erosion of joint surfaces and destruction of bone), myeloma (punched out lesions), ankylosing spondylitis (bamboo spine), secondary depositis (osteolytic or osteosclerotic for prostate), Paget's disease (sclerotic white vertebrae). Clinical indications for bone densitometry include personal history of low trauma, X-ray evidence of osteopenia or vertebral collapse, maternal history of hip fracture, low BMI, corticosteroid treatment, oestrogen deficiency, and conditions predisposing to secondary osteoporosis, including malabsorptive syndromes, organ transplantation, eating disorders, chronic renal failure, primary hyperparathyroidism, hyperthyroidism, Cushing's syndrome, prolonged immbolisation, male hypogonadism. A Chest X-ray is useful for looking for a primary tumour.

Also
- MRI (location of a disc lesion, spinal tumour, spinal compression).
- Ultrasound abdomen for aortic aneurysm and renal lesions. CT scan (pancreatic lesions).

Management

General management of back pain includes pain relief, physiotherapy or bed rest. Correct any infection either medically or surgically (if there is an abscess). Surgical microdistectomy is a potential option for a prolapsed disc. Treatment options for osteoporosis include bisphosphonates, SERMs, HRT, calcium and vitamin D3 supplementation.

Dizziness and Funny Turns

Points in the History

Symptoms including:
- Frequency and timing of episodes,
- Detailed description of what was observed by the patient (and others) before, during and after the attacks,
- Any associated fall,
- Any associated loss of consciousness,
- Any associated symptoms and their duration,
- Is dizziness precipitated by movements of the head (BPPV, labrynthitis, head injuries),
- Features of hypoglycaemia (nausea, vomiting, tinnitus, palpitations, aura, hunger, blurred vision, light-headedness, sweating), and possible causes of hypoglycaemia (e.g. endocrine, mesenchymal/ sarcomatous tumours and hepatic disease, relief of symptoms when glucose is raised again),
- Features of adult onset epilepsy (previous birth trauma or head injury, symptoms of space-occupying lesion such as headaches, past history of hypertension, alcohol intake. Ask about tongue biting and loss of sphincter control).
- Features of imbalance (Vertigo: An illusion of movement often rotatory of the patient and of his surroundings).

Dizziness + vertigo may suggest possible causes:
- Benign positional vertigo where there are recurrent acute episodes of vertigo in response to head movement, worse in the morning, very short-lived, often associated with cervical spondylosis),

- Meniere's disease (unilateral deafness is usually the first symptom accompanying tinnitus),
- Vestibular nerve damage for example ototoxicity, vestibular neuronitis, acoustic neuromas, brainstem pathology (e.g. ischaemia, demyelination, infarction), cerebellopontine tumours, epilepsy.
- Vertebrobasilar ischaemia causes dizziness and limb weakness, loss of vision, diplopia, ataxia, perioral numbness and dysarthria.

Dizziness without vertigo:
- Hypotension,
- Anaemia (ask about any bleeding),
- Cardiac arrhythmia (ask about palpitations),
- Endocrine (myxoedema),
- Systemic infection,
- Psychological (anxiety, ask about hyperventilation),
- Carotid artery stenosis,
- Tumour of the cerebellopontine angle,
- Carotid sinus hypersensitivity (elderly, moving neck, hanging washing),
- Vasovagal syncope which is provoked by emotion, pain, fear or standing two long and is due to reflex bradycardia with/without peripheral vasodilatation, TIAs).

Drug history including recreational drugs insulin regimen for diabetics, home monitoring, diet, use of snacks, β-blockers, diuretics and other antihypertensives. Also enquire specifically about ototoxic drugs (aminoglycosides and frusemide).

Social history (e.g. whether the patient lives alone, whether he would like an emergency lifeline system, steepness of stairs if dizzy, shift-pattern of work), alcohol and smoking, factitious overdosing of drugs, fear of family.

Differential Diagnosis

Blood tests, including glucose, LFTs, U&E, bone function tests, resting ECG, 24 hour tape, blood pressure, carotid Doppler ultrasound, CT, EEG, audiometry (loudness recruitment is impaired in Meniere's disease, neuronitis). Realistic goals, e.g. about glycaemia, insulin qds or rapidly acting insulin analogues for hypoglycaemia, lifestyle changes.

Investigations: Hb, WCC (infection), 24-hour ECG, Carotid Dopplers, CT and MRI.

Double Vision

Particular points to note in the history include:
- When first noticed, direction, associated ptosis,
- Any squint (convergent, concomitant, incomitant): Consider the causes of a neurogenic squint (IIIrd due to severe trauma, posterior communicating artery aneurysm or diabetes; IVth due to birth trauma, trauma, hypertension and diabetes; and VIth nerve palsy).
- Other symptoms including tiredness, weakness and fatiguability, weakness of other groups (e.g. snarl, dysphagia, dysarthria), respiratory muscle weakness.
- Past history of autoimmune disorders, features suggestive of neoplasm.
- Drug history (e.g. D-penicillamine, aminoglycosides for myasthenia gravis).
- Impact of symptoms on patient.

Differential Diagnosis

Monocular (originates from cornea or lens, e.g. cataract), or binocular (cranial nerve palsies (III, IV, VI), internuclear ophthalmoplegia, extraocular muscle disease (dysthyroid eye disease, myasthenia gravis, ocular myopathy, ocular myositis), orbital fracture).

Investigations

Anti-AChR assay, Tensilon test, LEMS, hyperthyroidism, botulism, intracranial mass lesions, thymectomy.

Headache

A common scenario.

Points in the History

A good "headache" history should include:
- Location (i.e. is it facial or headache pain) and radiation,
- Any prodromal symptoms,
- Associate symptoms (including signs of meningism),
- How recently did the attacks begin and have they changed over time,
- Frequency of attacks (episodic or unremitting) [a headache diary is often useful] details about the onset (presence of aura, time of day, associated sleep disturbance, after intercourse or exertion), associated symptoms, relevant psychosocial details.

- The duration of each headache, character and intensity, location of pain and radiation, whether constant or intermittent, does the pain wake the patient up?
- Particular triggers (for migraine, relaxation after stress, missing meals, missing sleep, long distance travel, alcohol, cheese, chocolate, caffeine, citrus fruit, sudden unaccustomed exercise); problems with teeth, sinuses, ear herpetic neuralgia, temporomandibular arthritis, temporal arteritis), nose sinus infection worse with coughing or sneezing, eye acute glaucoma, temporal arteritis.
- Relieving factors including dark rooms, family history of headache, what does the patient do during the headache?, investigations and treatments from the past, and the state of health in between attacks. Symptoms suggestive of depression or anxiety.

Differential Diagnosis

Broadly speaking, the causes are of an **acute** or **chronic** headache.
- An acute single episode may be a feature of meningitis, encephalitis, tropical illness, subarachnoid, sinusitis or head injury. Acute recurrent attacks include migraine, cluster headache, and glaucoma (mostly elderly long-sighted people with markedly reduced vision in the affected eye, nausea and vomiting. Attacks may be precipitated by sitting in the dark).
- A chronic headache may be due to tension headache, cluster headache, migraine, idiopathic intracranial hypertension, or analgesia overuse. Other causes include neck spondylitis (check if movement of the neck exacerbates the headache), sinus disease (ask about localized tenderness/fever), nitrate-induced (after spray or taking medication), carbon monoxide poisoning (consider if several members of the family are unwell), and raised intracranial pressure (typically worse on coughing/straining). Consider also trigeminal neuralgia (paroxysms of intensive, stabbing pain lasting seconds, in the trigeminal nerve distribution. The face may screw up with pain. Pain can recur many times during the day and night).

Management

According to the type of headache, e.g. tryptan or β-blocker (+ amitryptiline or pizotifen) for migraine (a triptan should be avoided if the patient is already taking ergotamine prophylaxis), lithium for prevention of cluster headaches; tension headaches normally managed with paracetamol. Urgent treatment is required for serious headaches include intracranial tumours (symptoms of raised intracranial pressure, e.g. morning headaches exacerbated by coughing), meningitis (fever, neck stiffness, altered consciousness), temporal arteritis (> 50 years, scalp tenderness), primary open angle (acute) glaucoma, idiopathic intracranial hypertension, subacute carbon monoxide poisoning.

Pins and Needles

Points in the History

Duration, hand/fingers, pain, numbness, clumsiness, feeling of heaviness, tingling, associated symptoms (tremor, muscle wasting, paraesthesia), previous medical history including metabolic disorders such as diabetes and vascular disease, history of trauma, drug history including isoniazid and nitrofurantoin, alcohol history, dietary history (B_1, B_6 and B_{12} deficiencies), features specifically concerning carpal tunnel syndrome (hypothyroidism, acromegality, hypothyroidism, obesity, arthritis, repetitive strain injury, previous fractures, vibrating tools), concerns of patient.

Differential Diagnosis

Peripheral neuropathy, peripheral nerve entrapment/compression (e.g. cervical rib, carpal tunnel syndrome, disc herniation), spinal cord disease (e.g. cord/nerve root compression, multiple sclerosis), cortical or thalamic lesions, hypocalcaemia (e.g. in respiratory alkalosis, hypomagnesaemia).

Investigations

NCS (sensory nerve action potentials), EMG for denervation.

Management

Treat underlying cause, nighttime splints, local steroid injections, surgical decompression.

Tremor

Points in the History

Time of onset of tremor, arms/hands, laterality, worse at rest or posture or intentional, examples of difficulty and type of disability produced, head nodding, blepharospasm, symptoms suggestive of Parkinson's disease, neurological changes, history of TIAs, drug medication (e.g. phenothiazines), alcohol effects (relief of tremor), symptoms suggestive of a thyrotoxic state (heat intolerance, oligomenorrhoea, eye problems, skin rashes), ingestion of xanthines (e.g. coffee, anti-asthmatics), family history.

Investigations

Neurology, e.g. CT, EEG or MRI, endocrine (e.g. thyroid), psychiatry (anxiety, dementia).

Differential Diagnosis

Idiopathic Parkinson's disease, benign essential tremor, Parkinsonian syndromes, physiological and exaggerated physiological tremor (thyrotoxicosis, alcohol, anxiety), Huntington's disease, ataxia, cortical dementias, dystonia, myoclonus.

Management

Treat underlying cause. Reassurance (and counselling to come to terms with disability), management (multidisciplinary team).

Weak Legs

Points in the History

Duration of symptoms, particularly since last completely well, nature of any pain (shooting pain typically of radiculopathy), sensory loss, pattern of weakness, evidence of falls, difficulty in getting out of chairs, other neurological symptoms (e.g. headache, diplopia, muscle wasting, sphincter problems, tremor, backache, paraethesia).

- Candidates would be expected to identify any pointers suggestive of cord compression, including an acute onset of weakness with sphincter disturbance and/or saddle anaesthesia, known history of lymphoma, breast cancer, choriocarcinoma, primary CNS tumour.
- Consider features also suggestive of multiple sclerosis: previous transient diplopia, vertigo, oscillopsia, sexual difficulties, or bladder dysfunction; prior weakness.
- Other possibilities include: myopathies (suggestive of Cushing's syndrome, thyrotoxicosis or severe hypothyroidism), neuropathies (diabetes mellitus, malignancy, GB syndrome), myaesthenia gravis – symptoms worse at the end of the day, ocular symptoms; intracranial mass lesion; myelitis – HIV, vasculitis, thromboembolic tendencies.

A full medical history should be elicited, including: Diabetes, spinal injury/trauma, neuromuscular disease, metabolic disorder (hyperthyroidism, Cushing's), TB, rheumatoid arthritis (atlantoaxial sublaxation), operations – thymectomy, diabetes mellitus, neck or spinal irradiation, STDs (syphilis and HIV). Drug history – steroids (reactivation of TB), warfarin, diuretics – diuretic or laxative abuse can cause hypokalaemia, oral contraceptive pill. Social history: Smoking and alcohol, occupation and nature of work. A systems review as part of a general history is essential, to look for evidence of an underlying neoplasm.

Differential Diagnosis

Demyelination, cord compression (extramedullary: Meningioma, neurofibroma and ependyoma), intramedullar lesion (e.g. glioma), hysteria, myelitis, myopathies, neuropathies, intracranial mass, sagittal sinus thrombosis.

Investigations

FBC, U&E, bone profile, LFTs, CXR, MRI, evoked potentials, lumbar puncture.

Management

Of underlying cause.

ENDOCRINE SYSTEM

Diabetes

Points in the History

A general history of diabetes includes:
- Mode of presentation,
- Duration,
- Type of diabetes,
- Symptoms of hyperglycaemia or hypoglycaemia,
- Frequency of admission to hospital,
- Level of knowledge of his/her level of contro,
- His knowledge of symptoms of complications – cardiovascular (knowledge of cardiac risk factors), renal, eye, foot, autonomic, sexual, his motivation and education with respect to treatment, and attendance at annual screening,
- Onset of any symptoms, for example, painful feet, lipohypertrophy, muscle weakness and wasting, backache, impact on life,

- Social history including smoking, alcohol history, exact meal patterns, exercise patterns (including sexual activity, if appropriate),
- A full drug history.

Consider also other causes of any symptoms offered, such as peripheral neuropathy, briefly, e.g. alcohol, vitamin deficiencies, thyrotoxicosis, Addison's disease, pernicious anaemia, myeloma, renal failure and/or uraemia, carcinoma, infections.

Management

- Education about diabetes mainly revolves around its complication, treatment types and goals, dietary advice, lifestyle advice, foot care monitoring, self-monitoring of urine and blood sugar, recognition and management of hypoglycaemia, intercurrent illness management, support groups such as "Diabetes UK" and driving: Patients on hypoglycaemic treatment have a responsibility to inform the DVLA.
- Drug treatments for glycaemic control include insulin (newer long-acting insulins have more predictable and sustained absorption from subcutaneous tissue) with short-acting boluses at mealtimes; sulponylureas precipitate insulin release and are generally used for type 2 patients who are not overweight (NB: Hypoglycaemia is an important side-effect), metformin increases peripheral sensitivity to insulin and is the drug of first choice for those who are overweight, thiazolidinediones activate peroxisome proliferators activated receptor gamma which are contraindicated in cardiac failure and liver disease. Overall glycaemic control is best measured by HBA1c measurmenent, and the benefit of good blood glucose control is 7%.
- Treatment of 'painful' diabetic feet includes pain relief, glycaemic control, TENS/pain relief pain. For vascular problems, emphasise need for treatment of underlying cause (inc. blood pressure, glycaemic control), multidisplinary tram, avoidance of infection, outpatient angiography (angioplasty, bypass), anticoagulation, temporary footwear, daily inspection of feet, good foot hygiene, avoidance of walking barefoot, prompt referral if abnormality, selection of footwear.
- Other methods of treatment include metatarsal bone resections to reduce the risk of high-pressure stresses, and debridement of non-viable tissue – to reduce the risk of infection (Lancet 1999; 354; 370-1).

Hypercalcaemia

Points in the History

Elicit relevant symptoms of hypercalcaemia (tiredness, mental confusion, constipation, malaise, depression, abdominal pain, renal colic, bony pain), as well as features suggestive of an underlying cause (e.g. sarcoidosis, peptic ulcer, hyperparathyroidism, thyrotoxicosis, malignancy – bone secondaries from breast and lung, or haematological malignancy, lymphoma, myeloma). A full history should also pay attention to a detailed drug history (e.g. vitamin D analogues, thiazides, lithium), family history (hypocalciuric hypercalcaemia), immobility, concerns of patient.

Differential diagnosis: As above

Investigations: Serum calcium, ECG – short QT.

Management: Treatment with hydration and bisphosphonate. Treat primary hyperparathyroidism with surgery. Preopoerative localisation: MRI, radioisotope subtraction scanning and the management of acute hypercalcaemia.

Hypogonadism

Points in the History

Look for other features of panhypopituitarism: Hyperprolactinaemia (galactorrhoea, reduced libido, headaches), growth hormone deficiency (lethargy, weight gain, depression reduced muscle mass, sleepiness), hypothyroidism.

Differential Diagnosis

Primary where serum testosterone is low and FSH/LH may be high (congenital: Klinefelter's, cryptochordism, varicocoele, myotonic dystrophy; Acquired: Mumps, radiation, alkylating and antineoplastic agents, trauma, torsion, autoimmune, cirrhosis, chronic renal failure), or secondary where testosterone is subnormal and FSH/LH are normal/reduced (Congenital: Kallman's, hypogonadotrophic hypogonadism, e.g. Prader-Willi, abnormal FSH/LH subunits; Acquired: Idiopathic, malignant tumours, infiltrative disorders (e.g. sarcoidosis and Langerhan's cell histiocytosis), meningitis, pituitary apoplexy, trauma, critical illness, glucocorticoid treatment, chronic narcotic administration).

Impotence

Points in the History

It is essential to take an adequate sexual history, including stress performance anxiety, history of morning erections/masturbation, drugs, trauma, neurological symptoms, claudication (a history of peripheral vascular disease especially buttock claudication is suggestive of Leriche's syndrome), symptoms of chronic renal failure (nausea, lethargy, peripheral oedema, dyspnoea, vomiting, hiccups and convulsions), and psychological history.

Differential Diagnosis

Psychological (patients may have morning erections), drugs (alcohol, anti-depressants, β-blockers, cannabis, diuretics, major tranquilizers, recreational drugs), endocrine disorders (hypogonadism/androgen deficiency, hyperthyroidism, prolactinomas, acromegaly), neurological (autonomic neuropathy, e.g. diabetes, uraemia, nerve damage after bladder neck/prostate surgery, multiple sclerosis), vascular disease (e.g. atherosclerosis).

Investigations

Endocrine, prolactin, testosterone, sex hormone binding globulin, FH/LSH, glucose, liver function tests.

Management

Knowledge of treatments and appropriate referral.

Polyuria

Points in the History

Chronological history of the polyuria, actual volume of urine passed (polyuria should be differentiated from frequency of micturition), volume of intake and types of fluid, colour of urine, appetite, weight, cough history), current and past psychiatric history (compulsive water drinking/psychogenic polydypsia). Attempts should be made to elicit the specific concerns of the patient.

Look for features of diabetes: Associated infection, lethargy, balanitis, blurred vision, positive family history and weight loss.

Look for features of hypercalcaemia: E.g. weight loss, polyuria, abdominal pain, constipation, vomiting. Look for causes of hypokalaemia: drug history, ACTH-secreting small cell carcinoma of the bronchus, prolonged diarrhoea.

Consider evidence of infections (TB, meningitis, cerebral abscess) consider the posssibility of a hypothalamic or pituitary tumour causing cranial diabetes insipidus, e.g. primary craniopharyngioma, ependymoma, hypothalamic pituitary glioma. Features of pituitary dysfunction (galactorrhoea, amenorrhea, hypogonadism, visual field defects, hypothyroidism, hypoadrenalism). This can result from severe, blunt, head injuries, cranipharyngiomas, pineal gland tumours, or as a transient postoperative complication following neurosurgery.

Consider the possibility of a nephrogenic diabetes insipidus (e.g. drug induced, lithium, glibenclamide) or features of chronic renal failure such as uraemia.

Features of pregnancy or thyrotoxicosis.

History of diuretic phase of acute renal failure.

Ask abpout therapeutic diuretics, for example used in hypertension or cardiac failure.

Obtain a detailed medical history: Including previous surgical procedures, previous radiotherapy, previous vascular events (haemorrhage, thrombosis), head injury. Obtain a drug history (including diuretics, as well as nephrotoxic drugs including aminoglycosides, ciclosporin, NSAIDs and ACE-inhibitors) and smoking/EtOH history.

Investigations

Blood urine, serum calcium, ACE, chest X-ray (carcinoma of the bronchus, sarcoid, eosinophilic granuloma), urea and electrolytes (K^+ and Ca^{2+}), MRI scan of head, bronchoscopy (granuloma), early morning paired plasma and urine osmolalities for cranial DI, water deprivation test. If the plasma osmolality low, consider compulsive water drinking and diabetes inspidus. Water deprivation produces only a small rise in urine osmolality in diabetes inspidus compared to compulsive water drinking. ADH will produce a concentrated urine in pituitary diabetes inspidus, no effect in nephrogenic diabetes insipidus.

Management

Treat the underlying cause.

Incontinence

Causes

- *Urinary tract infection:* This should always be considered in patients presenting with urinary incontinence.
- *Constipation:* This may cause urinary incontinence by causing bladder outlet obstruction or by reducing bladder capacity.
- Drug induced diuresis
- Poorly controlled Diabetes Mellitus
- Renal failure
- Excessive fluid Intake
- Nocturnal diuresis (this may be due to autonomic dysfunction)
- Loss of awareness of bladder filling
- Patients with severe dementia and/or psychiatric illness may exhibit severe behavioural disturbances which include inappropriate urination, (and defaecation).
- *Unstable bladder:* Patients with bladder instability experience strong detrusor contractions during bladder filling which may be followed by involuntary expulsion of urine. This may be preceded by the sensation or urgency but often no bladder sensation is experienced. They are common in patients with global cerebral disease, e.g. dementia, cerebrovascular disease. Patients with autonomic dysfunction may also exhibit bladder instability.
- Urge incontinence is present when the interval between the desire to urinate and involuntary expulsion of urine is very short. Patients with urge incontinence usually have an unstable bladder. Environmental and physical factors may contribute towards urge incontinence. Immobile patients take longer to reach the toilet, especially when there are stairs to negotiate (When they reach the toilet they may be unable to unfasten their clothes quickly enough.
- *Stress incontinence:* The underlying problem in female patients with stress incontinence is either pelvic floor muscle or urethral sphincter weakness. Stress leakage occurs with increases in intra-abdominal pressure as a result of standing or coughing especially when the bladder is full. Pelvic floor muscle weakness may occur due to damage of their innervation during childbirth or as result of chronic straining at stool. Vaginal prolapse may also be present in these patients. Urethral sphincter weakness may be due to atrophic urethritis which is often associated with pruritus vulvae and frequency of micturition. In the elderly, this is usually due to oestrogen deficiency.

Assessment and Investigation

- Rectal and vaginal examination.
- *MSSU/Urine cytology:* Cystoscopy is indicated if haematuria is present without urinary infection.
- *Incontinence chart:* Keep record chart initially for 48 hours.
- Fluid intake (aim for 1500-2000 ml/day).
- *Urodynamic assessment:* In most elderly patients it is possible to diagnose the cause of incontinence from the history and examination findings. Urodynamic assessment is indicated when there is difficulty making precise diagnosis, when treatment has not been successful or when surgical treatment is being considered.
- Pelvic floor muscle assessment.

Management

- Review medication and stop offending drug(s) if possible or use an alternative drug. When diuretic therapy is required a short acting diuretic with a predictable effect should be used, e.g. loop diuretic.
- *Urinary tract infection:* Antibiotic medication as indicated from urine culture sensitivity results.
- *Constipation:* Use laxatives or enemas.
- Urge incontinence/unstable bladder.
- Environmental adjustment (including commode).
- Modifications to clothing, e.g. velcro fastenings.
- *Anticholinergic drugs:* Oxybutynin (3 mg b.d.- 5 mg t.d.s.), for example, may be used to increase bladder capacity and reduce the distending volume at which urgency and/or unstable detrusor contractions occur.
- *Stress incontinence:* Pelvic floor exercise programme and electrical stimulation of the pelvic floor-techniques for the electrical stimulation of pelvic floor muscles are being developed to augment pelvic floor exercises. The main benefits, however, appear to be due to pelvic floor muscle exercises and until further evidence is available, electrical stimulation should only be used in a research setting.
- *Oestrogen for atrophic vaginitis:* Traditionally this has been given in the form of pessaries or vaginal cream.
- *Bladder neck repair:* This is indicated for patients with stress in continence who do not respond to the above treatment and are fit for an anaesthetic.

- Vaginal ring pessaries to control vaginal prolapse are usually ineffective in the treatment of stress incontinence.
- The treatment of choice for prostatic enlargement is transurethral prostatectomy)
- *Nocturnal diuresis:* (Autonomic dysfunction) - additional treatment possibilities include 10 degrees head up tilt at night and possibly fludrocortisone or antidiuretic hormone (DDAVP) at night for resistant cases.
- Patients with incontinence secondary to dementia should be managed by toileting at planned regular intervals.
- Control aids are used for patients with intractable incontinence and for selected patients undergoing treatment for their incontinence, including pads and pants and underpants. Catheterisation is also a possibility.

Weight Gain

Points in the History

Ask about basic details of weight gain, distribution of weight gain, recent changes in diet including "junk foods", types of physical exercise undertaken, previous attempts at weight loss. Elicit specifically symptoms suggestive of Cushing's (change in appearance, symptoms suggestive of hypothyroidism, skin changes, hair growth/acne, proximal myopathy, depression, amenorrhoea/oligomennorhea, poor libido, poor sleep, hypertension, diabetes, osteoporosis, bone fractures), or polycystic ovarian syndrome (menstrual irregularities, hirsutism, obesity). Obtain also a history of cardiovascular disease (hypertension, dyslipaemia), cardiac failure (fluid may lead to weight gain), history of renal failure, a history of snoring (obstructive sleep apnoea), any history of DVT, gallstones, back pain, previous pregnancy or anaesthetic complications. A full medical history should also include a family history, a social history (including alcohol history), a drug history (especially any intake of steroids). Finally, the candidate should address the patient's own perceptions (particularly effects on self-esteem, expectations of the patient).

Investigations

This should include weight and height measurements, waist circumference, blood pressure and urinalysis for protein. Other useful investigations are disptix the urine (+++ glucose in Cushing's, protein +++ in nephrotic syndrome), U&Es, thyroid function ests, dexamethasone suppression tests and a 24-hour urinary free cortisol collection, and the possibility of scans (MRI of pituitary, adrenal; u/s abdomen and pelvis).

Management

Options generally include brisk walking, swimming or cycling, reduction of fat intake, drug therapy when other therapies have failure, inhibiting appetite pathways. Selective transphenoidal resection is the treatment of choice for Cushing's disease with low-dose cortisol replacement post-operatively for up to 12 months.

RHEUMATOLOGICAL SYSTEM

Cold and Painful Fingers

Points in the History

Frequency of attacks, precipitating factors especially the cold, other associated symptoms including peripheral vascular disease, cervical spine problems, syringomyelia, carpal tunnel syndrome, trauma (vibrational injury), medical history (such as β-blockers), family history of Raynaud's disease, concerns (incl. job).

Consider features suggestive of secondary causes, e.g. connective tissue disease, peripheral vascular disease, drug-induced, neurological, trauma-induced, blood dyscrasias. Smoking cessation, nifedipine.

Differential Diagnosis

Idiopathic, occupational (vibrating tools), connective tissue disease (scleroderma, SLE, Sjogren's syndrome, rheumatoid arthritis, dermatomyositis), cold agglutinins, cryoglobulinaemia, macroglobulinaemia (Waldenstrom's), cervical rib, drugs (β-blockers), vascular disease.

Management

General measures such as wearing gloves, no long term damage usually.

Weak or Painful Shoulders

Points in the History

The candidate should identify:
- Which joints are affected (and in particular whether the joints are large joints or small joints)?

- Which part of the arm is weak (if any)?
- Is there any swelling and, if so, what the type of swelling is (synovial is soft and boggy, bone swelling has little associated heat and redness, fluctuant swelling is caused by fluid and may feel hot, but is not compressible)?
- How long the swelling has been present?
- Is the swelling associated with radiation, morning stiffness, skin rash, nodules, sensory loss. Is there joint stiffness as well as pain? Stiffness is the inability to get the joints moving again after a period of rest. The length of time that stiffness lasts is related to the severity of the inflammation. Morning stiffness improving with exercise is typical of inflammatory arthropathy. Typically, these symptoms improve as the day progresses. Pain that gets worse during the day is likely to be due to degenerative change.

Further questions could elucidate the following:
- Enquire about symptoms relating to systemic disorders (e.g. malaise, fatigue, fever, headache, tenderness of scalp, eye changes, respiratory and neurological changes).
- Enquire about occupational factors (trauma, repetitive strain).
- Ask about functional disability, e.g. lifting cups, doing up buttons, writing.
- Enquire about symptoms suggestive of particular underlying disease. A history of rheumatoid disease might symmetrical arthropathy in both hands, morning stiffness > 1 hour, various joints are affected, nodules). For SLE enquire about rashes, sunlight sensitivity, mouth ulcers, features of Raynaud's phenomenon, chest pains, seizures or depression. Cervical myelopathy (head movement restriction, pain along the distribution of the dermatomes in the arms, wasting of the small muscles of the hands). Associated neurological symptoms (e.g. headache, blurred vision, dysphasia, dysphagia, loss of consciousness, vomiting, seizure, confusion). History of hypothyroidism.
- Enquire about if there is deformity which is often the end result of an arthritic process. Disability is frequently also a result, and ascertain how much the disease interferes with his/her life. The sort of questions you will need to ask depend on the patient's daily activity and whether he/she can carry out their normal job.
- Past medical history (e.g. palpitations, connective tissue, vasculitis, autoimmune disorders, infections, GI, skin).
- Drug history (e.g. thiazides precipitating gout, long-term steroid use, procainamide, hydralazine).

- Social history (smoking, alcohol history, domestic circumstances including characteristics of house, including stairs, access to front door, toilet, kitchen facilities).

Differential Diagnosis

Muscles: Polymyalgia rheumatica, fibromyalgia, polymyositis, myopathy, myeloma, drug-induced; *Joints:* Rheumatoid arthritis, seronegative arthropathies, osteoarthrosis.

Investigations

Bloods, serology, X-rays, imaging, physiotherapy, ESR, immunoglobulins, muscle enzymes, EMG/biopsy for a muscle disorder. If the history is suggestive of TIAs, full investigation includes 24HT, carotid artery Doppler and CT head. Anticoagulation may be necessary. Patients < 65, consider aspirin. Patients > 75 consider warfarin if not contraindicated. Treatment of rheumatoid disease may be relevant, including the use of methotrexate, infliximab and symptomatic relief by COX-2 inhibitors.

GENERAL

Collapse and Loss of Conciousness

Points in the History

Diagnosis here is reliant important upon a good history.
- Firstly, distinguish between dysfunction of the central nervous system and a mechanical fall.
- Secondly, distinguish between the two main types of brain dysfunction: Syncope (transient reduction of blood flow) and epilepsy. Consider the common causes of syncope. Postural hypotension – falls after standing up. Cough syncope – in chronic bronchitis and emphysema. Micturition syncope – usually elderly men who pass urine standing up. Carotid sinus hypersensitivity– turning head, syncope with tight colours.
- Thirdly, consider other causes such as metabolic disturbance (hypoglycaemia, drug effect, intoxication).

An adequate history of collapse should include attempts to:
- Find out the circumstances in which the collapse happened,
- Any prodromal symptoms,
- Whether the patient lost consciousness,

- The last thing they remember doing,
- The next thing they remember,
- How they felt during the attack,
- Whether they bit their tongue, became incontinent, or became stiff and shaking,
- Any other attacks and their similarity to the present one, and relevant risk factors.
- The presence of warning symptoms are important (e.g. light headnessness, chest discomfort, palpitations, dyspnoea suggest a cardiovascular aetiology; headache, confusion, hyperexcitability, olfactory hallucination and 'aura' suggest a neurogenic aetiology)
- The identification of precipitants such as exertion (e.g. aortic stenosis, HOCM or exercise-induced arrhythmia), standing (orthostatic hypotension, vasovagal syncope), cough/micturition (decreased vasomotor response) or neck extension (vertebrobasilar insufficiency).

Consider Particular Causes

- A history of sudden, transient loss of consciousness suggests a global problem such as a seizure. Is there any prone to sleep (e.g. narcolepsy)?
- Any evidence of anxiety? (Panic attacks may precipitate vaso-vagal syncope).
- Any loss of memory during an attack? (Transient global amnesia).
- Abnormal illness behaviour? (Munchhausen's syndrome).
- In adult onset epilepsy, care must be taken to search for and exclude a structural pathology, i.e. mass lesion, neoplasm, bleed, infection, inflammation). Look for localizing features – motor, sensory or cerebellar symptoms, personality change, diplopia resulting from a sixth or third cranial nerve palsy. The candidate should establish risk factors of epilepsy by actively asking about any history of previous head injury or birth trauma, symptoms of cerebral space occupying lesion such as headaches, past history of hypertension, alcohol intake.
- A quick recovery is usual after cardiac syncope, although nausea and malaise may last a few minutes after vasovagal attacks. Consider relatioship to food, and in particular, hypoglycaemia (Diabetes, liver disease, hypopituitarism, hypoadrenalism, insulin/sulphonylurea treatment, reactive hypoglycaemia after a meal, thyrotoxicosis, post-gastrectomy). Prolonged recovery time (> 5

minutes) with drowsiness, headache and focal neurological signs suggest neurogenic syncope. Loss of consciousness is highly unusual in TIA, except in a small number of cases of vertebrobasilar TIA.

A full medical history should include previous medical history, drug history (sedatives, hypnotics, hypotensives) and social history (e.g. flashing lights, illicit drugs, risk factors of HIV, occupation). Travel history: E.g. histoplasmosis.

Investigations

Investigations should be guided by the history and examination and include:

- Bloods including blood glucose during an attack, GGT, calcium, liver function tests, serum and urinary toxicology screens, HBA1C, 24 hour ECG if symptoms are frequent and may be required if the ECG is non-diagnostic (usually the indication for a permanent pacemaker is so compelling, it may add little information).
- Echocardiogram for structural heart disease, ECG (to see previous MI, LVH, sick-sinus syndrome, heart block, atrial fibrillation).
- CXR (calcification in the cardiac silhouette, especially if focussed around the aortic valve; cardiomegaly and pulmonary plethora).
- Tilt testing is used for diagnosing vasovagal syncope (studing the haemodynamic response to prolonged upright posture).
- Imaging including CT head.
- EEG (with photic stimulation, sleep deprivation and hyperventilation), thyroid function. Measure lying and standing BPs.
- If neural infection suspected, lumbar puncture (also useful for subarachnoid haemorrhage), HIV test, Mantoux test, Toxoplasma serology, serum ACE.

Management

Treat the underlying cause. A detailed social history and premorbid condition are essential to determine subsequent management. Consider loose flooring at home. Alcohol. Driving issues.

FALLS

There is an increasing incidence of falls with age. Approximately 25% of 70-years-olds experiencing at least one fall per year rising to 35% in the over 75s. In the over 65s falls are the sixth commonest cause of, and account for 5% of all deaths. Although only 5% of falls result in fractures and 5% soft tissue injuries, the remaining 90% may result in loss of confidence. Causes of falls can be summarised as:

- Impaired balance due to ageing
- Environmental factors
- Medical factors.

Medical factors can be divided into non-specific illness and specific diseases.

- *Neurological and vision:* Confusion (acute and chronic), cerebrovascular disease, Parkinsonism, epilepsy, visual impairment, vertigo.
- *Drugs:* Alcohol, drug-induced Parkinsonism, drug-induced hypotension/postural hypotension (e.g. GTN, phenothiazines, prazosin), drug-induced electrolyte disturbance (e.g. hyponatraemia, hypokalaemia).
- *Cardiovascular:* Postural hypotension, arrhythmias, aortic stenosis.
- *Other causes of syncope:* Micturition, cough, vaso-vagal, carotid sinus syndrome.
- *Locomotor:* Arthritis, muscle weakness/myopathy, foot problems, and footwear.

Management

It is essential to take a good history, particularly with regard to loss of consciousness, position or activity at the time of the fall and specific symptoms such as chest pain. It is important to know how long the patient was on the floor and, if possible, to obtain an eye-witness account. Full examination with particular reference to lying and standing blood pressure, any neurological disorders, vision and gait should be performed. Investigation is guided by history and examination. All identifiable causes such as polypharmacy or untreated Parkinson's disease should be treated. Rehabilitation and the multidisciplinary approach will not only restore confidence but also increase stability and ensure safety if falls occur. A home visit is mandatory when patients present with recurrent falls and will identify environmental risks and help provide a safe environment for the patient.

Discussion

There are a number of important reasons why the elderly are susceptible to falls. Maintenance of man in an erect posture requires balancing a large mass over a very small base. Mechanisms involved include ocular, vestibular and proprioceptive receptors. The whole process is initially learned in childhood. Under normal circumstances the body sways from a fixed point with women having a greater sway than men. Sway also increases with normal ageing.

- *Ocular mechanisms:* We all require visual clues to help prevent falls. In the elderly, both visual acuity and the threshold for light stimulation is reduced. This coupled with poor environmental lighting increases the likelihood of falls.
- *Vestibular mechanisms:* The vestibule is involved with rotatory movements of the head. These mechanisms become relatively inefficient as patients age.
- *Proprioceptive mechanisms:* The main receptors are situated in the cervical interfacetal joints in the neck. Impulses generated in the neck are coordinated in the cerebellum with the efferent pathway being via the medial longitudinal fasciculus. Cervical spondylosis or the wearing of a cervical collar renders these receptors inefficient. Additionally, vascular problems in the carotid may lead to balance disturbances.

Confusion or Personality Change

Dealing with a confused patient may also be the focus of a **Communications Skills and Ethics** station.

Points in the History

A collaborative history from relatives is paramount.

- Find out when the symptoms were first noted, the degree of the patient's insight, orientation in time and place, behavioural problems (personality, mood, sleep, concentration, disorientation), differences in thinking (slow and muddled, problems in memory), differences in perception (delusions or hallucinations), speech, features of depression, personal hygiene.
- A medical history should try to identify any endocrine disorder (diabetes, thyroid disorders), history of malignancy (cerebral metastasis or hypercalcaemia of malignancy), history of trauma, seizures, vascular symptoms, (anti-convulsant therapy or non-convulsive status).
- A full drug history is vital in a patient with confusion especially to look for any compliance issues or any inadvertent overdose, e.g. benzodiazepines, barbiturates. Ask also about any intake of illicit drugs.

- A social history with risk assessment (e.g. gas) is needed, including the impact of the patient's symptoms on family. Also relevant is previous chronic exposure to carbon monoxide, excessive alcohol intake.

Differential Diagnosis

Drugs (opiates, anticonvulsants, L-dopa, sedatives, recreational), alcohol withdrawal, metabolic (hypoglycaemia, uraemia, liver failure, anaemia), hypoxia, vascular (stroke, MI), space occupying lesions, epilepsy (status epilepticus, post-ictal states), trauma/head injury, nutritional (thiamine, nicotinic acid, B_{12} deficiency).

Investigations

BM stix, blood glucose, oxygen saturation (to look for hypoxia), ABGs (hypercapnaea), Dementia screen (including FBC, U&Es, LFTs, TFTs, vitamin B_{12} and folate, folate, CT, MRI, cardiology, syphilis serology), referral to memory clinic if necessary, CXR (bronchial or lobar consolidation), CT scan (cerebral metastasis, stroke, headinjuries), sputum, urine and blood cultures, EEG, plasma drug levels (for anti-depressants and anti-convulsants), lumbar puncture (if meningitis is suspected).

Management

Important principles include reducing distress, and minimizing medication. Multidisciplinary team assessment, involvement of relevant community agencies.

Allergy and Facial Swelling

Points in the History

Features of a rudimentary "allergy" history include:
- Ask about any history of weals, atopy, urticaria (well-circumscribed erythematous weals which could also be a presenting feature of an underlying disorder such as SLE/thyrotoxicosis/lymphoma).
- Enquire about previous response to antihistamines and prednisolone.
- Find out about other symptoms (e.g. laryngeal oedema – stridor, dyspnoea), systemic disorders (fever, arthralgia, myalgia), pain (e.g. jaw pain in neoplastic lesions of the jaw; carcinoma of the sinuses is associated with a blocked nose and bloodstained

discharge). Puffiness around the eyelids usually indicates renal failure.

- Enquire about precipitating factors (e.g. trauma, local pressure, emotional stress, allergen, food allergy, extreme cold, jewellery).
- A full medical history should include a family history of atopy or angioodema, and alcohol, social and occupational history.
  If nephrotic syndrome is suspected, ask some focussed questions:
- Ask about the circumstances of the onset of the oedema,
- Elicit urinary symptoms including frequency, haematuria, pigmentation,
- Enquire about constitutional symptoms (lethargy is often associated with renal failure).
- Ask questions relating to the cause: Glomerulonephritis (autoimmune–joint pain, rash, eye symptoms), recent bacterial infection (streptococcal), risk fators for hepatitis B and C or episodes of jaundice, recent foreign travel (malaria), malignancy (particularly myeloma), diabetes (longstanding or new onset – thirst, polyuria, nocturia, weight loss), amyloid (altered bowel habit).
- Also ask questions relating to complications of disease (venous thrombosis, pneumococcal sepsis due to loss of immunoglobulins, symptoms of renal failure–lethargy, urinary symptoms). In taking a history of nephrotic syndrome, a full previous medical history is essential, including diabetes, malignancy, autoimmune disease.

Obtain, as usual, a drug history (e.g. penicillamine, gold, allergies), a social history including alcohol intake, and a travel history (any history of travel to areas of endemic malaria).

Differential Diagnosis

Causes of a facial swelling include:
- Allergy, contact sensitivity, atopic dermatitis, cutaneous mastocytosis and systemic mastocytosis (episodic flushing with or without urticaria but no angioedema)
- Hereditary angioedema (deficiency of C1 esterase inhibitor, with angiooedema not urticaria)
- Nephrotic syndrome
- Hypoalbuminaemia
- Infection: Orbital/periorbital cellulitis, dental/sinus infection
- Hypo/hyperthyroidism
- Dermatomyositis
- Caroticocavernous fistula, cavernous sinus thrombosis

- Subcutaneous emphysema
- SVC Obstruction
- Neoplasm (parotid, sinuses, jaw, mediastinal tumours)
- Cushing's syndrome, obesity
- Drug-induced (steroids).

Investigations

General useful investigations include FBC (malignancy, infection), ESR, U&Es (renal failure), skull X-rays (fractures, sinusitis, malignancy), CXR (tumour), swab for infection. For allergy, skin prick and RAST tests are commonly used. For nephrotic syndrome, useful investigations include: Complement levels, 24-hour protein level, EDTA for GFR, FBC, ESR, CRP, U&E, LFTs, glucose and HBA1c, Hepatitis B and C serology, HIV test, serum electrophoresis and immunoglobulins, cholesterol, ANA, dsDNA, C3, C4, ASO titre. *Also:* Throat swab. Urine microscopy for red-cell casts–glomerulonephritis, Other tests would be for specific causes outlined above.

Management

If allergy, reassurance, avoid aspirin and opiates, non-sedating histamines, laryngeal swelling will require admission to hospital for urgent treatment and observation. If a nephrotic syndrome, the general principles of treatment are: treat the underlying cause, dietary sodium restriction, diuretics, prophylactic antibodies against streptococcal infections, anticoagulation, high protein diet.

Fever of Unknown Origin

This is quite a common history station.

Points in the History

Useful aspects of the history include:
- Pattern of fever (e.g. fever-free patterns in Pel-Ebstein fever; intermittent (e.g. malaria), remittent fever (fever returns to normal for a time but it is always elevated, e.g. abscess formtion, tuberculosis and carcinoma).
- Presence of drenching sweats (e.g. malignant and infective causes, typically at 1-3 am often waking the patient up), and rigors in abscesses.

- Joint and muscles pains (e.g. connective tissue disease or vasculitis).
- Skin rashes (e.g. SLE and infective endocarditis).
- Ask about any changes in weight and lymphadenopathy. Relevant respiratory, cardiovascular, gastrointesinal and neurological symptoms (including headache and neck stiffness). Also enquire about recent surgical history.
- Obtain a full drug history. Enquire about recent travel abroad (malaria prophylaxis and compliance: 1 week before the trip and for 4 weeks after returning), and note especially sexual history.

Differential Diagnosis

Infective and malignant causes constitute 55% of cases. (1) Infective (abscess, TB, infective endocarditis, malaria, TB, urinary tract, tropical, EBV, CMV, Q fever, toxoplasmosis, brucellosis), (2) Cancer (lymphoma, epithelial tumours, leukaemia, renal cell carcinoma, hepatocellular carcinoma), (3) Connective tissue disease (SLE, polyarteritis, PMR, rheumatoid), (4) Miscellaneous (drug, factitious, Meditteranean fever, Crohn's disease, sarcoidosis).

Investigations

Basic screening investigations are: (1) Haemoglobin, red cell indices and blood film (e.g. anaemia, severe anaemia suggests malignancy; iron-deficiency suggesting gastrointestinal malignancy; normochromic and normocytic in infection, malignancy and chronic diseases), (2) White cell count (hallmark of pyogenic infection is leucocytosis with immature granulocytes and toxic granulation), leukaemoid reactions (pyogenic infection, or acute leukaemia), (3) ESR (raised in most causes of FUO), (4) Chest X-ray (abscess, pneumonia, bronchiectasis, empyema, pulmonary infiltrates, PCP, sarcoidosis, histoplasmosis, TB and follow-up (e.g. bronchial lavage), (5) Examination of urine (heavy proteinuria is suggestive of renal disease, whether inflammatory or neoplastic), (6) Cultures (sterile pyuria of TB, sputum, blood cultures, HIV test), (7) Ultrasound/CT scan for a lesion particularly abdomen, (8) Blood tests for connective tissue disease (e.g. antibodies to DNA, rheumatoid factor), (9) Other: e.g. temporal artery biopsy, (10) Urinary dipstix, (11) Tumour markers, (12) Echocardiogram, (13) White cell scan.

Management

Treat the underlying cause.

Loin Pain and Haematuria

Points in the History

Features (frequency, position, time span, radiation, nature, relieving/exacerbating factors), associated symptoms (dysuria, haematuria, history of prostatism), if no symptoms (IgA nephropathy, recurrent haematuria, Henoch-Schonlein purpura with cutaneous lesions and joint symptoms; benign familial haematuria; Alport's syndrome with bilateral sensorineural deafness), the nature of the haematuria (whether visible throughout the stream, at the beginning of micturition clearing towards the end of the stream or at the end of micturition), passage of any stones, other urinary symptoms such as dysuria, poor stream, postmicturition dribbing, past history of haematuria and prostatism, previous history of renal stones or renal disorders (e.g. cystic disease), history of acromegaly and activity (visual field defects, sweating, headaches) and possible link with renal calculi, respiratory symptoms for haematuria (e.g. cough, haemoptysis, fever, sputum), GI (changes in bowel habit per rectum), cardiovascular (palpitations, chest pain). Smoking and alcohol history, impact on patient. Travel history (e.g. schistosomasis).

Differential Diagnosis

(1) Tumours of kidney, bladder, ureter or prostate, (2) Glomerular pathology (IgA nephropathy, Henoch-Schonlein purpura, glomerulonephritis, vasculitis), (3) Renal medullary disorders (papillary necrosis due to sickle cell disease, analgesics, diabetes or medullary sponge kidney), (4) Infection (pyelonepritis, cystitis, prostatitis, tuberculosis, schistosomiasis), (5) Stones and trauma, (6) Coagulation disorders, (7) Factitious.

Investigations

If there is no other renal or urinary symptom, culture urine, renal and uterine ultrasound, consider cystoscopy; if there are deformed red cells and/or casts and/or proteinuria, then consider renal biopsy; if there not, renal ultrasound, and consider haemoglobin electrophoresis.

Loss of Weight

Points in the History

The first thing is to know how rapid the weight loss is. If rapid, this suggests organic disease.

In the evaluaton of weight loss, the next most important factor is loss of appetite. If the appetite is excellent with weight loss, consider thyrotoxicosis and steatorrhoea. Two conditions commonly associated with serious causes of weight loss are anaemia and fever, and these must therefore be specifically excluded, including malignancy, endocrine disease, malabsorptive states and diarrhoea.

Enquire whether clothes are looser, how much weight lost, timing of symptoms and whether they are deteriorating, whether intentional, current dietary intake (including cereals, ryes, wheat, barley or coeliac disease), previous history of weight loss, previous body weight.

Important features are:

- Enquire about associated gastrointestinal symptoms, e.g. abdominal pain, nausea/vomiting, gastrointestinal bleeding including blood in stool. There may be altered bowel habit (e.g. suggestive of carcinoma of the large bowel). The differential diagnosis of weight loss and diarrhoea includes: Malabsorption, including coeliac disease, bacterial overgrowth, tropical sprue, pancreatic disease, infective (bacterial includes *Shigella* and *Yersinia*), protozoan (amoebic dysentery), tuberculosis, parasitic (Strongyloides), small bowel Crohn's disease causing malabsorption, colonic neoplasm.
- Enquire about specific features suggestive of an infection (e.g. miliary TB, chronic HIV infection).
- Ask about asociated endocrine symptoms (e.g. thyrotoxicosis, tremors, increased appetite, diarrhoea, palpitations, eye symptoms; adrenal insuffiency, weakness, dizziness, excessive sweating), drug history (diet pills, laxatives, amphetamines).
- Associated psychological factors (e.g. anorexia nervosa, anxiety and depressive states).
- Relevant medical history (gastrointestinal surgery, autoimmune disorders including thyroid disease, IDDM, fibrosing alveolitis, rashes), coeliac disease, gut, neoplasia, DM).
- Impact of symptoms on life.

Differential diagnosis: As outlined above.

Investigations: FBC, U&Es, LFTs, iron, folate, vitamin B_{12}, calcium, autoantibodies for antireticulin and endomysial.

Microcytic Anaemia

A common complaint whose history can easily be messed up.

Points in the History

History should concern iron deficiency anaemia, thalassaemia, and congenital sideroblastic anaemia. The majority have iron deficiency. Causes of iron deficiency anaemia include blood loss including menorrhagia or GI bleeding from oesophagitis, peptic ulcer, carcinoma, colitis, diverticulitis or haemorrhoids. Poor diet may be a cause, or malabsorption. Ask specifically about melaena or haematemesis. In elderly women, oesophagitis due to gastrointestinal reflux is a common cause and often asymptomatic. Bruising and bleeding from sites such as the gums and urinary tract are serious symptoms suggestive of thrombocytopaenia or bleeding from local malignancy as a reason for iron deficiency. Anaemia of chronic disease may be hypochromic).

Investigations

These include blood film, serum iron and ferritin. In iron deficiency, there will be pencil cells, anisocytosis and poikilocytosis. Serum iron and ferritin will be low. In anaemia of chronic disease, there is hypochromia, and low serum iron, but there is no rise in transferrin. If serum iron is normal, the diagnosis may be sideroblastic anaemia or thalassaemia. Sideroblastic anaemia may be idiopathic, or occur in anaemia, carcinoma, leukaemia or nutritional disorders. The blood film may exhibit anisocytosis, and the bone marrow appearance with ring sideroblasts is normal. Thalassaemia is usually demonstrated in a blood film with target cells and basophilic cells, and diagnosis is by haemoglobin electrophoresis which shows a moderate increase in HbA_2. Oral iron, but can cause black stools and constipation. Hb should rise by 1g/dl/week with a modest reticulocytosis.

Continue until Hb is normal and for at least 3 months to replenish stores.

Consider further investigation of an iron deficiency anaemia, i.e. gastroscopy, colonoscopy, barium swallow and meal.

Management

Treat the cause.

Macrocytic Anaemia

See the initial comment for microcytic anaemia.

Points in the History

Useful aspects of the history of a macrocytic anaemia are:
- Ask about associated symptoms, such as skin changes (e.g. haemorrhagic manifestations and follicular hyperkeratosis of vitamin C deficiency),
- Obtain a full GI history, especially loss of weight, small bowel disease symptoms (e.g. steatorrhea, ileal disease, bacterial overgrowth, tropical sprue, malignancy), jaundice, sore tongue in pernicious anaemia (glossitis), dietary history, vegan, systemic history (heart failure, SC degeneration of spinal cord, autoimmune disease). Obtain a past history of GI surgery (gastrectomy, ileal resection),
- Obtain a drug history (antifolate drugs, e.g. phenytoin, methotrexate, trimethoprim).
- Obtain a family history of autoimmune disorders including pernicious anaemia, alcohol history, concern of patients.
- Take a full social history including activity at home, any tiredness or dyspnoea, poor diet or appetite.

Differential Diagnosis

Causes: (1) Lack of vitamin B_{12}, due to dietary intake poor (strict vegetarians, fish tapework), lack of intrinsic factor (pernicious anaemia, total gastrectomy, partial gastrectomy), due to failure of intestinal absorption (disease or resection of terminal ileum; stagnant loop syndrome; tropical sprue) or (2) Lack of folic acid (due to inadequate intake, e.g. dietary deficiency, pregnancy, chronic haemolytic anaemia, or lack of absorption, e.g. coeliac disease, tropical sprue, anticonvulsant drugs).

Investigations

Vitamin B_{12} and folate levels, LFTs bilirubin, parietal cell antibodies, bone marrow examination, Schilling test if serum B_{12} is low with and without intrinsic factor to be confirmed with antiintrinsic factor and antiparietal cell antibodies. If a patient is found to be folic acid deficient, investigation of any steatorrhoea will be needed.

Management

Treat vitamin B_{12} deficiency with hydroxocobalamin (please note that this is parenteral treatment (IM) to total of 5 mg over 3 weeks then 1 mg im every 3 months for life). Folate replacement, if folate deficient.

Pain

Pain may be a feature of any history referred by a GP, and it is important not to approach this symptom in a haphazard fashion.

Points in the History

Consider the characteristics of the pain – character (quality of pain for example, neuropathic pain feels burning, stabbing or shooting, and bone pain may be described as aching or throbbing, and variation of the pain), location, duration and alleviating factors, any decreased mobility, sensory symptoms.

A full social history is essential: Where does he live and with whom? Severe pain may disrupt sleep and cause insomnia, anxiety and depression. Ask about stairs/stairlift at home, any help at home, any help with shopping, washing and cooking. Ask also the patient whether he/she is able to leave house or not. Obtain the patient's perception of the pain (misconceptions can lead to the patient's suffering; the patient's insight and understanding can be ascertained).

Management

Treat the underlying cause (e.g. antibiotics for cellulitis, surgical fixation for a pathological fracture).

In pharmacological treatment, the principles of a "pain ladder" of analgesic use are used. Prescribe regularly, and use the oral route for the majority of patients. One starts with simple analgesia (NSAIDs, paracetamol), moving onto weak opiods (codeine, dihydrocodeine, tramadol) compound preparations (co-dydramol), eventually moving onto opiates (e.g. morphine, diamorphine) but laxatives and antiemetics may be needed. Morphine should initially be given every 4 hours to titrate the dose, the starting dose being 2.5–5 mg; once a stable dose has been achieved it is switched to a 12-hour, slow-release preparation of morphine sulphate. The route should be oral, unless the patient cannot take drugs by mouth. Patients in pain do not become addicted and morphine does not also result in clinically significant respiratory depression; the dose may need to be increased with time due to tolerance. Monitor frequently.

Also consider non-pharmacological methods for pain and multidisciplinary input may be useful (e.g. TENS, local blocks, relaxation techniques, cognitive behavioural therapies).

Painful Shins

This is seen often by GP's, and therefore could easily be referred on. Therefore, examiners would expect you to deal with this in a reasonable methodological fashion.

Points in the History

Site, shape, size, colour, raised/flat, painful/painless, systemic symptoms, symptoms suggestive of sarcoidosis, recent infection especially. TB, myocoplasma, *Yersininia, campylobacter, Salmonella,* tuberculosis, streptococcus, drug history especially OCP, penicillin, sulphonamides, other inflammatory conditions (including thyroid disease and inflammatory bowel disease) travel abroad, impact on life.

Diagnosis

Erythema nodosum (females, arthralgia, fever, malaise, blue-red nodules, lower limbs and shins).

Causes

Sarcoidosis, infection (Bacterial: Streptococcus, Chlamydia, TB, Yersinia, Rickettsia, leprosy, leptospirosis; Viral: EBV; *Fungal:* Histoplasmosis, coccidiomycosis, histiomycosis; *Protozoal:* Toxoplasmosis), drugs (e.g. sulphonamides, penicillins, OCP, salicylates, dapsone), pregnancy, malignancy (lymphoma and leukaemia), inflammatory disorders (inflammatory bowel disease), sarcoidosis, Behcet's disease.

Investigations

CXR, ESRs, sputum, bacteriology (anti-streptolysin O titre, sputum or early morning urine), Mantoux test, serum ACE.

Management

Treat with bedrest and NSAIDs, oral steroids, stop OCP.

Pruritus

A common complaint, and you should be guided initially by the GP referral letter. The author is aware of one history in the real examination where the examiners were looking for dermatitis herpetiformis in the context of coeliac disease, in a lady who had been unable to adhere to a gluten-free diet, but the patient wished to know why her children were itching too, but as it happens the locum GP had previously already diagnosed the condition as as scabies.

Points in the History

Timing, parts of body affected, relieving actors or provoking factors (bath oils, stress, depression, drugs, foods, hot baths as in polycythaemia), effects on sleep and work, whether localised or not (e.g. scabies infection, urticaria, dermatitis herpetiformis, pruritus vulvae and pruritus anae), associated skin rashes, living conditions and contact history (e.g. scabies), occupational exposure (e.g. fibre-glass).

Ask about associated features (haemoptysis, chronic cough and weight loss may be suggestive of a bronchial carcinoma; night sweats and weight loss may suggest Hodgkin's disease).

Ask about the usual features of thyroid disease and renal failure (e.g. lethargy, anorexia, oliguria, polyuria, haematuria, proteinuria, skin fragility, oedema and bone pains).

Enquire about psychiatric features, and systemic symptoms (e.g. tiredness, jaundice for PBC and haemochromatosis), fever, weight loss (malignancy, lymphoma), features of thyroid disease, chronic renal failure, history of HIV, Enquire also about drugs including herbal remedies and recreational/domestic agents, e.g. biological washing powders, alcohol and smoking history.

Ask about the impact of symptoms of the pruritus on life.

Differential Diagnosis

(1) Obstructive liver disease, (2) Haematological disorders (iron-deficiency anaemia, polycythaemia; consider whether the pruritus is worse after a hot bath or shower), (3) Endocrine (hyperthyroidism, hypothyroidism, diabetes mellitus), (4) Chronic renal failure through calcium-phosphate product, (5) Malignancy (internal malignancy and lymphoma), (6) Drugs (e.g. morphine), (7) Others, e.g. pregnancy and senility, (8) *Malabsorption:* In steatorrhoea (especially with that of gluten-sensitivity), (9) Collagen disorders (e.g. scleroderma).

Management

Treat underlying cause, e.g. cholestyramine and ursodeoxycholic acid for PBC.

Purpuric Rash

Points in the History

Ask about the concerns of the patient. Useful factors to consider for 'purpura' are:

- How long have the symptoms been present for (e.g. early in life, adolescence, adulthood)?
- Distribution of the rash.
- Description (size, shape, circumscribed, itchy, blanching).
- Ask about any enciting cause (e.g. dental extraction, cut, site, mucosa or joint).
- Ask about operations and tooth extractions, and past attacks of joint swelling. Haemophiliacs usually notice their symptoms when they run around and hurt themselves. Ascertain the extent of the bleeding.
- Ask about haemarthrosis, a feature of many bleeding disorders, e.g. haemophilia A and B, and polyarthritis may accompany diseases in which bleeding is a feature, e.g. purpura, SLE, and drug sensitivity.
- Associated symptoms (malaise, febrile symptoms common in leukaemia and acute thrombocytopaenia, epistaxis, weight loss (leukaemia, secondary malignancy)).
- Ask about other haematological symptoms that might suggest bone marrow disease: Platelet disease (e.g. melaena, haematuria, haemoptysis), red cell disease (ankle swelling, breathlessness), white cell disease (increased susceptibility to infection).
- Relevant past medical history of lymphadenopathy, liver disease or viral infections, bleeding/coagulopathies.
- A full drug history (includes anticoagulants, steroids, sulphonamides, chloramphenicol, non-prescription drugs, gold, carbamazepine, substance abuse).
- Dietary history (vitamin C deficiency).
- Family history of haematological disease or organ-specific autoimmune disease.
- Systems review (abdominal pain, malabsorption, arthralgia, pruritus).

Differential Diagnosis

Bone failure (e.g. leukaemia, infiltration by secondary malignancy), coagulation deficiency (TTP, DIC, HUS), drug-induced (e.g.

sulphonamides, chloramphenicol, steroids), infection (e.g. EBV, CMV and toxoplasmosis) and others such as Henoch-Schonlein purpura.

Investigations

Full blood count for thrombocytopaenia, liver function tests, and blood film (if leukoerythroblastic, this is suggestive of marrow infiltration, causes of which include carcinoma, lymphoma or myelofibrosis). Consider causes of thrombocytopaenia: (1) Bone marrow infiltration includes acute leukaemias, CLL and CML, (2) Bone marrow depression (e.g. drug, toxic, uraemic), (3) Increased platelet destruction (ITP), (4) Intrinsic platelet defects (e.g. myeloprolifertive disorders). Other causes to consider: (1) Cryoglobulinaemia and paraproteinaemias, (2) Vitamin K and specific factor deficiencies, (3) DIC. The most important next investigation is bone marrow aspiration or trephine. Other investigations include blood urea, radiological skeletal survey, protein electrophoresis or ANF.

Management of ITP

(Women, 20-40, abrupt fall in platelet count, thromboytopaenia, platelet antibodies, consider EBV serology for splenomegaly). Treatment with IVIG. Emergency splenectomy for desperately ill.

Tiredness

Points in History

Whatever the aetiology of the tiredness, it is useful to ask a few detailed questions.
- What does the patient actually mean by "tiredness"?
- Are the symptoms episodic?
- Do they occur at specific times of the day (for example, rheumatoid arthritis causes morning stiffness which improves with activity).
- What is the duration of lethargy?
- What is the effect on routine activities (in particular, how the tiredness affects work and home wife, and whether or not there are any factors the patient can identify which contribute to the way he/she feels).
- Ask about social factors (e.g. sleep deprivation which may be self-induced, noisy neighbours, new work and domestic pressures, new child).

- Past history of neoplasm, viral illness, thyroid disorder or surgery, diabetes mellitus or psychiatric illness, psychological symptoms (stress/anxiety/depression), occupational and smoking history, drugs including anxiolytics and benzodiazepines, concerns of patient. Investigation and management according to cause.

Enquire about symptoms which might suggest important causes:
- Haematological, e.g. anaemia, pallor, per rectal or vaginal bleeding;
- Endocrine, e.g. hypothyroidism–preference for warmth, weight gain, dry skin, hair thinning) Addison's disease (postural dizziness),
- Respiratory, e.g. obstructive sleep apnoea (snoring), chronic lung disease, lung cancer (cough, haemoptysis).
- Cardiovascular heart failure (dyspnoea),
- Gastrointestinal inflammatory bowel disease (changing bowel habit), colorectal cancer (changing bowel habit),
- Infection, (e.g. infectious mononucleosis lasting a few weeks, tuberculosis, Lyme disease),
- Neurological, (e.g. myaesthenia gravis, proximal myopathy specifically causing muscle fatigue).
- Psychiatric depression (sleep disturbance, change in appetite or weight), chronic fatigue syndrome (fatigue after minimal activity, associated with aching muscles).
- Others, iatrogenic (β-blockers), renal failure, limb weakness (including the very rare cause of periodic paralysis).
  Say that you would also try to obtain a history from a relative.

Investigation

As above, including a chest X-ray, FBC, ESR, monospot, liver function tests, thyroid function tests, calcium.

Management

Treat the underlying cause.

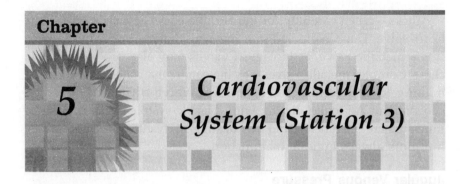

Chapter

5
Cardiovascular System (Station 3)

INTRODUCTION TO EXAMINATION TECHNIQUE

INSPECTION

General inspection is specifically stated on the marksheet, and this is because of its relevance to the overall cardiological examination.

Look for signs, whilst introducing yourself/repositioning, of certain systemic disorders:

Acromegaly: Spade-like hands, widely-spaced teeth, protruding tongue, coarse facies.

Marfan's syndrome: Tall-thin habitus, spindle fingers (arachnodactyly), wide arm span, high-arched palate.

Ankylosing spondylitis: Question-mark posture, aortic incompetence seen in approx 1% of patients.

Specific

Breathlessness – High respiratory rate,

Failure to maintain semi-recumbent position,

Identify finger clubbing (loss of nail bed angle, increased transverse curvature, drumstick appearance increased angle between nail plate and posterior nail fold; causes, cyanotic congenital heart disease, infective endocarditis), cyanosis (right to left cardiac shunts) and stigmata of endocarditis (Osler's nodes, Janeway lesions, splinter haemorrhages, digital infarcts).

Look for abnormalities of complexion: Anaemia – pallor/ koilonychias (causing heart failure, tachycardia), polycythaemia. Malar flush – signs of pulmonary hypertension, seen with mitral stenosis and primary pulmonary hypertension.

A visible earlobe crease is stastically correlated with coronary artery disease, especially in the Asian population.

Clicks – listen carefully for the audible clicks of a clean prosthetic heart valve. Don't be fooled into thinking that the audibility implies it is a metallic valve, as biological valves may also produce audible clicks. Complex metallic valves may have more than one metallic sound, making identification of the replaced valve difficult. Similarly, concomitant AF makes timing with diastole-systole difficult. Systolic murmurs are often heard and do not suggest dysfunction but diastolic murmurs always indicate malfunction.

Jugular Venous Pressure

The candidate is expected to inspect the JVP. The right internal jugular vein should be used in preference to the left. The JVP is the vertical height of the pulse above the sternal angle. With the patient semi-prone, assess the character of the waveform (canon a wave, CV waves seen in time with the arterial pulse hence the alternative term systolic), X and Y descents of pericardial tamponade; frequently the earlobe may be seen to oscillate, with tricuspid incompetence (very prominent CV waves). Time "A" (atrial contraction) and "V" wave (tricuspid valve drawing away from the right atrium; synchronous with the carotid pulse).

Specific patterns of jugular venous pressure in relation to certain valvular abnormalities:

Tricuspid incompetence X descent is lost and replaced by very prominent right systolic waves, synchronous with the carotid pulse called systolic V waves.

Pulmonary stenosis, pulmonary hypertension, tricuspid stenosis large a waves.

Constrictive Pericarditis

Paradoxical rise in the JVP on inspiration (Kussmaul's sign), prominent X descent and sharp Y descent.

Complete Heart Block

'Giant A' or 'cannon' waves when the atrium contracts on a closed ventricle. They are therefore found in patients with ventricular pacemakers and in patients with complete heart block or ventricular extrasystoles.

Atrial flutter 'A' wave is lost because effective atrial contraction is lost.

Chest Wall

Chest wall shapes: See Station 1: Respiratory system.

Operation scars: Median sternotomy (CABG or prosthetic heart valve replacement; check vein graft sites), left lateral/inframammary thoracotomy (closed mitral valvotomy) may be missed under the left breast unless specifically sought for, pacemaker/AICD implant (infraclavicular scar with the device often palpable): Note that pacemakers are usually inserted on the non-dominant side (handedness-wise) for convenience of the patient. Never mistake a mastectomy scar for an inframammary scar. Don't miss the scars of an AV fistula in the ante-cubital fossa.

Oedema: Look down to ankles, expose if covered. Check for pitting; depress for 3 seconds and release finger. When examining posterior lung fields, check for the presence of sacral oedema.

PALPATION

Pulse

The candidate is expected to check the pulse, and derive as much information as possible.

At the radial artery, determine the rate (count for 15 seconds), rhythm (sinus, irregular), character (weak/bounding). Ideally, the carotid artery should be palpated to determine the character of the pulse. Different types of pulse that should be recognised are stated clearly in the **MRCP Clinical Guidelines**.

Characteristics of the Pulse

- *Slow rising pulse:* Or plateau or anacrotic pulse, delayed percussion wave, palpable judder on the upstroke, narrow pulse pressure.
- *Sharp upstroke jerky pulse:* May be a sign of hypertrophic cardiomyopathy, ventricular ejection stops and starts. Pulse may be jerky if a large volume of blood regurgitates into the left ventricle with reduced systolic ejection time.
- *Small volume collapsing pulse:* Associated with ventricular run-off states such as mitral regurgitation or ventricular septal defect. There is a quickly rising small percussion wave.
- *Collapsing pulse:* To examine for a collapsing pulse, place the three middle fingers across the strongest brachial impulse and then slowly lift up the arm, after establishing whether the patient has

any shoulder discomfort, above the level of the heart. Simultaneously feel the other radial pulse to note any radio-radial delay (pre-subclavian coarctation, cervical rib). Brisk upstroke with collapse following, occurs in av fistula, aortic regurgitation, patent ductus arteriosus; if large volume, consider thyrotoxicosis, Paget's disease, severe anaemia.

- *Low volume:* Aortic stenosis.
- *Pulsus alternans:* Alternating large and small beats, sign of left ventricular failure, common in aortic stenosis.
- *Paradoxical pulse:* Excessive fall in pulse pressure > 10 mm Hg during inspiration, which may occur physiologically, cardiac tamponade, peripheral constriction, acute severe asthma.
- *Sinus bradycardia:* Causes: Fitness, ageing, MI, drugs, hypothyroidism, obstructive jaundice, raised intracranial pressure, hypothermia, hyperkalaemia. Temporary/Permanent Pacing if symptomatic 2nd or 3rd degree heart block, complete heart block, symptomatic bradycardia.
- *Sinus tachycardia:* Causes: Fever, anaemia, heart failure, thyrotoxicosis, phaeochromocytoma, carcinoid syndrome, drugs such as nifedipine and theophylline.
- *Atrial flutter- fibrillation:* Look for malar flush, mitral valvotomy, elevated JVP without a waves. *Differential:* AF, multiple ventricular ectopics, AF with variable block, complete heart block. *Causes:* Mitral valve disease, IHD, thyrotoxicosis, constrictive pericarditis, chronic pulmonary disease, hypertensive heart disease, cardiomyopathy, acute infections (particularly lung), local neoplastic infiltration (particularly lymphoma).
- *Radio-femoral delay:* Coarctation of the aorta.
- *Absent radial pulse:* Absent radial artery, abnormal position of the radial artery, catheterization of the brachial artery with poor technique, subclavian artery stenosis, Blalock-Taussig shunt, A-V shunt for dialysis, embolism into the radial artery, Takayasu's arteritis.

Apex Beat

Move swiftly to the precordial region and localise the apex beat by starting out in the axilla and then moving medially (showing the examiner that you are considering left ventricular enlargement). Be seen to be counting down the rib spaces with the other hand, keeping the localising hand still. A displaced apex beat has a number of important causes: Volume overload, aortic regurgitation, mitral regurgitation. Determine the character of the apex beat as this may help determining the dominant pathology in patients with mixed valvular disease. Additionally, by placing the flat of the hand over the line of the lower heart border and by placing the hand over the precordium (left parasternal area), you may be able to detect any palpable heaves.

The candidate should be able to distinguish different types of apex beat:

- *Double impulse:* May be a sign of hypertrophic cardiomyopathy.
- *Tapping apex:* Palpable equivalent of loud S1 (mitral stenosis).
- *Hyperdynamic/Thrusting apex:* Aortic incompetence.
- *Sustained apex:* Aortic stenosis.
- *Heaving apex:* Left ventricular hypertrophy.

Impulses

The candidate should test for and recognize abnormal cardiac impulses such as:

- Right ventricular parasternal lift/right ventricular heave/left parasternal heave: Usually a consequence of pulmonary hypertension.
- Left ventricular dyskinesia.
- *Palpable heart sounds:* Thrill at apex, consider mitral regurgitation; upper parasternal thrill, consider aortic stenosis (right parasternal edge) or pulmonary hypertension (left parasternal edge).

Measurement of Blood Pressure

The candidate should be famililar with the technique of measurement of arterial blood pressure with a conventional syphgmomanometer using standard or large cuffs. Phase V recordings are acceptable as diastolic blood pressure.

Percussion

Percussion of the cardiac border or area of dullness adds little to the clinical assessment in modern practice.

Auscultation

Candidates should remember that the examiners will have agreed. the signs that they are expected to elicit, using standards appropriate for the level of competence required.

CHARACTERISTICS OF HEART SOUNDS

Loud S1: Tachycardia, hyperdynamic circulation, short PR interval, mitral stenosis with mobile valve.

Wide expiratory splitting: When right ventricular emptying is slow (pulmonary stensosis/RBBB) or left ventricular emptying is fast (mitral regurgitation).

Reverse splitting: When right ventricular emptying is fast (right ventricular pacing) or left ventricular emptying is delayed (e.g. LBBB, aortic stenosis, HOCM).

Fixed splitting: Wide fixed splitting in ASDs.

Loud S2: Tachycardia, systemic hypertension (loud A2), pulmonary hypertension (loud P2).

Ejection click: Aortic stenosis or pulmonary stenosis.

Opening snap: Mitral stenosis (high pitched sound caused by high left atrial pressure snapping open the valve).

S3: Rapid left ventricular filling in early diastole, hyperdynamic states, heart failure and mitral regurgitation.

S4: Vigorous atrial contraction on a stiff ventricle, systemic hypertension, aortic stenosis, left ventricular hypertrophy–always pathological.

> *Mid systolic click:* Mitral valve prolapse.
> Metallic prosthetic sounds (see below).

Auscultation Technique

The candidate should be familiar with the surface markings of the four valve "areas" and be able to time murmurs to diastole and systole (e.g. mid, late or pansystolic) or continuous. The loudness/intensity of the murmur should be described. The candidate may use a grading system. If appropriate, auscultation should be performed with the patient in different positions. A murmur is heard, the candidate should also auscultate the carotid arteries, lateral chest, and the posterior chest to assess the radiation of the murmur and basal crepitations (for left ventricular failure). The candidate should also be able to differentiate between innocent murmurs and murmurs related to significant valvular lesions.

Complete the examination by offering the blood pressure, peripheral pulses, sacral or peripheral oedema, assessment of the lower limb pulses, urinalysis and fundoscopy for signs of hypertension.

ENDOCARDITIS PROPHYLAXIS

This is subject to change but please check with the British National Formulary at time of publication.

Common Cases

Once the abnormal signs have been elicited, they need to be presented correctly. The signs should be interpreted correctly within the context of a diagnosis or differential diagnoses. Common cardiology cases are listed below, along with related discussion of investigation and sequence, therapy and management.

IRREGULAR PULSE/ATRIAL FIBRILLATION

This man feels fine and has been referred by his GP due to an abnormality found on his cardiovascular examination. Please examine that system and report any abnormal findings.
– Pulse is chaotic both in rhythm and volume "irregularly irrregular".
– Radial pulse is less than apical "pulse deficit".
– JVP – No 'a' wave.
– Apex – Normal unless other disease, e.g. mitral senosis.
– Auscultation – S1 varies in intensity and S2 is normal.
   Consider the aetiology, e.g. features of mitral valve disease or thyrotoxicosis.

Symptoms: Usually none, paroxysmal palpitations, fatigue and dyspnoea, presyncope and dizziness, embolic symptoms – clinical features of mitral stenosis, symptoms of the underlying cause.

Aetiology: Ischaemic heart disease, mitral valve disease, hyperthyroidism, hypertension, pulmonary embolism, cardiomyopathies, alcohol, constrictive pericarditis, sick-sinus syndrome, lung pathology, e.g. carcinoma, pneumonia.

Differential diagnosis: Ectopic beats–atrial or ventricular. Unifocal ectopics have a constant compensatory pause after the beat. Dropped beats are followed by a normal RR interval. Multifocal ectopics can result in a truly chaotic pulse. Wenckenbach AV block has a progressively lengthening RR interval, followed by a dropped beat.

Sinus Arrhythmia

Investigations: Treat the underlying cause. Is this paroxysmal, persistent or established AF? Does the patient warrant anti-coagulation? In paroxysmal or persistent AF, the aim is cardioversion, and then maintenance of, sinus rhythm; if this is unattainable, aim to minimise the duration and frequency of AF. Atrial systole may contribute up to 25% of cardiac output by increasing the LVEDV, and may be symptomatically critical in patients with poor LV function.

Cardioversion is either chemical or electrical. Warfarin is the anticoagulant of choice, to give the INR between 2.0 and 3.0. In patients, where rate control is preferable to conversion to sinus rhythm, digoxin, β-blockers and calcium channel antagonists are all effective. Urgent DC cardioversion is the treatment of choice in the haemodynamically compromised patient. In those patients with AF of less than 48 hours, cardioversion can be generally undertaken without the need for prior anticoagulation with warfarin, although hepatin cover is advisable. Transoesophageal echocardiogram is often employed to exclude intracardiac thrombus.

METALLIC PROSTHETIC VALVE REPLACEMENT

This patient has recently been treated for shortness of breath. Please examine his cardiovascular system, and discuss what precautions (if any) are needed for an upcoming routine dental extraction.

An Extremely Common Cause

Clinical symptoms: Prosthetic valve endocarditis (any unexplained malaise, fever, weight loss, dyspnoea; any dental treatment in the last 6 months with no antibiotics; change in valve sounds; new symptoms); systemic embolization (commonest with mechanical valves, approximately 1% per year even with ideal anticoagulation); dyspnoea associated with a failing valve – this is a predictable feature of biological valves which fail more rapidly than mechanical valves; haemolysis, valve thrombosis, valve dehiscence, myocardial failure and arrhythmias may occur.

Clinical signs: Audible prosthetic clicks (metal) on approach and scars on inspection. The closing sound is the dominant one with both valves. Disc valves tend to produce a 'clicking' noise on opening or closing while ball and cage valves have a characteristic 'plopping' sound.

Aortic valve prosthesis: 1st heart sound normal, ejection click, ejection systolic murmur, click at the second heart sound.

Mitral valve prosthesis: Click at 1st heart sound, opening click in diastole. A regurgitant murmur should be regarded as pathological and indivative of valve failure.

Note that tricuspid valve prostheses tend to be bioprosthetic, as the risk of clot due to the nature of flow on the right-side of the heart is slower.

Extra points: Bacterial endocarditis signs, valve failure, stigmata of anti-coagulation (bruises, metal valve) or embolic disease, anaemia. Inspect the teeth – meticulous dental care is vital.

The opening and closing sounds of either ball or disc should be clear and sharp and not muffled. Vegetations may muffle the sounds or restrict movement.

Cause: Multiple valve murmurs/replacements; rheumatic fever; saphenous vein harvest scars: aortic valve replacement more likely.

Choice of Valve Replacement

An advantage of a metallic valve is that it is comparatively durable. However, warfarin is needed. Metallic valves are indicated for young patients, Porcine valves, in contrast, do not require warfarinisation of the patient, but they are less durable. They are most suitable for elderly people or those at risk of haemorrhage. Note however, that the choice of the valve is ultimately the patient's choice. Even young women who wish to become pregnant may have a metallic valve inserted because of the option of low-molecular weight heparin as the mode of anti-coagulation. Currently the operative mortality is around 3-5%, with survival @ 10 years, 50%.

Late complications: Thromboembolus 1-2% per annum despite warfarin, bleeding 1% per annum on warfarin, prosthetic dysfunction and LVF; haemolysis (mechanical destruction against the metal valve); valve regurgitation; infective endocarditis.

Types: Ball-and-cage ball devices (e.g. Starr-Edwards), pivotal single tilting disc (e.g. Bjork-Shiley) and double leaflet valves: All require anti-coagulation for life. More durable, but greater risk of thromboembolism than xenografts. The partner can be disturbed by the audible clicks.

Midline sternotomy scar, metallic S1/S2.

Complex metallic valves may have more than one metallic sound, making identification of the replaced valve difficult.

Biological valves: Homografts (cadaveric) and xenografts (porcine or pericardium mounted on a frame). Most prosthetic mitral valves are inserted in patients with AF, who thus require anticoagulation. Xenografts are less durable and need replacing in 8-10 years; they are less durable in younger patients, but better in the elderly. Homografts are the first choice in a young patient needing an aortic valve, but they may degrade with time. Historically, women of childbearing age received bioprostheses due to theoretical concerns of fetal abnormalities with warfarin.

Features of decompensation: Thromboembolic sequelae, infective endocarditis, leakage, dehiscence, ball embolus, valve obstruction due to thrombosis and clogging, haemolysis with anaemia, fracture, poppet escape, calcification. Mechanical valves are increasingly preferred to biosynthetic valves because of lower re-operative rates. Endocarditis risk is higher. Bioprosthetic valves may be more suitable for patients where anticoagulation is a risk/patients unlikely to live longer than the prosthesis, patients over 70 requiring AVR as the rate of degeneration is slow.

Investigations: CXR, refer endocarditis to a prosthetic valve to a cardiothoracic centre, endocarditis (cultures, ESR, CRP, FBC, echo, 24-hr tape for transient arrhythmia).

Management: The guidelines on oral anticoagulation (3rd edition, 1998) state 3.5 as the target INR for mechanical prosthetic valves (not indicagted for bioprosthetic valves where aspirin can be used for the first few months). An effective relatively low intensity regimen (INR 3.0 – 4.0) is supported by the latest analysis of a large Dutch study equating actual INRs to events (Cannegieter et al. 1995). Different valves have different targets, according to some clinic (e.g. bileaflet valves need an INR of 2.0 – 3.0), whereas, Starr-Edwards valves need an INR of 2.5 – 3.5.

HYPERTROPHIC OBSTRUCTIVE CARDIOMYOPATHY AND PACEMAKER

This young man has complained of palpitations whilst playing football. Examine his cardiovascular system.

Caused by mutations in contractile proteins.

Symptoms

- Often asymptomatic;
  - Chest pain (around 50%);
  - Palpitations (associated with WPW syndrome);
  - Syncope (15-25%) or sudden unexpected death; dizziness;
  - Angina can occur even with normal coronary arteries;
  - Dyspnoea on exertion can be due to a stiff entricle in diastole, thus reducing atrial transport.

Exercise often exacerbates these symptoms and may induce syncope.

Signs: Prominent pressure-loaded double apical impulse and pansystolic murmur at the apex due to mitral regurgitation, and ejection systolic murmur at the left sternal border starting well after S1 towards the axilla (across the outflow tract obstruction), accentuated by squatting. Pulse jerky in character with large tidal wave. The murmur is accentuated by forceful expiration or the Valsalva manoeuvre (raising the intrathoracic pressure), and is diminished by deep inspiration or the Muller manoeuvre. Atrial impulse can often be felt – the double apex. Systolic thrill – present at the lower left sternal edge.

Differential diagnosis: Aortic stenosis, subvalvar mitral regurgitation, VSD. Up to 70% of cases are inherited as an autosomal dominant condition, with a variable degree of penetrance and equal sex distribution. There is a large degree of genetic heterogeneity which accounts for the wide spectrum of HCM. Mutations on the gene coding for Troponin T at 1q3 carry the worst prognosis. The identification of the gene in an individual of the gene in an individual or family may enable an earlier and more precise diagnosis, and enable more useful prognostic information to be given.

Associations: Associated mitral valve prolapse (MVP), family history of Fredreich's ataxia or myotonic dystrophy, family history.

Investigations: ECG: LAD, LVH, large Q waves (V1-V3) and inverted T waves (V1-V3). Normal in 25%. ST-T and T-wave changes and tall QRS in mid-precordial leads, WPW syndrome, ventricular ectopics. Q wave in inferior and lateral precordial leads. Exercise ECG, 24hr ECG (ventricular tachycardia). CXR: Normal unless heart failure. Echocardiogram is diagnostic and to assess left ventricular structure and function, valvular regurgitation and atrial dimensions.

Characteristic finding is of systolic anterior motion of the mitral valve (SAM) on M-mode. Mid-systolic aortic valve closure. Cardiac catheter – echocardiography has reduced the need to pass a catheter into the excitable and unstable LV, which often induces VT. But it does document the withdrawal gradient, any MR and blood flow in the coronary arteries; it is also used for electrophysiological studies in the WPW syndrome.

Treatment: Nitrates should be avoided for angina as they increase the outflow obstruction; β-blockers are the mainstay of treatment for giddiness, syncope, angina and dyspnoea; amiodarone is given for SVT; infective endocarditis may occur. Genetic testing, but the genotype-phenotype correlation is uncertain. Dual-chamber pacing with depolarisation from the RV apex alters septal motion and is a promising alternative to surgery. Dual-chamber pacing is required as atrial transport is so important in HCM. Surgical myotomy or myomectomy through the aortic valve effectively reduces the left ventricular outflow tract gradient more than pacing but with a higher mortality risk. Implantable cardioverter defibrillators should be considered in those at risk of sudden cardiac death.

PERICARDITIS AND PERICARDIAL EFFUSION

This man is short of breath. Please examine his cardiovascular system and suggest why.

Features of a constricted perdicardium: Pericardial rub, raised JVP, prominent X and Y descents, non-pulsatile heapatomegaly.

Causes: Viruses, TB, SLE, malignancy, Dressler's, renal failure. Look for signs of SLE and other immune disease and weight loss (for TB or malignancy).

Pericarditis may lead to pericardial effusion and even tamponade (small volume pulse, hypotension, raised JVP). ECG shows small complexes.

Echocardiogram: Volume of fluid, cardiac contractility, guide pericardiocentesis.

AORTIC STENOSIS

This man is short of breath. Please examine his cardiovascular system and suggest why.

Aetiology: Either valvar, subvalvar or supravalvar.

Valvar stenosis is the commonest (congenital in 7% M:F 4:1, bicuspid aortic valves are present in 1% of the population); it is the commonest cause of AS in the 40-60 year age group. Inflammatory – rheumatic fever causing AS and AR. Arteriosclerosis in type Ia hypercholesterolaemia; gross atheroma can involve the aortic wall, the major arteries, coronary arteries and aortic valve.

Subvalvar: Discrete fibromuscular ring, HCM.

Supravalvar: A constricting ring of fibrous tissue at the upper margin of the sinus of Valsalva–associated with Williams' syndrome (hypercalcaemia, giant 'a' wave in JVP, PA stenosis – RVH, P thrill, elfin facies, mental retardation) due to mutations in the elastin gene.

Associations: Coarctation, angiodysplasia.

Symptoms: Left ventricular hypertrophy occurs with a compensatory enlargement of the coronary circulation. There is a relatively fixed cardiac output, and thus the heart is at its maximum output at rest.

- *Angina:* The increased muscle mass and increased pressure in the heart muscle, in both systole and diastole, increase oxygen demand while decreasing supply.
- *Dyspnoea:* The increased pressure within the LV increases further with exercise.
- Paroxysmal nocturnal dyspnoea and orthopnoea supervene as the LV function deteriorates.
- *Giddiness and syncope:* On exertion, the relatively fixed cardiac output cannot increase further.
- Sudden death can occur.
- *Emboli:* Can arise from the calcified valve.
- Symptoms of infective endocarditis can be seen.

Features: Pulse is regular, low volume with delayed upstroke ('judder'), slow rising pulse, narrow pulse pressure, undisplaced heaving apex beat, systolic thrill over apex area; S4; S3. harsh ejection systolic (crescendo-decresendo) murmur radiating to neck. The carotids may be difficult to palpate in severe disease.

Venous pressure is not elevated.

Systolic blood pressure is low normal.

Signs of severe aortic stenosis: Pulsus alternans, narrow pulse pressure, slow rising pulse, soft S2, reversed S2, aortic systolic thrill/heave in the second right intercostals space, left ventricular failure, S4, cardiac failure, dispalced apex (Note, in real life, the pulse pressure can be wide in view of the rigid peripheral circulation).

Echocardiogram: The definition of aortic stenosis is based on the valvular area, the normal area being around 3 cm^2. Aortic stenosis is normally graded as mild, moderate or severe. Mild valve area > 1.5 cm^2, moderate valve area > 1.0 to 1.5 cm^2, severe valve area < 1.0 cm^2, critical area < 0.75 cm^2.

Progression is manifest as a reduction in valve area and an increase in transvalvular systolic pressure gradient. Some factors of significance in rapid progression are aortic jet velocity, degree of valvular calcification, hypercholesterolaemia, renal impairment, hypercalcaemia.

Differential diagnosis: HOCM, VSD, aortic sclerosis (normal pulse character and no radiation of the murmur), aortic flow murmur, innocent flow murmur (pregnancy, fever, anaemia, thyrotoxicosis), ASD, VSD.

Investigations: ECG (usually shows LVH – found in 85% of patients with significant aortic stenosis – and possibly left axis deviation, ST-T changes, LBBB or CHB), CXR (cardiac enlargement and poststenotic aortic dilatation, pulmonary oedema and LVF), echocardiogram (bicuspid valve, calcifiation, LVH and function, AR, gradient assessment), not exercise testing. Cardiac catheter to confirm and clarify diagnosis, gradient, LV function, aortic root size, and assess coronary circulation prior to surgery.

Complications: (a) Endocarditis (splinters, Osler's node, Janeway lesions, Roth spots, temperature, splenomegaly, haematuria, petechial rashes on the skin and conjunctivae, conjunctivae for anaemia, immune complex phenomena manifest through glomerulnephritis or neuropsychiatric complications), (b) Left ventricular dysfunction: Dyspnoea, displaced apex, bibasal crackles, (c) Conduction problems – Acute (endocarditis) or chronic (calcified valve); ventricular arrythmias are more common than supraventricular arrhythmias, and heart block may occur because of calcification of conducting tissues, (d) Sudden death.

In the late stages of aortic stenosis, when cardiac failure and low cardiac output supervenes, the murmur may become markedly diminished in intensity.

Treatment: Symptoms (syncope, chest pain or dyspnoea), asymptomatic with mean gradient > 50 mmHg. This figure is only a guide and operation may be indicated with a lower gradient if the cardiac output is low. Valve replacement is required as valvuloplasty offers limited benefit in adults. Age alone is not a contraindication. Asymptomatic: Regular review 6/12, antibiotic prophylaxis for dental, genitourinary and colonic investigations or treatments. Nitrates and ACE inhibitors should be avoided as they increase the gradient across the valve (reduce afterload). Critical coronary lesions should be bypassed at the same time. The average survival (without surgery) once symptoms of angina/syncope occur is 2-3 years in patients with angina/syncope, and 1-2 years in heart failure without surgery. The mortality of surgery is < 5%. If coronary disease or LVF is present, it rises to 10-20%. Calcific aortic stenosis is increasingly common and, due to the proximity of the atrioventricular node, may be associated with atrioventricular nodal block, particularly in the post-surgical population. *Emergency treatment:* Admit the patient with heart failure and treat with diuretics.

Aortic sclerosis: The carotid pulse is normal, the apical impulse is just palpable and not displaced. There are no thrills. There is an ejection systolic murmur which is not usually harsh or loud and is audible in the aortic area but only faintly in the neck. The aortic component of the second sound is well heard. The blood pressure is normal (or may be hypertensive).

AORTIC INCOMPETENCE

This man is short of breath. Please examine his cardiovascular system and suggest why.

Symptoms: Dyspnoea is the main symptom. However, initial symptoms in patients with chronic aortic incompetence often related to the augmented stroke volume with complaints of a forceful heartbeat and pulsations in the neck. Angina and syncope are much less common than in AS. It can be well tolerated if gradual compensation occurs. Conversely, if the onset is rapid (e.g. dissection or infective endocarditis), then LVF or CCF can rapidly supervene.

Causes: Primary disease of the valve (congenital valve lesions, connective tissue laxity as in Marfan's syndrome or Hurler's syndrome), aortic root dilatation and stretching of the valve ring (hypertensive root dilatation and dissection), or secondary – infective endocarditis, prosthetic paravalvular leak, rheumatic heart disease, ankylosing spondylitis, cystic medial necrosis, seronegative arthritis, rheumatoid disease, quaternary syphilitic aortitis (note acute causes include infective endocarditis, trauma, failure of prosthetic valve, and rupture of sinus of Valsalva).

Signs: The signs are peripheral signs of increased stroke volume. Corrigan's sign (visible carotid pulsation which may be seen with harmonious head nodding), Quinke's sign (capillary pulsation of nail beds), De Musset's sign (head bobbing). Duroziez's sign – femoral diastolic murmur. One may ask the examiner to listen over the femoral arteries for pistol shots synchronous with the pulse (Traube's sign). Pulse is regular of good volume and collapsing in nature ("waterhammer"). HS normal, apex displaced and forceful, third heart sound, early diastolic rumbling murmur audible at the left sternal edge which is loudest with the patient sitting forward in expiration, ejection-systolic flow murmur across the aortic valve displaced apex beat towards 5th intercostal space. Carotid pulse has a rapid upstroke with no dichrotic notch; if the stroke volume is large, there may be a judder. Systolic blood pressure is usually high.

Signs of severe AR: Wide pulse pressure, soft S2, EDM, S3/left ventricular failure, Hill's sign (systolic bp legs > arms), Austin-Flint (mid-diastolic murmur at apex) murmur. As the regurgitation becomes more severe, the length of the murmur increases.

Investigations: ECG (left ventricular hypertrophy/strain and left atrial hypertrophy), CXR (aortic valve calcification is rare in pure AR, LVH and venous congestion, the aortic arch may be prominent in hypertension or dissection, or aneurysmal in Marfan's syndrome or syphilis), echocardiogram (LV function and dimensions, aortic valve thickening or vegetations, fluttering of the anterior mitral valve leaflet with prominent mitral valve closure), exercise testing, cardiac catheter (essential when coronary artery disease suspected and when the severity of the regurgitation is doubted, anatomy of the aortic root, LV function, coronary artery and ostial anatomy, other valve disease), syphilis serology, ANA/rheumatoid factor, sacroiliac XR and HLA B27 haplotype.

Other causes of a collapsing pulse: pregnancy, patent ductus arteriosus, Paget's disease, anaemia, thyrotoxicosis.

Treatment: Competitive sport should be discouraged, surgery to halt volume overload, replace valve (aortic root reconstruction) before LVESD > 55 mm or concomitant angina/severe AR; nifedipine in asymptomatics with severe AR, long-term vasodilator not recommended. In young, metallic prostheses are used as more durable. The indications for surgery are symptomatic (dyspnoea and reduced exercise tolerance), or if the following criteria are met: (a)

Pulse pressure > 100 mmHg, (b) ECG changes, (c) Postinfective endocarditis not responding to medical management, and (d) LV enlargement on CXR. Ideally replace the valve prior to significant left ventricular dilatation and dysfunction. Medical management is the treatment of heart failure and endocarditis prophylaxis.

A REMINDER ABOUT MARFAN'S SYNDROME

Tall with long extremities (arm span > height; pubis-sole>pubis-vertex).

Arachnodactyly: Can encircle their wrist with thumb and little finger.

Hyperextensible joints: Thumb able to touch ipsilateral wrist and adduct over palm with its tip visible at the ulnar border.

Face: High-arched palate with crowded teeth.

Eyes: Iridodonesis (with upward lens dislocation)

Chest: Pectus carinatum or excavatum, scoliosis, scars from cardiac surgery.

Other features: Aortic incompetence (collapsing pulse), mitral valve prolapse, blue sclerae, underdeveloped muscles, pectus excavatum, multiple spontaneous pneumothoraces, kyphoscoliosis, aneurysm tendency, coarctation.

Abdominal: Inguinal hernia and scars.

CNS: Normal IQ.

Differential diagnosis: Homocystinuria (mental retardation and downwards lens dislocation).
   Autosomal dominant, chromosome 15. Defect in fibrillin gene.

Management: Surveillance (monitoring of aortic root size with annual trans-thoracic echo), treatment with β-blockers to slow aortic root dilatation and pre-emptive aortic root surgery to prevent dissection and aortic rupture.

MIXED AORTIC VALVE DISEASE

This man is short of breath. Please examine his cardiovascular system and suggest why.
   May have some/all features of both pathologies and the candidate must determine which lesion dominates.

There may be a bisferiens pulse (notch halfway up the upstroke). Aortic systolic and diastolic murmurs, maximal down the left sternal edge.

Determine the dominant lesion: A small volume pulse with a narrow pulse pressure favours AS; a large volume, collapsing pulse with a wide pulse pressure favours AR.

Investigations: Echocardiogram (confirms LVH, measures the LV cavity size and so gives an idea of the severity of regurgitation from the stroke volume, confirm or exclude the presence of rheumatic valve disease) and CXR (moderate cardiac enlargement).

Management: The indications for surgery remain the same as that for pure stenosis or regurgitation.

Table 5.1: Factors pointing to a predominant lesion in mixed aortic valve disease

	Aortic incompetence	*Aortic stenosis*
Pulse	Mainly collapsing	Mainly slow rising
Apex	Thrusting, displaced	Heaving, not displaced much
Systolic thrill	Absent	Present
Systolic murmur	Not loud, not harsh	Loud, harsh
Blood pressure	High	Low
Pulse pressure	Wide	Narrow

MITRAL STENOSIS

This man is short of breath. Please examine his cardiovascular system and suggest why.

Usual Symptoms

* Dyspnoea on exertion, orthopnoea and PND as secondary pulmonary hypertension develops.
* Pulmonary oedema may be precipitated by AF, pregnancy, exercise, a chest infection or anaesthesia.
* Fatigue–because of the low cardiac output in moderate to severe stenosis.
* *Haemoptysis:* Alveolar haemorrhage, bronchial vein rupture, pulmonary infarction because of the low cardiac output and immobility, bloody sputum with chronic bronchitis due to bronchial oedema.
* Systemic emboli occur in 20-30% of cases, e.g. cerebral, mesenteric, saddle or iliofemoral.
* Chest pain: RVH and normal coronaries.
* Palpitations and paroxysmal AF.

- Right heart failure with TR and hepatic angina, ascites and oedema.
- Dysphagia from left atrial enlargement.
- Infective endocarditis is unusual.

Causes: Congenital, rheumatic heart disease, SLE, carcinoid, rheumatoid disease, malignant carcinoid, left atrial myxoma.

Features: Left thoracotomy scar, atrial fibrillation (irregularly irregular pulse) or chaotic low volume pulse, malar flush, prominent 'V' wave in JVP if triscuspid regurgitation secondary to right ventricular hypertension, undisplaced, tapping apex beat, undisplaced, left parasternal heave, loud S1, maybe loud S2 if pulmonary hypertension is present, low-pitched rumbling mid-diastolic murmur loudest at the apex in the left lateral position in held expiration and accentuated by exertion, giant v waves due to tricuspid incompetence, signs of previous valvotomy. Murmur is accentuated by exercise (increase in heart rate). May be accompanied by early diastolic murmur of pulmonary regurgitant murmur (Graham-Steel), if there is concomitant pulmonary hypertension.

Extra points: Haemodynamic significance (pulmonary hypertension, functional tricuspid regurgitation), endocarditis, embolic complications (stroke and absent pulses), other rheumatic valve lesions.

Aetiology: Rheumatic valvular disease is by far the commonest cause – Lancefield Group A streptococci cell wall antigens cross react with the heart valve structural glycoproteins causing inflammation and non-commissural fusion; non-rheumatic disease is very rare, for example, Congenital: Mucopolysaccharidoses, endomyocardial fibroelastosis, malignant carcinoid.

Differential diagnosis: Inflow obstruction (left atrial (LA) myxoma, ball-valve thrombus), mid-diastolic murmur can be mimicked by flow through an atrial septal defect (ASD) but the presence of a widely, fixed second heart sound, together with the absence of a loud S1, tapping apex beat and no opening snap in the latter distinguishes the two conditions; left atrial myxoma; Austin-Flint murmur–associated with aortic regurgitation (AR), collapsing pulse, volume-loaded ventricle and early diastolic murmur at the left sternal edge.

Severity determined by signs of pulmonary hypertension and/or recurrent thromboembolism, shorter interval between S2 and the opening snap (0.04 – 0.10 s after opening snap is usual), the longer the diastolic murmur. A guide to severity on auscultation is: Mild (opening snap is late around >100 ms after A2), moderate (about 80 ms after A2) and severe (about <60 ms after A2). A tight stenosis is defined on area (< 1 cm^2).

Tricuspid regurgitation is common in advanced stenosis. The presence of atrial fibrillation also favours the existence of mitral stenosis. Evidence of decompensation include pulmonary hypertension, thromboembolic disease, signs of infective endocarditis, Ortner's phenomenon.

Complications: Left atrial enlargement, pulmonary hypertension, right heart failure, systemic embolization, tricuspid regurgitation, right heart failure.

Investigations: ECG (bifid P wave/P mitrale, AF, low voltage in V1, progressive right ventricular hypertrophy), chest X-ray (congested upper lobe veins, Kerley B-lines, enlarged left atrium, large carinal angle, straight heart border, upper lobe diversion, horizontal left main bronchus), echocardiogram (necessary for differential diagnosis and to calculate the valve area, as well as to measure the PAP), valve area and stenosis, transmitral gradient), cardiac catheter (not initially, unless previous valvotomy, other valve disease, prior to surgery, angina or valve calcification on the CXR).

Treatment: Medical treatment involves digoxin, verapamil (rate-limiting calcium antagonists), or β-blockers andanticoagulation for AF, diuretics for fluid retention, antibiotics for chest infections, prophylactic antibiotics for all dental manipulations and potentially septic procedures, warfarin if previous emboli.

Surgical treatment involves severe symptoms, recurrent emboli, pulmonary hypertension, pulmonary oedema in pregnancy, haemoptysis, tight = <1 cm^2, percutaneous or open surgical valvotomy, transvenous balloon valvuloplasty = closed commisurotomy (rather than mitral valve replacement), prosthetic heart valve, anticoagulation and antibiotic prophylaxis during procedures, rate control (for atrial fibrillation). Valvotomy (open or transcatheter) are for mobile valve and absence of mitral incompetence.

It is embarrassing that, having given rheumatic fever as a cause of mitral stenosis, candidates sometimes give the impression that they do not know much about it. Immunological cross-reactivity between Group A β-haemolytic streptococcal infection, e.g. Streptococcus pyogenes and valve tissue. Duckett-Jones diagnostic criteria. Proven β-haemolytic streptococcal infection diagnosed by throat swab ASOT or clinical scarlet fever **plus** 2 major *or* 1 major and 2 minor: *Major:*

Chorea, erythema marginatum, subcutaneous nodules (Aschoff nodules), relapsing polyarthritis (not polyarthralgia), carditis, *Minor:* Raised ESR, raised WCC, arthralgia, previous rheumatic fever, pyrexia, prolonged PR interval.

MITRAL INCOMPETENCE

This man is short of breath. Please examine his cardiovascular system and suggest why.

Causes: Severe left ventricular dilatation of any cause, rheumatic heart disease, connective tissue disease, mitral valve prolapse, coronary artery disease, infective endocarditis, cardiomyopathy, connective tissue disorders complication of mitral valvotomy, papillary muscle rupture.

Signs: Chaotic small volume pulse, displaced laterally forceful/thrusting apex beat, left parasternal heave, apical thrill, soft S1, S3 may be present due to rapid ventricular filling, apical blowing pansystolic murmur at the apex radiating to the axilla growing through S2, the loudness of the murmur is of no significance, signs of cardiac failure.

Extra points: Pulmonary oedema, endocarditis, other murmurs, e.g. VSD.

Aetiology

- Functional (commonly secondary to dilatation of the mitral valve annulus in severe left ventricular dilatation, either an ischaemic left ventricle or dilated cardiomyopathy). In elderly, females>males, calcification of the annulus is seen, this can extend to involve the cusps, causing MR or it may be benign. It is associated with diabetes mellitus and Paget's disease and doubles the relative risk of embolic stroke.
- Structural (valvular regurgitation is caused by rheumatic fever or infective endocarditis).
- MV prolapse.
- Papillary muscle dysfunction (ischaemia, infarction or other degenerative disease of the chordae tendinae).

Differential diagnosis: Aortic stenosis, mitral valve prolapse (midsystolic click), hypertrophic cardiomyopathy, ASD, mitral regurgitation, tricuspid regurgitation, and ventricular septal defect.

Investigations: ECG–P mitrale, atrial fibrillation, left ventricular hypertrophy ± right ventricular hypertrophy; CXR–pulmonary congestion and large heart, echocardiogram: anatomy of mitral valve apparatus, LA and LV size and function; cardiac catheter needed to confirm the diagnosis, and for coexistent coronary artery or aortic stenosis disease, size of jet, vegetations or ruptured papillae. The LA/ pulmonary wedge V wave pressure gives a measure of severity.

Severity: Larger left ventricle dilated with a displaced thrusting apex, S3.

Complications: LV failure, AF, infective endocarditis, pulmonary hypertension, RV failure, thromboembolism, sudden death.

Treatment: Management of AF with digoxin, antibiotic prophylaxis during procedures followed by serial echos, digoxin to slow ventricular response, anticoagulation is withheld unless there is a history of emboli, prosthetic MVR or coexistent MS with a low cardiac output, treatment of heart failure though diuretics (to decrease pulmonary venous congestion and LV preload) and ionotropes.

Acute MR is managed as cardiogenic shock-sodium nitroprusside reduces afterload.

Major consideration should be given to surgery if LVEF < 55 – 60% or patients with enlarging left ventricular dimensions, and a threshold LVSD and cardiomegaly despite medical therapy.

Moderate to severe symptoms (NYHA III/IV should be offered surgery provided left ventricular function is adequate, or NYHA II and LV enlargement on CXR, or increasing dyspnoea. Valve repair (preferable) or replacement. Aim to operate when symptomatic, prior to severe LV dilatation and dysfunction.

If surgical repair is possible, it should be considered in all patients < 75 years who have a flail leaflet or persistent AF.

Prognosis: Often symptomatic for > 10 years, mortality 5% per year in symptomatic patients. 60% of patients with chronic MR are alive at 10 years. Prognosis depends on the LV function. Poor prognostic features are symptomatic history at < 1 year, AF, > 60 years of age, LVEF < 50% dilated LV, and echo LV size at end-systole > 5 cm, end-diastole >7 cm.

MIXED MITRAL VALVE DISEASE

This man is short of breath. Please examine his cardiovascular system and suggest why.

May have some/all features of both pathologies and the candidate must determine which lesion dominates.

Determining the dominant lesion:

- AF favours MS rather than MS but the latter can also cause AF.
- Raised JVP.
- Left parasternal heave is present.
- Loud S1 and tapping apex favours MS.
- Soft S1 favours MR.
- Opening snap is either soft or absent.
- Mitral regurgitation causes the pansystolic murmur.

The delayed diastolic murmur is not of full length, but may be loud, or even palpable indicating the increased left ventricular stroke volume.

May have ankle oedema or even ascites due to fluid retention, although these are rather unusual in the absence of tricuspid regurgitation.

The presence of S3 suggests that accompanying MS is not severe.

Features of pulmonary hypertension (malar flush; loud P2; accompanying TR; Graham-Steel murmur) favours MS rather than MR.

Investigations

ECG: AF, LVH

Echocardiogram: Reduced diastolic closure rate with anterior movement of the posterior cusp during diastole confirms the presence of rheumatic valvular disease. Left ventricular cavity size may be increased. The extent of disease of the valve cusps and subvalve apparatus is apparent.

CXR: Cardiomegaly with selective enlargement of the left atrium. In mixed mitral valve disease, the LA may be very large with a volume up to three litres. The lung fields may show similar changes to those of pure mitral stenosis.

Management: Valvotomy/valvuloplasty is unlikely to be appropriate.
Mitral valve replacement is probable.

Dominant abnormality: Mitral stenosis – small volume pulse, non-displaced/tapping impulse, loud S1, absent S3. Mitral incompetence – small abbreviated pulse, displaced thrusting apex, loud S1, S3 present.

Table 5.2: Factors pointing to a predominant lesion in mixed mitral valve disease

	Mitral stenosis	Mitral incompetence
Pulse	Small volume	Sharp and abbreviated
Apex	Not displaced; tapping impulse present	Displaced; thrusting
First heart sound	Loud	Soft
Third heart sound	Absent	Present

MIXED AORTIC AND MITRAL VALVE DISEASE

This man is short of breath. Please examine his cardiovascular system and suggest why.

Most commonly mitral regurgitation together with aortic stenosis.

MR with mid/late systolic murmurs may mask the AS murmur. If the apex beat is displaced, MR dominates.

Tricuspid Incompetence

Examine this patient's cardiovascular system. He has been complaining of abdominal discomfort.

Symptoms: Abdominal discomfort and distension; hepatic angina; jaundice; peripheral oedemal fatigue and dyspnoea.

Examination: Pulse chaotic and of low volume, V waves or giant systolic 'CV' waves in the JVP, right ventricular/left parasternal heave, palpable S2, atrial fibrillation, pansystolic murmur at LSE louder on inspiration, S3, hepatic pulsation, ascites, peripheral oedema including ascites and ankle oedema. One must proceed to examine the lungs for a cause of pulmonary hypertension (and features, including RV heave, loud P2), as well as the abdomen and beyond, for the peripheral signs of tricuspid regurgitation: Peripheral and central cyanosis, ascites and other signs of chronic liver disease, tender pulsatile hepatomegaly, peripheral oedema.

Important to look for multiple venepuncture sites (mainline drug addiction) and facial telengectasias (carcinoid syndrome).

Aetiology: Functional (secondary to pulmonary hypertension), organic (infective endocarditis, floppy tricuspid valve associated with a floppy mitral valve associated with congenital heart disease), rheumatic tricuspid valve disease in association with aortic and mitral valve area; right sided endocarditis; right ventricular infarction; endomyocardial fibrosis; rarer causes include carcinoid syndrome and secondary to the centrally acting appetite suppressants phentermine, fenfluramine and dexfenfluramine all of which have been withdrawn.

Investigations: ECG – AF, P pulmonale and RV hypertrophy; echocardiogram – dilated or hypertrophic RV, functional TV disease, vegetations, magnitude of regurgitant jet on Doppler ultrasonography; cardiac catheter.

Management: Management of the underlying lung disease, diureics, fluid restriction, surgery, annuloplasty and plication, valve replacement (rarely).

MITRAL VALVE PROLAPSE

This young lady is short of breath.

Please examine her cardiovascular system and suggest why.

Mitral valve prolapse is most prevalent in young females who present with atypical chest pain or paroxysmal arrhythmias.

Common especially in tall young women.

Common, 2–10% population, associated with Marfan's syndrome. Ehler Danlos, rheumatic heart disease, ostium secundum, ASD, Ehler-Danlos/pseudoxanthoma elasticum, psoriatic arthropathy, congenital heart disease, congestive cardiomyopathy, HOCM, myocarditis, mitral valve surgery, Fabry's disease, osteogenesis imperfecta, SLE, Ebstein's anomaly.

Pulse may have ectopics.

Apex is undisplaced, normal character.

Murmur is a systolic mid- or even pan-systolic; the clicks may be multiple and there may be a systolic squeak or honk at the apex. With posterior leaflet prolapse the murmur may radiate to the left sternal edge.

The duration of the murmur is reduced by short squatting exercises (the click is brought closer to S2), and increased by standing from squatting or performing a Valsalva manoeuvre. This decreases the cardiac volume and as a result the click and murmur occur earlier during systole and the murmur is prolonged. Increasing cardiac volume (squatting) has the reverse effect.

ECG may show T wave inversion.

Complications: Small risk of emboli, severe mitral regurgitation, arrhythmias, atypical chest pain, TIAs, infective endocarditis, sudden cardiac death. Rx: Reassure asymptomatic patient, prophylaxis if murmur, atypical chest pain treat with painkillers or β-blockers, aspirin for TIAs, antirhythmics, endocarditis prophylaxis. Palpitations are usually due to benign ventricular ectopy and generally respond well to beta blockade if symptoms are troublesome.

PULMONARY HYPERTENSION

This woman is short of breath, and has been reported by her GP as having a blood pressure around 90/55 most of the time. Please examine her cardiovascular system and suggest why.

Presentation is usually with dyspnoea, fatigue, syncope, oedema, palpitations; in the discussion offer a discussion without offending the patient for OCP and fenfluramine, HIV history; large a waves JVP, left parasternal heave, loud P2, ejection click in the pulmonary area, early diastolic murmur. CXR: Enlarged pulmonary arteries; ECG: RVH, right atrial hypertrophy. VQ scan to exclude thromboembolic disease. Echo. Rx: Diuretics, anticoagulants, prostaglandins, sildanefil.

PULMONARY STENOSIS

This patient has a long standing cardiovascular problem, but he is generally well. Please examine his chest and report your findings.

Extra points: Noonan's syndrome: Phenotypically like Turner's syndrome but male sex, other valve lesions, right ventricular failure (ascites and peripheral oedema). Noonan's syndrome is on 12q24.

Other aetiological factors: Rheumatic fever, carcinoid syndrome.

PR invariably results from dilatation of the pulmonary annulus, which may occur with pulmonary hypertension. RVH and right atrial hypertrophy may develop.

Both mild PS and mild PR are asymptomatic. More severe disease may present with a low cardiac output and right heart failure.

Clinical signs: Raised JVP with giant a waves, left parastenal heave, thrill in the pulmonary area. Auscultation reveals an ejection systolic murmur loudest in the pulmonary area in inspiration. Pulmonary regurgitation is characterized by a decrescendo early diastolic murmur in the pulmonary area (Graham-Steell murmur).

Investigation: ECG–normal, p pulmonale, RVH, RBBB, CXR – oligaemic lung fields and large right atrium, TTE–gradient calculation. *Management:* Pulmonary valvuloplasty, pulmonary valvotomy, if gradient > 70 mmHg or there is RV failure.

POOR LV FUNCTION

This man is short of breath. Please examine his cardiovascular system and suggest why.

Hypertension, fluid retention, cold clammy skin, low blood pressure, displaced apex beat, right ventricular heave; aetiology–valvular disease, hypertension, atherosclerosis, severe anaemia, pathological arrhythmia, generalized myopathy. Ix: CXR, echo. ECG: cause, left ventricular hypertrophy, arrhythmia, pathological Q waves. Blood tests for associated renal/liver disease, metabolic causes, thyroid, sarcoid, amyloid (electrophoresis, rectal biopsy), nuclear imaging. 24 Holter for ventricular arrhythmia.

Congestive cardiac failure is a cause of a raised JVP. Other causes are cor pulmonale, pulmonary hypertension, constrictive pericarditis, and a large pericardial effusion.

CONGENITAL HEART DISEASE

The congenital heart diseases are:

Basic classification of congenital heart disease

Cyanotic	Acyanotic
Tetraology of Fallot	Atrial septal defect
Eisenmenger's syndrome	Ventricular septal defect
Transposition of the Great Arteries	Patent ductus arteriosus
Ebstein's anomaly	Coarctation of the aorta

The following are complications of chronic cyanosis:
1. Polycythaemia causing hyperviscosity symptoms
2. Abnormal haemostasis and haemorrhagic risk
3. Paradoxical embolism causing cerebral abscess or stroke.

ACYANOTIC HEART DISEASE

Ventricular Septal Defect

This 26-year-old lady was found to have a murmur on routine examination by her GP. Please examine her cardiovascular system and suggest your management.

Symptoms: Small VSDs are common and asymptomatic. As pulmonary hypertension develops, fatigue, dyspnoea and symptoms of right ventricular failure occur.

Pulse: Normal

Left parasternal heave (if there is RV enlargement).

Absence of the normal splitting of S1 suggests that the left and right ventricle pressures are equal.

A loud, harsh pansystolic murmur and associated thrill at the left sternal edge should also be heard.

Perhaps mid-diastolic murmur at the apex due to high flow through the mitral valve.

As VSD becomes larger, both left and right ventricular hypertrophy occur and the pulmonary arteries may become palpable. Both the murmur and the thrill become softer. The jet veloity of the VSD and the pressure gradient between the ventricles is smaller, the larger the defect. As pulmonary hypertension becomes prominent the murmur may disappear as the ventricular pressures equalise. Eventually, Eisenmenger complex (a right-to-left shunt) may develop.

Extra points: Other associated lesions: AR, PDA (10%), Fallot's tetraology and coarctation.

Pulmonary hypertension: Loud P2 and RV heave.

Shunt reversal: Right to left (Eisenmenger's syndrome), cyanosis and clubbing.
    Feaures of endocarditis.

Causes: Congenital, or acquired (post-MI). May be associated with a syndrome (tricuspid atresia, pulmonary atresia, transposition of the great arteries, coarctation), or be an integral part of the syndrome (Fallot's tetraology, double-outlet right ventricle, truncus arteriosus).

Differential diagnosis: Mitral valve regurgitation, AS, HCM, tricuspid regurgitation, PS.

Investigations: ECG (LAH, left or right ventricular hypertrophy in a large defect), CXR (cardiomegaly, pulmonary plethora, prominent pulmonary arteries in a large defect as pulmonary plethora), echocardiogram for pressures and cardiac catheter for oxygen saturations.
    QRS axis may shift to the right in pulmonary hypertension.
    The pulse volume may be small if there is a large left-to-right shunt.
    Magnetic resonance scanning can demonstrate the defect and enable the shunt to be measured. Catheterisation confirms the step-up in oxygen saturation in the RV, quantitates the shunt, and diagnoses the site. Aortography will check the valve and exclude PDA or coarctation. RV angiography checks the RV outflow tract.

Complications: Endocarditis (possibly recurrent; look for splinter haemorrhages), biventricular cardiac failure, aortic regurgitation, pulmonary hypertension eventually leading to Eisenmenger's syndrome.

Treatment: Surgery, if a large defect with a pulmonary: Systemic flow of >2:1 and right ventricular overload, medical therapy has failed, symptomatic +++ or infective endocarditis; patients who survive to adulthood usually have left ventricular failure or pulmonary hypertension with associated right ventricular failure. Surgical closure of such defects is recommended. Medical treatment: Many (30-50%) small VSDs close spontaneously, and although the surgical morbidity and mortality surrounding correction of small defects is low, surgery is usually unnecessary; all types require IE prophylaxis, there are septal closure devices available that may be placed at the time of cardiac catheterisation. Post-MI VSDs require urgent surgery.

Note on congenital heart disease: Acyanotic heart disease: ASD, VSD, Aortic coarctation, PDA; Cyanotic: Fallot's (VSD with right to left shunt, pulmonary stenosis, RVH, aorta overriding septal defect), Transposition of Great Arteries, Eisenmenger's syndrome. A small defect may produce a loud murmur (*Maladie de Roger*). Eisenmenger – centrally clubbed and cyanosed, left parasternal heave, palpable pulmonary valve closure.

ATRIAL SEPTAL DEFECT

This young woman complains of cough and occasional palpitations. Examine her cardiovascular system.

Features: Presents with dyspnoea, productive cough indicating recurrent pulmonary infections, symptoms of paradoxical emboli, palpitations (indicating atrial arrhythmias), fatigue and ankle swelling (indicating heart failure).

Examination: Diffuse or normal apical impulse, left parasternal heave (prominent right ventricular impulse), ejection systolic flow murmur in left second and third intercostals space, wide fixed split second heart sound, atrial fibrillation, 'A' and 'V' waves in raised JVP.

Look for signs of pulmonary hypertension (Eisenmenger complex: Centrally cyanosed and clubbed; pulse volume usually small; second heart sound is loud and single, there may be a right ventricular fourth heart sound). When an ASD is suspected, go onto carefully listen for a murmur of mitral stenosis which, if present with ASD, is called *Lutembacher's syndrome.*

Types-of ASD: Ostium secundum defect accounts for around 70% of cases, and the defect is in the middle portion of the atrial septum.

Primum is nearest the atrioventricular valve apparatus. ECG often shows right axis deviation and incomplete right bundle branch block.

CXR demonstrates prominent pulmonary arteries (large pulmonary conus) and shunt vascularity, progressive aortic enlargement, small aortic knuckle. *ECG:* Right axis deviation, RBBB (left axis deviation in ostium primum defects), atrial arrhythmias. *Echocardiogram:* Micro-bubble contrast is used to visualize shunting.

Complications: Atrial arrythmias (atrial fibrillation is most common), pulmonary hypertension, paradoxical embolus, infective endocarditis (in patients with ostium primum defect only), recurrent pulmonary infections, Eisenmenger syndrome with reversal of shunt. *Management:* Surgical closure between 5 and 10; in adults, small ASDs can be left alone but large shunts large enough to give clear physical signs should be closed.

Management: Drug treatment has a role only in the management of the complications of the defect such as atrial fibrillation (digoxin), right ventricular disease (diuretics), and infective endocarditis (antibiotis). "Umbrella" devices may be placed at the time of cardiac catheterisation. Left-to-right shunt saturations of 1.5:1 or more require surgical closure to prevent right ventricular dysfunction. Otherwise, ostium secundum ASDs whilst having been traditionally closed in or before the third decade may be little gained from surgery in asymptomatic adults.

Associations: Down's syndrome: Endocardial cushion defect causes a primum ASD and other atrioventricular valve abnormalities.

COARCTATION OF THE AORTA

This man is hypertensive. Please examine his cardiovascular system and suggest why.

Large volume asymmetric pulses, vigorous carotid pulsation, radiofemoral delay, ejection systolic murmur loud posteriorly over the praecordium, visible scapular collaterals, visible arterial pulsations and bruits over scapulae and anterior axillary areas and left upper thorax in general, heaving/thrusting apex due to left ventricular hyptertrophy. Request permission to take blood pressure measurements in upper and lower limbs. Coarctation is usually distal to the left subclavian artery near the insertion of ligamentum arteriosum. Early clues to the lesion on inspection may be greater development of the upper extremities and thorax than the lower extremities.

Associations: Cardiac: VSD, bicuspid aortic valve and PDA; Non-cardiac: Turner's syndrome and Berry aneurysms.

Decompensation: Hypertension and its consequences, bicuspid aortic valve, cerebral aneurysms, infective endocarditis.

Investigations: ECG LVH, CXR – rib notching, dilated descending aorta, a "figure of three" sign due to indentation of the aorta of the site of coarctation with pre- and post-stenotic dilatation. Note that rib notching is not a specific sign as it may occur in neurofibromatosis or inferior vena cava obstruction. Echo: Visualize.

Treatment: Treatment for transcoarctal pressure > 30 mmHg through balloon dilatation/surgical resection. Hypertension may continue after surgery.

Patent Ductus Arteriosus

This patient is to have a routine dental extraction. Examine his cardiovascular system, and suggest whether any precautions need to be taken.

Definition: Aortopulmonary shunt, high to low pressure, with a continuous machinery pansystolic murmur due to increased blood flow through the lungs best heard at the end of systole in expiration which may preclude S2, radiating to the left clavicle and heard posteriorly, location left upper sternal edge, associated thrill in the second intercostal space, large defects may be associated with a collapsing pulse, apex displaced inferolaterally,

History: Low birth weight baby, baby born prematurely, baby borne at altitude, 1st trimester rubella in mother.

Symptoms: If small, picked up routinely or coincidentally in a well pink thriving child. If large shunts, they become systematic with heart failure.

Differenetial diagnosis: Pulmonary AV fistulas, coronary AV fistulas, venous hum (young children), MR and AR, VSD with AR.

Investigations: ECG N or LVH, CXR normal or left ventricular/left atrial enlargement, echocardiogram to visualize DA, cardiac catheter.

Common complications: Heart failure, infective endocarditis, pulmonary hypertension, death, rupture. Signs of decompensation: Untreated pulmonary hypertension, Eisenmenger's complex.

Treatment: Infective endocarditis is extremely rare on very small PDAs and these can be left alone. Larger PDAs need treating – to avoid failure and endocarditis. Medical therapy is necessary to treat failure (which can occur for the first time in adult life). Definitive treatment is with ligation or duct occlusion: many of the problems of ligation have been obviated by the use of duct occluders implanted in patients in the catheter laboratory. Irreversible pulmonary hypertension causing Eisenmenger's syndrome is rare, around 5%.

CYANOTIC HEART DISEASE

Eisenmenger Syndrome

This young woman aged 26 has had learning difficulties. Please examine her cardiovascular system and comment on her potential management.

Symptoms: Failure to thrive, impaired growth, intellectual impairment (if severe).

Limited exertional dyspnoea, haemoptysis and frequent chest infections are symptoms of cyanotic heart disease.

Cerebral abscesses, paradoxical emboli, polycythaemia, bleeding diathesis and gout occur.

Signs

- Centrally cyanosed and plethoric,
- Digital clubbing,
- Pulse – regular and small volume,
- Venous pressure – normal (or raised if RV failure has developed) and the 'a' wave is prominent (the atria are contracting against a raied RV pressure); there may be a prominent 'V' wave (if tricuspid regurgitation).
- Left parasternal heave.
- Pulmonary arteries – may be palpable, as may P2.
- There is no thrill (there is insufficient pressure differential to create one). S2 - single and loud (pulmonary hypertension has developed, thus P2 is loud); there may be a (right ventricular) P2.
- Possible pansystolic murmur over the tricuspid area (TR, if the valve cusp has been dilated consequent upon RV failure), as well as an early diastolic murmur over the pulmonary valve (similarly, PA dilatation causing PR – the Graham-Steell murmur).

Aetiology

- Large non-restrictive ventricular septal defect (a single S2),
- Primary pulmonary hypertension,
- Atrial septal defect (S2 is widely split and does not vary with ventilation – A2 precedes P2; P2 does not move, as the increased stroke volume does not vary with ventilation),
- Patent ductus arteriosus (S2 is normal, i.e. A2 precedes P2 and P2 moves with ventilation; there may be differential cyanosis, pink fingers and blue, clubbed toes).
- Other complex congenital heart disease,
- Fallot's tetraology.

A palliative procedure involving redirection of the venous return has been successful in the presence of the great arteries, VSD and severe pulmonary vascular disease.

Investigations: FBC – polycythaemia; ECG: P pulmonale, RAD, tall R waves, inverted T waves in the right precordial leads (right ventricular strain pattern), atrial arrhythmias; CXR: PA dilatation, pruning of the peripheral vessels, prominent pulmonary arteries; echocardiogram – underlying anatomical defect will be localized, flow seen with Doppler ultrasonography; catheter – measures PA pressure and looks for evidence of right-to-left shunting. The response to pulmonary vasodilators should be tested.

Management: If Eisenmenger's syndrome has developed, it is too late for correction of the cardiac anomaly. As a consequence of the increased pulmonary blood flow, the pulmonary vascular resistance rises. When the pulmonary pressure exceeds the systemic pressure, the left-to-right shunt reverses to become right to left, and Eisenmenger's syndrome develops. Heart-lung transplantation offers the only hope for a few young selected patients. Give endocarditis prophylaxis. Pregnancy should be avoided. Perform venesection – to keep the haematocrit below 0.45. Avoid anticoagulants. A poor prognosis is associated with syncope, signs of RV failure, low cardiac ouptut and severe hypoxaemia.

TETRALOGY OF FALLOT

This man is short of breath. Please examine his cardiovascular system and suggest why.

This is an acyanotic congential heart disorder which comprises four separate defects.

- Ventricular septal defect with reversal of the shunt
- Right ventricular hypertrophy
- Pulmonary stenosis
- Aorta that overrides the VSD.

Signs: Cyanosis, clubbing, RV heave, inaudible P2, normal S1.

Investigations: ECG (right ventricular hypertrophy and R-axis deviation), CXR (boot shaped heart).

Complications: Ventricular arrhythmias, AF or atrial flutter, pulmonary regurgitation, recurrent VTOTO.

Eisenmenger's syndrome is the reversal of flow through a shunt, resulting in cyanosis as the pressures from the right heart exceed those of the left heart. This is most often seen in the context of shunts through VSDs, e.g. in Tetralogy of Fallot but can occur in any shunt situation.

Blalock-Taussig shunts: Corrects the Fallot's abnormality by anastamosing the subclavian artery to the pulmonary artery. Currently complete surgical correction is standard.

Other causes of an absent radial pulse. Acute: Embolism, aortic dissection, trauma, e.g. cardiac catheter, and death. Chronic: Coarctation, Takayasu's arteritis.

TRANSPOSITION OF THE GREAT ARTERIES

This man is quite short of breath. Please examine his cardiovascular system and suggest why.

The aorta arises anteriorly from the right ventricle (the systemic ventricle) and the pulmonary artery from the left (so the two circulations are separate). A communication (foramen ovale, patent ductus arteriosus or septal defect) between them is necessary for survival.

Clinical presentation is with cyanosis from birth, and LVF in infancy if the left-to-right shunt is large.

Signs are of cyanosis and a single loud S2.

The ECG may show right axis deviation and RVH. Look for cardiomegaly and increased pulmonary vascularity on the chest radiograph.

The treatment was previously by atrial switch (venous returns are re-routed through the atria). Currently, treatment is by arterial switch in neonates.

EBSTEIN'S ANOMALY

This man was found have an enlarged liver clinically, later verified on ultrasound. Please examine his cardiovascular system and suggest why.

The tricuspid valve is displaced into the right ventricle, leaving a small functional ventricle. 80% of these have a ASD or PFO and a right-to-left shunting occurs if the right atrial pressure rises.

There is a wide spectrum of presentation, from incidental finding to severe venous congestion and cyanosis.

Signs: Cyanosis, tricuspid regurgitation, hepatomegaly.

Investigations: ECG – tall/broad P waves, RBB, first-degree heart block, delta wave.

Treatment: Diuretics and digoxin for LV failure, anti-arrhythmics or ablation for arrhythmics and tricuspid repair/replacement and surgical closure of ASD.

Complications: Atrial arrhythmias and/or accessory pathways (Wolff-Parkinson-White syndrome).

6 Central Nervous System (Station 3)

INTRODUCTION TO EXAMINATION TECHNIQUE

This title of this station is really a misnomer, as much of the station potentially can focus on the peripheral nervous system. Anyway, neurology appears to be everybody's favourite nightmare. It becomes easy when approached in a logical fashion, but practice is required, and you must fulfil the requirements of the task within the time allowed.

Tips for the Examination

- **Always** introduce yourself properly.
- Ask the patient if he/she is comfortable, and **ask whether or not he/she is in pain** before you touch the patient regardless of what you are about to examine.
- Always adequately expose the patient, e.g. if you are to examine the upper limbs ensure that jumpers and shirts are removed to expose the entire limb including the shoulder girdle.
- Position the patient in the correct position.
- Ensure that there is adequate lighting.
- Observe the surroundings, e.g. look for the wheelchair, walking stick, glasses.

Examination of the Limbs

The approach to the examination should **always** be systematic and methodical. Regardless of what you think the diagnosis is, you have to approach all cases systematically. This will demonstrate that you can demonstrate the signs to your examiner and also it is important that you do not miss other pathology. Approaches to the neurological differential diagnosis include: Pattern recognition inferred from a specific constellation of symptoms and signs – requires accurate recall of details; hypothesis testing such that from a patient's initial complaints a diagnostic hypothesis is generated; and anatomical diagnosis, i.e. the site of the lesion with a pathological differential diagnosis (the advantage of this approach is that it requires basic knowledge to organise the signs and symptoms into the major anatomical systems involved. The neurological findings become manageable, when put into the appropriate anatomical compartments: Upper motor neurone (UMN), lower motor neurone (LMN), root lesion, nerve lesion, neuropathy (distal distribution), myopathy (proximal distribution). Neurology requires a good understanding of the functional anatomy of the nervous system.

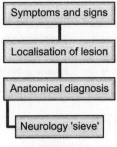

Figure 6.1

COMMON FOCAL NEUROLOGICAL SIGNS AND THEIR LOCALISATION

A lot of neurology, like the rest of medicine, is pattern recognition. The summary Table 6.1 gives some common neurological signs and their localisation.

Table 6.1: Pattern recognition in neurology

Hemiparesis and facial weakness, hemisensory loss, aphasia, or hemianopia	Contralateral hemisphere
Hemiparesis without any other findings	Lacunar infarct pons/contralateral hemisphere
Hemiparesis with contralateral cranial nerve	Brainstem
Bilateral pain and temperature loss, LMN signs level of the lesion sacral sparing	Central cord syndrome
Hemiparesis with contralateral loss of pain and ipsilateral loss of vibration and position sense	Hemicord syndrome (Brown-Séquard syndrome)

Contd...

Contd...

Bilateral motor weakness and loss of pain and temperature-sense, sparing vibration and position-sense	Anterior cord syndrome
Bilateral loss of vibration and position sense	Posterior columns
Paraparesis	At or below thoracic cord parasagittal lesions
Monoparesis (most muscles of a limb)	Brachial or lumbar plexus, exclude cerebral infarct
Loss of pain and temperature in a saddle distribution, sphincter and sexual dysfunction/motor signs	Conus medullaris
Bilateral, asymmetrical motor and sensory loss L & S segments, sphincter and sexual dysfunction	Cauda equina syndrome
Weakness of isolated muscles	Spinal root lesion or peripheral neuropathy
Bilateral distal numbness ± weakness – reflexes	Peripheral neuropathy
Bilateral proximal limb weakness w/o sensory signs	Muscle / NMJ / GBS

PHYSICAL EXAMINATION

In examination of the upper or lower limbs, the marksheet explicity states that the candidate should assess motor function in limbs (including tone and power) and sensory function (including pinprick, vibration sense, propioception and temperature), as well as coordination and cerebellar function.

APPEARANCE

Appearance of the limbs is very important.

Look for evidence of muscle wasting and hypertrophy – look at all the muscle groups: note any atrophy or dystrophy and whether this is generalaised (systemic cause) or focal (localised cause), proximal (muscle disease) or distal (conduction problem – peripheral nerve/ root). Muscle wasting tends to be symmetrical in the case of a muscle disorder.

Look for any evidence of deformity, there may be deformity as a result of neurological imbalance, with gross discrepancies in the size of limbs (infantile hemiplegia, childhood polio). The pseudo-hypertrophy seen in both Duchenne and Becker muscular dystrophy is due to replacement of muscle by fatty/fibrous tissue. The classical 'inverted champagne bottle' (greater muscle loss distally than proximally), appearance attributed to hereditary sensorimotor neuropathy be seen in any longstanding peripheral neuropathy, as can the often co-existent pes cavus and hammer toe deformities (also Refsum's disease and Fredreich's ataxia). The deformity of a spastic upper motor neurone syndrome should not be missed (flexed upper limb, extended lower limb), as often this sole finding when unilateral puts the site of the pathology within the cerebral cortex.

Look for fasciculation: Look closely at the thigh and deltoid muscle groups for any twitching or fasciculation (look for at least 30 seconds).

Elicit any pronator drift: Ask the patient to hold out their arms in front, with the palms facing the ceiling. If the arm starts to dtift (often first) and pronate, there is a high chance of detecting other signs of an upper motor neuron (UMN) syndrome.

TONE, POWER, REFLEXES AND COORDINATION

Tone: Tone is resistance to passive movement at a joint.

Two ways of checking it in the legs:

1. *Lift up the knee quickly and watch the foot:* If there is increase in tone, the heel will lift off the bed, as the knee does not bend. A lot of people argue that this is an unpleasant way of testing, and if there is a diabetic ulcer on the heel.

2. *Roll the whole leg backwards and forwards and watch the foot:* The foot should flop at the ankle. With increased tone it moves as a stiff extension of the lower leg.

Two types of increased tone:

Spasticity: UMN sign of pyramidal tract damage. Commonest form seen after the stroke. Resistance is high in the early range of movement, but eases suddenly when this is (gently) overcome.

Rigidity: Extrapyramidal sign, virtually always related to Parkinson's disease. Resistance is maintained throughout the range of movement, a bit like bending a lead pipe (which we do regularly in our department). If there is associated tremor, this results in "cogwheeling". Best tested at wrist and elbow simultaneously. "There is waxy resistance to passive movement, which is maintained throughout the range of movement."

Clonus: It is easiest to perform the test for clonus at this stage for two reasons. Firstly, if present, it implies there is an upper motor neurone problem and hyper-reflexia should be present and secondly it is often forgotten about, if left until later to perform. Clonus is best elicited at either ankle or knee joint.

MRC Classification of Power

This is a subjective assessment. Be gentle and compare the corresponding groups of both sides before moving to the next group, i.e. left biceps, right biceps, left triceps, right triceps, etc. Ideally you should test the patient's dominant and therefore stronger side with your dominant side.

0 – no movement,

1 – flicker/fasciculation,

2 – movement on the bed surface but no anti-gravity power,

3 – anti-gravity power but no more (cannot overcome resistance),

4 – reduced power against resistance,

5 – normal power, for all the major flexor/extensor pairs as well as small muscles of the hand.

It will be expected that, at any point during the examination, the examiners may ask the candidate for the muscle being tested, the root value and the action of that particular muscle.

Upper Limbs

"Hold your arms out to your sides. Now keep them up". Deltoids C5 Shoulder abduction.

"Now push them in towards you and don't let me stop you". Pectoralis C6, 7, 8 Shoulder adduction.

"Pull your arms up towards you and don't let me stop you". Biceps C5 Arm flexion.

"Now push me away" Triceps C7 Arm extension.

"Clench your fists and bend your wrists up towards you" Wrist flexors C7.

"Now push the other way" Wrist extensors C7.

"Put your hand down flat like this and point your thumb towards your nose. Now, keep it there and don't let me push it down" Abductor pollicis brevis/Median nerve C8/T1.

"Spread your fingers wide apart and don't let me push them together". Finger abduction/dorsal interossei/ulnar nerve. T1

"Now hold this piece of card between your fingers and don't let me pull it away". Finger adduction/palmar interossei/ulnar nerve T1.

Reflexes - with the tendon hammer held perpendicular to the line of the tendon, strike the tendon gently by holding the hammer by its length. The reflexes should be graded against the MRC standard 0 – areflexia, 1 – with reinforcement only, 2 – physiological, 3 –

hyperreflexive, 4 – clonus. Plantar response: The Babinski response is present, if a contraction in the quadriceps is seen, even if the toes don't fan or extend.

Upper limbs: Biceps C5/6, Supinator C5/6, Triceps C7.

Coordination: If performed early, valuable information can be sought even before power is assessed. This is particularly useful, as occasionally the examiner will cut short your examination if he/she feels that too much time has been taken up by power assessment and an assessment of coordination cannot even be made. However, it is extremely unlikely that an examiner will ask you to finish prior to assessing the power. Secondly, if the patient is unable to lift his arm or leg in order to assess coordination, then all that remains to be done when assessing power, is to determine to what degree the loss of power is. In the upper limb, perform the finger-nose test and in the lower limb perform the heel-shin test.

Lower Limbs

"I'm going to test the strength of some of the muscles in your legs. Keep your leg straight and lift it up into the air. Now, keep it up and don't let me stop you." Hip flexion. L1,2. Iliopsoas.

"Now push your leg down into the bed and don't let me stop you". Hip extension. L4,5. Gluteus.

"Push out against my hand". Hip abduction. Glutei. L4,5.

"Push in against my hand". Hip adduction. Adductor group. L2,3,4.

"Bend your knee and pull your heel up towards you: don't let me stop you." Knee flexion. Hamstrings. L5,S1.

"Now straighten your knee out". Knee extension. Quadriceps. L3,4.

"Pull your foot up to you and don't let me stop you." Ankle dorsiflexion. Tibialis anterior and long extensors. L4,5.

"Push your foot down against my hand". Ankle plantar flexion. Gastrocnemius. S1.

"Push your foot out against my hand". Eversion of foot. Peroneus. S1.

"Push your foot in against my hand". Inversion of foot. Tibialis anterior and posterior. L4.

Reflexes: See above.

Lower limbs: Knee L4, Ankle S1.

Coordination: See above.

SENSORY TESTING

It is important that you are confident about the dermatome distribution in the upper and lower limbs, bearing in mind that the clearest delineation is distally, rather than proximally, and that you are clear in your instructions to the patient.

For this reason, start distally and assess sensation (start with the orange stick if available, rather than your finger) in the dermatome distribution, working your way proximally. Explain "I'm going to move this down your arms/legs, tell me if it feels sharp/soft", then say "now shut your eyes", compare one dermatome on the right with the corresponding one on the left, and move down the dermatomes – try to define the sensory level or glove and stocking peripheral neuropathy. Useful levels are: T4 – nipple, T10 – umbilicus, T12 – above the inguinal ligament, and L1 – below the inguinal ligament. Test pinprick sensation using appropriate sharps which do not penetrate the skin. Pinprick sensation using appropriate sharps which do not penetrate the skin. Also remember to check the back of the patient to determine whether the abnormality is actually dermatomal or not.

If you are asked to examine to perform a sensory neurological examination of the lower limbs, the first thing is to rule out is a peripheral neuropathy.

Cotton-wool to touch and not drag the stimulus along the surface of the skin. "I want you to say YES if you feel me touch you with this piece of cotton wool". Avoid hairs on legs where you can, tickle is transmitted in the spinothalamic tract.

Joint position sense: Upper limb drift with eyes closed. "I'm going to move your finger up and down; this is up and this is down. Now close your eyes and tell me whether I am moving your finger up or down".

Place a ringing tuning fork on the superior aspect of the manubrium. Establish what the patient recognises as normal (i.e. reference at the top of the manubrium sterni), and ask him/her to confirm whether they next feel the same again. Start distally on *bony prominences*: For the legs, 1st MTP joint (bunion), medial malleolus, tibial protuberance (knobble below patella), anterior superior iliac spine.

Temperature: This is rarely tested. If pinprick is impaired, test temperature sensation with a tuning fork (cold) and your hand (warm).

The lateral spinothalamic tract carries sharp pain and temperature. The dorsal columns carry soft touch (most of it), deep pain (pinch Achilles tendon) and joint position sense.

Dermatomes

Remember to perform Romberg's test: Ask the patient to stand with his feet together and tell the patient you are ready to catch him if he falls. If he stands with his eyes open and falls with his eyes closed, this is loss of joint position sense (Romberg's test is positive), as with a posterior column lesion in the spinal cord or peripheral neuropathy. If he is unable to stand with his eyes open and feet together, then this is severe unsteadiness, most commonly due to cerebellar syndromes and central and peripheral vestibular syndromes.

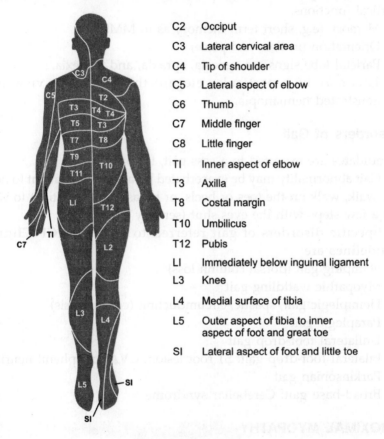

C2	Occiput
C3	Lateral cervical area
C4	Tip of shoulder
C5	Lateral aspect of elbow
C6	Thumb
C7	Middle finger
C8	Little finger
TI	Inner aspect of elbow
T3	Axilla
T8	Costal margin
T10	Umbilicus
T12	Pubis
LI	Immediately below inguinal ligament
L3	Knee
L4	Medial surface of tibia
L5	Outer aspect of tibia to inner aspect of foot and great toe
SI	Lateral aspect of foot and little toe

Figure 6.2: Dermatomes

In testing sensation, the candidate should show understanding of the need to move from areas of reduced to normal sensation when cutaneous sensitivity.

It is sensible to think whether the pattern fits a dermatomal distribution or a peripheral neuropathy. If the sensory loss looks as if it is in a glove and stocking distribution, start at the tips of the fingers and toes, and work up until you find a sensory level.

Sensory abnormalities that suggest non-organic (functional) loss: This is suggested by a non-anatomical distribution of sensory deficit frequently with inconsistent findings.

Features which suggest a cortical basis for the sensory loss, e.g. sensory suppression, asterognosis.

Disorders of Higher Cortical Function

Where appropriate, the candidate should be able to assess higher cortical functions:

Memory (e.g. short term memory as in MMSE)

Orientation (in time and place)

Parietal lobe signs are agnosia, apraxia, and dyslexia.

This may be a particular elegant thing to do in view of a demonstrated hemianopia.

Disorders of Gait

Candidates are expected to assess gait, if appropriate.

Gait abnormality may be exacerbated by asking the patient to heel-toe walk, walk on the toes or heels, or by asking the patient to walk for a few steps with the eyes shut (sensory ataxia).

Specific disorders of gait referred to in the **MRCP Clinical Guidelines** are:

- Stamping gait (dorsal column loss)
- Myopathic waddling gait
- Hemiplegic gait/spastic/circumducting (cord paresis)
- Paraplegic gait
- Unilateral foot-drop gait
- Bilateral foot-drop gait: S1 root lesion, CVA, peripheral neuritis
- Parkinsonian gait
- Broad-base gait: Cerebellar syndrome.

PROXIMAL MYOPATHY

This 45-year-old woman has weak legs. Please examine her legs and elucidate why.

Causes of a proximal myopathy:

- *Inherited:* Myotonic dystrophy, muscular dystrophy.
- *Endocrine:* Cushing's syndrome, hyperparathyroidism, thyrotoxicosis, diabetic amyotrophy.
- *Inflammatory:* Polymyositis, rheumatoid arthritis, dermatomyositis.
- *Metabolic:* Osteomalacia.
- Polymyalgia rheumatica.
- Periodic paralysis due to channelopathies.

- *Malignancy:* Carcinoma, paraneoplastic, Lambert-Eaton myaesthenic syndrome.
- *Drugs:* Alcohol, steroids.
- Uraemia.

Investigations: EMG – no denervation, repetitive discharges; CK; muscle biopsy; ESR, CRP; thyroid function tests; dexamethasone suppression test; anti-AChR antibodies; CXR – thymoma, lung malignancy.

HEMIPLEGIA

This 45-year-old woman has weak legs. Please examine her legs and elucidate why.

Having elicited the signs in the limbs, test for sensory inattention, visual inattention and hemianopia, and ask if you may test the patient's speech. Show that you are considering the aetiology by feeling the patient's pulse (atrial fibrillation), auscultation for valve lesions and carotid bruits, and taking the patient's blood pressure. There is a sided upper motor neurone weakness of the facial muscles, with increased tone and hyper-reflexia. The plantar is extensor, and abdominal reflexes are diminished. The most likely causes are cerebrovascular accident due to cerebral thrombosis, haemorrhage or embolism; brain tumour. A right-sided hemiplegia associated with dysphasia woulod suggest that the causative lesion is affecting the speech centres in the dominant hemisphere as well as the motor cortex (precentral gyrus) and if there are sensory signs the sensory cortex (postcentral gyrus). If cerebrovascular in origin, the causative lesion is likely to be in the carotid distribution.

PARKINSONISM/PARKINSON'S DISEASE

This 55-year-old man has found himself with walking problems. Examine his upper limbs and elucidate why.

An Extremely Common Causes

The three features are tremor, rigidity and bradykinesia. In latter stages, postural instability is the fourth feature.

Causes of Parkinsonism: Idiopathic Parkinson's disease, Parkinson Plus syndromes (Multiple system atrophy, progressive supranuclear palsy: Steele-Richardson-Olsewski, cortical Lewy body disease), drug-induced, particularly phenothiazines, anoxic brain damage from anoxia, neurosyphilis, post-encephalitis, MPTP toxicity ("frozen addict syndrome").

Pathology: Degeneration of the dopaminergic neurones between the substantia nigra and basal ganglia.

- Monotonous tone/dysarthria/dysphonia.
- Withdrawn facies (expressionless face with absence of spontaneous movements); dribbling of saliva.
- Supranuclear gaze palsy.
- Asymmetrical resting tremor; tremor disappears on voluntary movement.
- This tremor is a coarse, pill-rolling tremor (4-6 cps) at rest is characteristic.
- Bradykinesia as demonstrated by thumb finger opposition/tapping one hand with the other/tapping foot on the floor. Cogwheeling rigidity marked with synkinesis.
- Muscle rigidity throughout the range of movement (tremor = cogwheeling).
- Festinant gait. Watch the difficulty when turning. Check righting reflexes by standing behind the patient and gently pushing them forwards and pulling them backwards.
- Stooped, flexed posture with loss of arm swing.
- Speech is slow, faint and monotonous.
- Facial expression
- Eye movements
- Micrographia and impaired dressing ability.
- Glabellar tap sign (on repeated tapping of the glabella, the Parkinsonian patient continues to blink).

Extra points: BP looking for evidence of multisystem atrophy (Parkinsonism with postural hypotension, cerebellar and pyramidal signs), vertical eye movements for progressive supranuclear palsy, dementia and Parkinsonism (Lewy-body dementia), ask for a medication history.

Diagnosis is made by clinical observation, a therapeutic trial of levodopa, or an apomorphine challenge. Other tests include MRI (abnormal hypointensity in the putamen of patients with multiple system atrophy), copper and caeruloplasmin measurements, testing of automonic function (including sphincter electromyography).

Treatment: Forge a therapeutic alliance between the patients, carer and specialists, assess disability and cognition, antmuscarinic medication where there is drug-induced parkinsonism, consider drugs when the condition is interfering with life, dopamine agonists, e.g. pergolide, ropinirole and pramipexone which are well tolerated.

Ropinirole carries a much lower risk of dyskinesia. Other medications include MAO-B inhibitors, e.g. selegiline, inhibit the breakdown of dopamine; anticholinergics are effective for reducing tremor, particularly drug-induced; L-dopa with a peripheral dopa-decarboxylase inhibitor, e.g. madopar (problems with nausea and dyskinesia, effects wear off after a few years so generally delay treatment as long as possible, end of dose effect and on/off motor fluctuation may be reduced by modified release preparations).

Levo-dopa without a decarboxylase inhibitor cause nausea and vomiting and postural hypertension so it is always combined with a decarboxylase inhibitor. Side effects of Levo-Dopa include involuntary movements, psychiatric disturbance, nightmares, hallucinations, frank psychosis, fluctuations in response including on/off syndrome. COMT inhibitors (e.g. entacapone) block breakdown of L-dopa outside the brain thus reducing motor fluctuations.

Surgery: Thalamotomy, pallidotomy, deep brain stimulation (e.g. pallidal) and fetal neural transplantation [this may be dependent on a referral to a tertiary centre, if necessary.] The next step is the addition of a COMT inhibitor; and apomorphine given as SC injection or infusion.

Other issues: Symptomatic treatment may be necessary (constipation with stool softeners, laxatives or enemas), bladder symptoms (look for the presence of a UTI; detrusor hyperactivity can be treated with oxybutinin), postural hypotension (a tilted bed or fludrocortisone). Patients can drive with PD provided that they are not severely disabled by their PD and do not have sleep attacks during driving (this may be drug-induced). Sophisticated vehicle adaptation is possible with joysticks and infrared controls.

Carers should be aware of the Crossroads scheme. The Parkinson's Disease Society provides support for patients and carers.

UNILATERAL FOOT DROP

This 45-year-old woman has weak legs. Please examine her legs and elucidate why.

Here the main differential diagnosis is between:

- Pyramidal lesion affecting lower limb (e.g. cerebrovascular accident, multiple sclerosis: Pyramidal weakness, hyperreflexia and upgoing plantar should make the diagnosis obvious).
- Common peroneal nerve palsy: Weakness of dorsiflexion of the feet and toes and of eversion of foot. Ankle jerk is intact and plantar

response normal; the ankle reflex is conveyed through the S1 root via the tibial branch of the sciatic nerve, and is therefore spared in a peroneal nerve lesion. Sensory loss often restricted to the dorsum of the foot (may extend to anterolateral aspect of the leg below the knee), including the first phalanges of the toes and the anterolateral aspect of the bottom half of the leg. Causes include compression or trauma at the fibula neck, diabetes mellitus, vasculitis, and leprosy (look also for thickening of peripheral nerves which become palpable, notably the greater auricular nerve).

- L5 lesion often due to prolapsed intervertebral disc. Weakness of dorsiflexion but not eversion of the foot (latter supplied by S1). Ankle jerk is intact, plantar response normal, sensory loss on dorsum of the foot often extending to the lateral aspect of the leg below the knee.

CEREBELLAR SYNDROME

This 46-year-old woman, with a previously treated breast lump, now finds herself with some problems buttoning her shirt. Please examine her cranial nerves and suggest why.

An Extremely Common Causes

Causes: Posterior fossa syndrome, alcohol, demyelinating disease, trauma, rare, inherited, e.g. Fredreich's ataxia (pes cavus, kyphoscoliosis, spastic paraparesis with extensor plantars, but areflexia due to an axonal neuropathy, spinocerebellar degeneration causes ataxia, diabetes mellitus in 10% of patients, cardiomyopathy), anti-epileptic medication, stroke, paraneoplastic cerebellar syndrome, severe hypothyroidism, ataxia-telengectasia, lesions at the cerebellopontine angle, congenital disorders such as a Dandy-Walker syndrome or Arnold-Chiari malformation.

Cerebellar dysarthria (slurred speech): Scanning dysarthria.

Finger-nose (dysmetria, intention tremor) and heel-knee-shin tests; dysdiadochokinesis in upper limbs.

Hypotonia/pendular knee jerk.

Overshooting phenomenon/rebound phenomenon.

Nystagmus. In a cerebellar lesion, the fast-phase direction is towards the side of the lesion, and maximal on looking towards the lesion. Check also for broken pursuit and slow saccadic movements.

Truncal ataxia characteristics from a vermal lesion (rather than limb ataxia).

Cerebellar ataxia (gait abnormality).

Differential diagnosis: Wilson's disease, Refsum's disease (pes cavus, retinitis pigmentosa, nerve deafness, anosma, cerebellar ataxia; autosomal dominant).

Investigations: MRI is better than CT in posterior fossa, LP if there is no space occupying lesion, phenytoin level, blood alcohol, gGT, LFT, thyroid function tests, HIV test, glucose, lipids. CXR – lung cancer causing paraneoplasic syndrome, or with multiple metastases. ECG.

Management: Is there anything to be repaired–tumour aneurysm? Ensure abstinence from alcohol. Give thyroxine replacement. Reduce phenytoin dose.

SPASTIC PARAPARESIS

An Extremely Common Cause

This 40-year-old man has weak legs. Please examine his legs and offer some explanations to the examiner why.

Never forget to demonstrate a sensory level and for absence of the abdominal reflexes. Tell the examiners that you would normally ask the patient about bowel and bladder function and test sacral sensation.

The hypertonia, clonus and hyperreflexia tell you that the lesion lies above L1 as the pyramidal tracts end there. Lesions below L1 can result in cauda equina compression. This too is a medical emergency: Flaccid paraparesis, saddle anaesthesia, reduced reflexes, downgoing plantars, sphincter disturbance.

History is crucial (trauma, malignancy, pain in the spine, onset).

Common Causes

- Cerebral palsy (check for intellectual impairment, behavioural problems, a history of birth injury),
- Demyelination/multiple sclerosis (commonest),
- Spinal cord compression (medical emergency, disc prolapse above L1/L2, malignancy, trauma, fracture of the vertebra), cervical myopathy,
- Trauma,
- Motor neuron disease (no sensory signs),
- Transverse myelitis,
- Anterior spinal artery thrombosis (dissociated sensory loss with preservation of dorsal columns),

- Syringomyelia with typical upper limb signs, subacute combined degeneration of the spinal cord,
- Hereditary spastic paraparesis,
- Fredreich's ataxia,
- Parasagittal falx meningioma,
- Cervical spondylosis,
- Infection (e.g. HIV, abscess, syphilis, Pott's disease of the spine, HTLV-1 (tropic spastic paraparesis),
- Radiation myelopathy,
- Vascular (arterial occlusion),
- Other inflammatory causes (sarcoid, SLE),
- Intrinsic cord pathology (vitamin B_{12} deficiency, AVM).

Clinical signs: Contractures, wheel-chair and walking sticks (disuse atrophy and contractures may be present if chronic), urinary catheter *in-situ*, bilateral symmetrical paralysis of the lower limbs, symmetrical lower limb hyperreflexia, bilateral extensor plantar responses, ankle clonus, wasting, sensory level to mid-thoracic region, scissoring "gait".

L2/3	Hip flexion
L3/4	Knee extension
L4/5	Foot dorsiflexion
L5/S1	Knee flexion, hip extension
S1/2	Foot plantar-flexion

knee jerk L3/4

ankle jerk S1/2

The term "level" is a very indescript term, but literally means sensory level, reflex, and motor level (both at the level), and tone (below the level). Any sensory level must be determined, particularly if the history suggests an acute or subacute onset with recent alteration in sphincter function. See Fig. 7 for a pictorial representation of the dermatomes.

Localisation of the level of the lesion can be achieved by:
- Spasticity of the lower limb alone: Lesion of the thoracic cord (T2 – L1)
- Irregular spasticity of the lower limbs with flaccid weakness of scattered muscles of lower limbs: Lesion of lumbosacral enlargement (L2 – S2).

Examine for a sensory level suggestive of a spinal lesion. Look at the back for scars or spinal deformity. Search for features of multiple sclerosis, e.g. cerebellar signs especially dysarthria, fundoscopy to look for optic atrophy. Ask about bladder symptoms and note the presence or absence of urinary catheter. State that a complete examination would include anal tone.

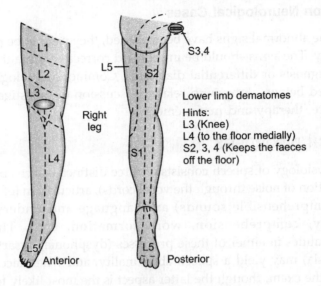

Figure 6.3: Dermatomes of lower limb

If allowed to proceed, you should examine the arms. You may be able to localise the lesion. Ask the examiner's permission to test the neck movements.

Investigations: Suspicion of spinal cord compression is a medical emergency. Once sphincter dysfunction has been present for 24 hours, it is irreversible. Therefore, the necessary investigations must be carried out as a matter of urgency–FBC, ESR, CXR, plain radiology of the spine, then either a CT myelogram or MRI. A neurosurgeon should be contacted. Depending on the likely differential diagnosis: Electromyography, nerve conduction studies, lumbar puncture (CSF for oligoclonal bands, culture, acid-fast bacilli, ACE), blood and CSF syphilis, blood culture, biopsy of masses, HIV test, vitamin B_{12} levels, CRP, autoantibodies and MRI of the central nervous system.

Management: This is dependent on the cause. Spinal cord compression with bladder or bowel involvement often requires surgical decompression. Stabilisation of the spine may be necessary. Dexamethasone and radiotherapy may suffice for malignant compression. The problem with benign tumours is that the paraparesis may be attributed to multiple sclerosis, despite the symptoms not being disseminated in time and place. With malignancy, the main danger is indecision; the condition is obviously incurable but surgical treatment at an early stage may relieve pain, minimise weakness and preserve bladder function.

Common Neurological Cases

Once the abnormal signs have been elicited, they need to be presented correctly. The signs should be interpreted correctly within the context of a diagnosis or differential diagnoses. Common neurological cases are listed below, along with related discussion of investigation and sequence, therapy and management.

SPEECH DISORDERS

The physiology of speech consists of three distinct aspects; phonation (generation of noise through the vocal cords), articulation (of the noise into comprehensible sounds) and language and understanding (fluency, comprehension, word formation, etc.). Therefore, abnormalities in either of these processes (dysphonia, dysarthria and dysphasia) may yield a speech abnormality, and when faced with a case in the exam, though the latter aspect is the most likely to require assessment, you must be able to assess speech in its entirety.

Dysphonia–can the patient generate the effort to push air through the vocal cords (myasthenia and other neuromuscular conditions–normal at first but starts to fade), or is there an obstruction within the larynx or the recurrent laryngeal nerve impeding adequate phonation.

Dysarthria–are the words fluent or stuttery? Can the patient pronounce vowels correctly "EE" or "AA" other useful ones are "P" and "B". Are there gross articulation problems when coordination of speech is tested "British constitution" (cerebellar). Does the articulation sound mumbling (Parkinson's – also dysphonia). Assessment of dysarthria:

1. Monotonous speech of Parkinsonism.
2. Staccato or broken speech of cerebellar syndrome.
3. Hot potato speech of pseudobulbar palsy: Usually bilateral pyramidal signs, spastic tongue, brisk jaw jerks.
4. Nasal speech of bulbar palsy: Flaccid and often fasciculating tongue, and other signs of MND.
5. Dysarthria (unclassified) usually following stroke with incomplete recovery.

Examine the motor system: LMN weakness (facial palsy, bulbar palsy), UMN weakness (hemiparesis, pseudobulbar palsy), cerebellar disease – nystagmus, intention tremor, hypotonia and ataxia, extrapyramidal disease (Parkinson's disease).

Dysphasia: This should be assessed in terms of object naming (nominal), fluency and repetition (expressive) and comprehension, e.g. by asking the patient to perform simple commands (receptive). Repetition can be performed by difficult words, e.g. statistican analysis, "No ifs ands or buts". Finally, remember that dysphasic speech problems usually imply a lesion in the left dominant frontotemporal region, and other complimentary signs should be sought (right hemiparesis). The presence of a dysphasia will also suggest a cortical lesion when faced with a patient that looks like a stroke, rather than a lacunar syndrome (internal capsule). Test the patient's inability to name objects (wrist watch, second hand and winder on watch). Difficulty in naming objects is found in both motor and sensory aphasia but is relatively selectively impaired in the rare nominated dysphasia (lesion on angular gyrus).

You may be asked the site of the lesion:

- *Broca's area:* Inferior frontal gyrus of the dominant hemisphere. This produces non-fluent aphasia. The content may be good, but the patient says little.
- *Wernicke's area:* Posterior part of superior temporal gyrus plus adjacent parts of parietal and occipital cortex of dominant hemisphere.

MOVEMENT DISORDERS

Resting tremor: Parkinson's disease.

Postural tremor (worse with arms outstretched): Benign essential tremor, anxiety, thyrotoxicosis, metabolic: carbon dioxide and hepatic encephalopathy, alcohol. Look for the signs of thyroid disease, and tell the examiner you would like to know if there is any family history of tremor, and if the patient is on any medications (e.g. salbutamol, lithium).

Intention tremor: Seen in cerebellar disease. Look for other cerebellar signs.

Dystonic posturing: Co-contraction of agonist and antagonist which may lead to an intermittent or persistent maintainence of abnormal pasture.

Chorea: Non-rhythmic movements of a rapid, jerky nature which frequently appear pseudo-purposeful.

Athetosis: Slower writhing, irregular movements predominantly in the hands and wrist.

Others (in cranial nerve territory): Hemifacial spasm
Myokymia
Blepharospasm
Orofacial dyskinesia.

MULTIPLE SCLEROSIS

This 30-year-old woman complains of double vision and incoordination with previous episodes of weakness. Please perform a neurological examination of her legs and suggest a likely diagnosis.

An Extremely Common Cause

Key signs: Optic neuritis (you may not be allowed to examine the eyes but you may ask "May I ask about eye problems"), internuclear ophthalmoplegia (frequently bilateral in MS), reduced visual acuity, and other cranial nerve palsy. In an internuclear ophthalmoplegia, on looking to the right, the right eye abducts normally but the left eye is unable to adduct; the right eye has nystagmus.

- *Peripheral nervous system:* Upper motor neuron spasticity, weakness, brisk reflexes, altered sensation.
- *Sensory alteration:* Often hot/cold appreciation is disturbed, or there is a history of Lhermitte's phenomenon–electric shock like pain on flexing the neck which shoots down the arms and legs and is caused by disease abutting the dorsal columns.
- *Higher cortical function:* Euphoria, depression and disinhibition.
- *Autonomic:* Urinary retention/incontinence, impotence and bowel problems.
- Signs of disseminated lesions in CNS.

Investigations: MRI is most useful to detect involvement and characteristic pattern of lesions, lumbar puncture is now less regularly used.

Visual evoked response is useful in a patient with an isolated lesion which may be due to multiple sclerosis to identify subclinical involvement and provide evidence for demyelination (SSEPs are used as well).

CSF shows an increase in total protein, and oligoclonal bands (not matched in serum).

Central nervous system demyelination causes neurological impairment that is disseminated in both time and space.

Benign course more likely if there is pure sensory presentation, infrequent relapses and long remissions, onset with optic neuritis or sensory or motor symptoms, or benign condition 5 years after onset.

Complications: Visual loss, paresis, tremor and incontinence; significant cognitive impairment may occur late.

Management: Supportive, including catheters, etc. as appropriate, methylprednisolone, be prepared to discuss interferon. *CSF:* Monoclonal IgG bands, *MRI:* Periventricular white matter plaques, visual evoked potentials: delayed velocity but normal amplitude (often even where there is no evidence of optic neuritis, indicating that there is some neuronal loss sustained). Diagnosis can be made clinically (e.g. 2 or more attack with 2 or more objective clinical lesions), or a combination of clinical and corroborative data (e.g. 2 or more attacks + 1 objective lesion + MRI / +ve CSF).

Treatment: Multidisciplinary team (nurse, physiotherapist, occupational therapist, social worker, and physician); disease-modifying treatments (β-interferon) and symptomatic treatments (methylprednisolone during the acute phase may shorten the duration of the 'attack' but does not affect propnosis), anti-spasmodics, e.g. tizanidine, clonazepam, dantrolene, baclofen, carbamazepine (for neuropathic pain), cognitive and emotional problems (emotionalism, depression using anti-depressant medication or psychological treatments such as cognitive behavioural therapy, anxiety), speech difficulties (specialist speech and language therapist), sexual dysfunction, laxatives and intermittent catheterisation/oxybutinin for bowel and bladder disturbance. *Consider the impairment, disability and handicap:* Arm paralysis is the impairment, inability to write is the disability, subsequent inability to work in a job is the handicap. Occupational therapy for rehabilitation.

The key points are outlined in the "National clinical guideline for diagnosis and management of multiple sclerosis in primary and secondary care" (The Royal College of Physicians, The Chartered Society of Physiotherapy).

DIABETIC AND PERIPHERAL NEUROPATHY

This patient has noticed generalised weakness/tingling of his fingers. Please examine the motor and sensory system in the upper limbs to establish the cause.

An Extremely Common Cause

- This is done quickest by assessing vibration loss with the vibrating tuning fork applied to the bony prominence of the metatarsal head, malleoli, patella and if required anterior superior iliac spine.

- If you cannot detect a peripheral neuropathy, then you must resort to performing an orthodox sensory examination as prescribed.
- Ensure that, if given the time, you perform sufficient tests to determine function in the two main sensory tracts (this usually means "pinprick" and "vibration" testing).
- If during the course of your sensory assessment, there is a gross sensory loss that is bilaterally symmetric then proceed to determine if a sensory level exists. Motor loss may be present in mixed motor/sensory neuropathies.
- *Sensory loss:* Look for foot ulcers, roughened thickened callous skin, tropic changes and Charcot joints (common causes of these: diabetes mellitus and syringomyelia).
- Palpate for tenderness of affected muscles which is common in diabetic or alcoholic polyneuropathy. Palpate for thickened peripheral nerves present in: Refsum's disease (cerebellar damage, peripheral neuropathy, deafness and retinitis pigmentosa), Amyloidosis, Leprosy, Dejerine-Sottas disease, Charcot-Marie-Tooth disease some thickening detectable in 25% of cases.
- *Glance briefly for clues as to the cause:* Insulin injection sites (diabetes mellitus), signs of chronic liver disease (especially alcoholic), anaemia and slight jaundice (B_{12} deficiency), cachexia (malignancy), pigmentation, anaemia and brown line on nails $\pm$ evidence of haemodialysis (uraemia), pes cavus (HSMN or Fredreich's ataxia), rheumatoid hands or butterfly rash of systemic lupus erythematosus.
- *Sphincter function:* You should enquire about bladder and bowel function by asking the examiner. Along with the obvious catheter tube, sphincter disturbances should be suspected in patients with impaired 'saddle region' anaesthesia.
- *Enquire about vision:* Causes according to sensory/motor: Predominantly sensory (carcinomatous neuropathy, diabetes mellitus, uraemia, alcohol, drugs, e.g. isoniazid and vincristine, vitamin deficiency, e.g. B_{12} and B_1); predominantly motor (Guillain-Barré syndrome and botulism acutely, lead toxicity, porphyria, HSMN). The broad areas of aetiology are acute symmetrical peripheral neuropathy, multiple neuropathy, and chronic symmetrical peripheral neuropathy.

Broad Classes of Causes

- *Mononeuritis multiplex:* Diabetes mellitus, connective tissue disease, e.g. SLE and rheumatoid arthritis, vasculitis, e.g. polyarteritis nodosa and Churg-Strauss syndrome,

- Infection, e.g. HIV, malignancy. Hereditary: E.g. HMSN-1 and -2
- *Inherited disorders:* Refsum's disease, Fredreich's ataxia.
- *Drug causes:* Isoniazid, nitrofurantoin, phenytoin, ciclosporin, vincristine, amiodarone, cisplatin.
- *Deficiencies:* Vitamin B_{12}, folate, thiamine (Wernicke's encephalopathy and Korsakoff's psychosis in alcohols) and niacin (pellagra).
- *Collagen vascular disease:* E.g. SLE, rheumatoid arthritis, polyarteritis nodosa, scleroderma.
- Malignant disease.
- Malignancy.
- Endocrine, e.g. diabetes mellitus, uraemia, hypothyroidism
- Others, e.g. porphyria and amyloidosis.
- Idiopathic.

Causes of a predominantly motor neuropathy: Carcinomatous neuropathy, lead, porphyria, Charcot-Marie-Tooth.

Investigations: Urine for glucose and protein, haematology (ESR, vitamin B_{12} level, folate, FBC), biochemistry (fasting blood glucose, renal function, liver function, TSH), neurophysiological tests, immunology (ANA, ENA, ANCA), chest X-ray, urine (Bence-Jones protein), CSF, immunology (anti-neuronal antibodies, anti-HIV), tests for Sjogren's syndrome, molecular genetics test, nerve conduction studies (diagnosis confirmed by slowing of motor or sensory conduction velocities, moderate in axonal type and marked in demyelinating type), CSF (in GBS/inflammatory neuropathies for raised protein level), nerve biopsy in progressive neuropathy or to identify vasculitis as the cause (sensory nerves are usually biopsied), imaging (screening for malignancy in patients with suspected paraneoplastic neuropathy; skeletal survey for myeloma; chest radiography for suspected sarcoidosis), DNA analysis (for hereditary sensorimotor neuropathies); bone marrow biopsy (for vitamin B_{12} deficiency or myeloma). *Management:* Tight control of diabetes, consider other related problems in eye and kidney, educate patient about the need to control foot inspection, etc.

Management: Directed towards the specific cause. Rigorous control of glycaemia, often with intensive insulin regimens, can improve diabetic neuropathy, particularly if the syndrome arose acutely. Simple analgesics, tricyclic anti-depressants, anticonvulsants (phenytoin and carbamazepine) may help. Autonomic neuropathy is difficult (postural hypotension: Fludrocortisone; vomiting: metoclopramide; bacterial overgrowth: Erythromycin). In deficiency, vitamin B$_{12}$ for subacute combined degeneration of the cord.

ULNAR NERVE PALSY

This 72-year-old lady with worsening osteoarthritis has difficulty using her hands. Please examine her upper limbs from a neurological perspective, and suggest why.

Usually due to lesion at the elbow; inspect for scars or arthritis.

The hand shows generalized muscle wasting and weakness which spares the thenar eminence. There is sensory loss over the fifth finger, the adjacent half of the fourth finger and the dorsal and palmar aspects of the medial aspect of the hand.

In a low ulnar nerve lesion, the hand is claw shaped – the metacarpophalangeal (MCP) joints of the ring and little fingers are hyperextended and the interphalangeal joints remain flexed. There is weakness in abduction and adduction of the fingers and thumb. Sensation is impaired over the medial sign of the hand, little finger and medial (ulnar) border of the ring finger. In a high lesion, the FDPs are also paralysed. The DIPs are not flexed, and so the clawing is less obvious. This is termed the ulnar paradox. Low lesions occur at the wrist, but high lesions occur in osteoarthritis and dislocations, commonly at the elbow.

Occasionally due to repeated trauma to heel of hand (no sensory loss in this case). Common causes are fracture or dislocation at the elbow, and osteoarthrosis at the elbow with osteophytic encroachment on the ulnar nerve in the cubital tunnel. Other causes are occupations with constant leaning on elbows (secretaries), excessive carrying angle at the elbow, injurie at the wrist or palm (e.g. occupations using screwdrivers, drills, etc.)

MEDIAN NERVE PALSY

This 72-year-old lady with worsening rheumatoid arthritis has difficulty using her hands. Please examine her upper limbs from a neurological perspective, and suggest why.

Carpal tunnel syndrome is a common case.

NB. Associations include pregnancy, myxoedema, rheumatoid arthritis, acromegaly, trauma. Remember that sensory loss is very variable since the palmar branch of the median nerve passes superficial to the flexor retinaculum.

(Please note that this would make a suitable case for Station 5 as well).

RADIAL NERVE LESION

This 30-year-old with a remitting alcohol dependence syndrome was referred from casualty because of problems with his hands. Please examine his upper limbs neurologically, and discuss with the examiners the possible diagnosis.

The commonest cause of this rare condition is 'Saturday night palsy' where the nerve is compressed against the middle 1/3 of the humerus and brachioradialis and supinator are also paralysed as well as the forearm muscles.

There is wrist drop and the patient is unable to straighten their fingers. There is sensory impairment over the 1st dorsal interosseus. Straightening of the fingers at the IP joints is made possible if the wrist is passively straightened because the intrinsic muscles of the hand supplied by the ulnar nerve (interossei and lumbricals) permit some extension. No extension is possible at the MCPs. Grip strength is impaired in a radial nerve lesion, not because any of the flexors are weak but because a degree of wrist extension facilitates good grip. Likewise, abduction and adduction of the fingers are both unaffected in a radial nerve palsy but may appear to be with a flexed wrist. Check elbow extension and check the triceps reflex. An intact triceps reflex indicates a lesion below the spinal groove. Triceps wasting and an absent reflex implies a high axillary radial nerve lesion or a C7 radiculopathy. C7 lesion causes weakness of shoulder adduction, elbow extension, wrist flexion and wrist extension, because it makes a significant contribution to both median and radial nerves. A radial nerve lesion cannot affect shoulder adduction or wrist flexion.

Management: The prognosis is good; in compression, recovery is over weeks. Even if the wrist requires splinting, muscle function starts to recover 4-8 months later. The wrist must be splinted in extension as must the MCP joints – the latter not rigidly.

CEREBROVASCULAR ACCIDENT / STROKE

Examine this patient's upper limbs neurologically and then proceed to examine anything else that you feel is important if time before discussing your findings with the examiners within the time allowed.

An Extremely Common Causes

Symptoms: The duration of onset is crucial for the differential diagnosis. An abrupt onset of neurological deficit with a tendency to improve, with or without preceding transient ischaemia, in the presence of cardiovascular risk factors. A protracted illness with a slowly worsening circadian headache, drowsiness, vomiting, symptoms attributable to focal brain damage and seizures suggest a space-occupying lesion. The nature of the lesion usually dictates the speed of onset, e.g. meningioma or breast cancer metastases.

Definition of stroke: Rapid onset, focal neurological deficit due to a vascular lesion > 24 hr.

Key signs: Vary dependent on stroke.

Inspection: Walking aides, nasogastric tube or PEG tube, posture (flexed limbs and extended lower limbs), wasted or oedematous on the affected side. Asymmetrical facial droop.

Pyramidal posture: The upper limb tends to be flexed at the elbow, pronated and internally rotated and internally rotated at the shoulder, and the lower limb extended at the hip and knee, with the foot inverted and plantar-flexed.

Pyramidal drift: Perhaps the only sign.

Weakness in the motor divisions of the cranial nerves ± homonymous quadrantanopia/hemianopia; there may be papilloedema. Check for gag reflex.

Dysphasia: Broca's area – anterior lesions causing an expressive dysphasia with non-fluent speech but intact understanding; the patient should be asked to write; Wernicke's area – posterior lesions causing a receptive dysphasia can be difficult to identify; the speech is fluent but mistakes made in syllables to talking fluent nonsense can occur.

Tone: Spastic rigidity, 'clasp-knife' (resistance to movement, and then sudden release). Ankles may demonstrate clonus (>4 beats).

Power: Hemiparesis.

Reflexes: Asymmetrical hyperreflexia.
Unilateral extensor plantar response.

Coordination: Reduced, often due to weakness (but can be seen in posterior circulation strokes)
Characteristic gait and paucity of movement.

Extra Points

Upper motor neuron unilateral facial weakness (spares frontalis due to its dual innervation).

Gag reflex and swallow to minimize aspiration.

Visual fields and higher cortical functions, e.g. neglect helps determine a Bamford classification.

Cause: Irregular pulse (AF), blood pressure, cardiac murmurs or carotid bruits (anterior circulation stroke).

Aetiology

Ischaemic stroke (cardiovascular disease and risk factors, prothrombotic tendencies, vasculitis, internal carotid dissection, foci for emboli), haemorrhage (hypertension, aneurysm, e.g. SAH, AVM, thrombocytopaenia or bleeding diatheses). *Differential diagnosis of a hemiparesis:* Space-occupying lesion (tumour, aneurysm, abscess, haematoma, granuloma, tuberculoma, toxoplasmosis, cysts).

Anatomical Territory

Anterior cerebral artery (ACA) syndrome causes contralateral leg weakness and sensory loss. Voluntary loss of micturition may be lost. Middle cerebral artery syndrome may be indistinguishable from internal carotid artery occlusion, leading to contralateral hemiparesis (weak arm, face and often leg), contralateral hemisensory loss, contralateral homonymous hemianopia, global dysphasia (if dominant cortex), and severe agnosias and apraxias. Posterior circulation strokes cause bilateral weakness or sensory loss, cerebellar signs, e.g. ataxic hemiparesis and diplopia.

Investigations

CT – new guidelines suggest within 24 hours. As 80-90% of strokes are ischaemic, a CT scan is not always necessary. However, it is definitely indicated if there is any suggestion of an intracranial haemorrhage or doubt about the aetiology. In practice, most patients have a CT scan. If there is swelling of cerebellar or brainstem disease, a CT scan is necessary as swelling in the posterior fossa can be rapidly life-threatening. CT ± contrast will identify a mass lesion.

Bloods: FBC, ESR (young CVA may due to arteritis), glucose, renal function.

Blood cultures if suspicion of infective endocarditis.

Do consider carotid and cardiac investigations – "I would like to know if the patient has ever had an irregular pulse or chest pain.

ECG: AF or previous infarction.

CXR: Cardiomegaly or aspiration.

Echocardiogram.

Carotid Doppler ultrasound.

MRI/MR angiography.

Tests looking for risk factors such as cholesterol, Hb for polycythaemia, diabetes. Thrombophilia screen (protein C and S, antithrombin III, factor V Leiden). ANA, dsDNA, C3, C4.

Bamford classification of stroke (Lancet, 1991).

- *Total anterior circulation of stroke (TACS):* Motor or sensory deficit (contralateral to the lesion), homonymous hemianopia (contralateral to the lesion), higher cortical dysfunction, e.g. dyspasia, dyspraxia and neglect.
- Partial anterior circulation (PACS) 2/3 of the above.
- *Lacunar (LACS):* Pure hemi-motor or sensory loss.
- *Posterior circulation stroke (POCS):* Isolated hemianopia, brainstem signs, cerebellar ataxia.

Dominant parietal lobe cortical signs: Dysphasia: Receptive, expressive or global; Gerstmann's syndrome (dysgraphia, dyslexia or dyscalculia), L-R disorientation, finger agnosia.

Non-dominant parietal-lobe signs: Dressing and constructional apraxia, spatial neglect.

Management

Readers are advised to familiarize themselves with the current National Guidelines for Stroke (from the Royal College of Physicians of London), prepared by the Intercollegiate Stroke Working Party.

- There is no single effective treatment for established stroke. However, patient management should include looking for reversible causes that may mimic stroke such as hypoglycaemia or over anticoagulation and ensuring patient safety with regard to the swallow reflex. Nursing in the unconscious position, assessing skin condition and ensuring an adequate fluid intake. The family should be interviewed early on and informed of the prognosis.
- Brain imaging should be undertaken as soon as possible, at least within 24 hours of onset. It should be undertaken as a matter of urgency if the patient has been having anticoagulant treatment, a known bleeding tendency, a depressed level of consciousness, unexplained progressive or fluctuating symptoms, papilloedema, neck stiffness or fever, severe headache at onset, or indications for thrombolysis or early anticoagulation. If the result of a CT scan is uncertain, MRI should be considered.

- Blood pressure should be recorded but patients with high blood pressure should not have this lowered in acute stroke as it may result in an extension of the condition.
- Complications such as pressure sores, aspiration, pneumonia, contractures, deep venous thrombosis should be prevented.
- Depression which is common in stroke patients and may occur in up to 40% of these patients should be screened for and treated as appropriate.
- Mobilisation should occur as early as possible and this is best achieved with a team approach directed by the physiothe rapist with instructions to nurses to carry this on in the ward. The occupational therapist is essential in the assessment and therapy of simple procedures such as dressing, feeding and cooking.
- Aspirin is indicated for any patient who suffers a transient ischaemic attack and as secondary prophylaxis after cerebral infarction unless there is a contraindication. Ideally, aspirin should be started within 48 hours. Anticoagulation is useful in patients under 80 who are in atrial fibrillation or any patient who has a clear source of cardiac emboli. Where treatment with warfarin is considered then cerebral haemorrhage must be excluded by a CT scan. Some patients will die as a result of their stroke and it is the responsibility of all members of staff to ensure a comfortable and dignified death. It is indicated for patients with atrial fibrillation, or ischaemic stroke associated with mitral valve disease, a prosthetic valve or within 3 months of a myocardial infarction.
- Intracranial haemorrhage requires an urgent neurosurgical opinion. Referral to a specialist stroke unit: Multidisciplinary approach (physiotherapy, occupational therapy, speech and language therapy and specialist stroke rehabilitation nurses). This team should ideally meet at least once a week.
- Consider statins, carotid endarterectomy if carotid stenosis > 70%, meticulous glycaemic control, low cholesterol diet, and physical exercise. A reduction in risk of recurrent CVA has been demonstrated for both hypertensive and normotensive patients using perindopril (the PROGRESS study).

Acute Stroke/TIA

[Please note that, in 2007, guidelines were published in the UK by the Royal Colleges of Physicians and NICE for an acute stroke.]

The NICE guideline covers the acute stage of a stroke or TIA, mainly the first 48 hours after symptoms start. TIA is defined as stroke symptoms and signs that resolve within 24 hours. There is evidence for stroke that rapid diagnosis, admission to a specialist stroke unit, immediate brain imaging and use of thrombolysis where indicated can all contribute to a much better outcome for patients. For people who have had a TIA, rapid assessment for risk of subsequent stroke allows appropriate treatment to be started quickly to reduce the chance of having another stroke.

Their key recommendations are that:

- All patients with suspected stroke should be tested with the FAST' (Face Arm Speech Test) or similar test to recognize symptoms of acute stroke.
- All patients with acute stroke should be taken to hospital as quickly as possible and transferred from A&E to an acute stroke unit.
- Immediate CT scanning should be available 24/7 for those who need it.
- High risk patients who have already had a TIA should receive a diagnosis, investigations and initial treatment within 24 hours.
- All patients should receive a swallowing assessment within 24 hours of assessment and before being given any oral food, fluid or medication.

[The quick reference guide, patient versions of the NICE guideline and the full NICE guideline at www.nice.org.uk/CG68].

MOTOR NEURON DISEASE

This patient was referred by the GP to a local hospital because he had appeared to have lost weight. Examine his upper limbs, and offer possible diagnosis.

MND is a progressive disease of unknown aetiology. There is axonal degeneration of upper and lower motor neurons. Motor neuron disease may be classified into three types: Amyotrophic lateral sclerosis (50%) affecting the corticospinal tracts affecting predominantly producing spastic paraparesis or tetraparesis, progressive muscular atrophy (25%) affecting anterior horn cells predominantly producing wasting, fasciculation and weakness (best prognosis), and progressive bulbar palsy (25%) affecting lower cranial nerves and suprabulbar nuclei producing speech and swallowing problems (worst prognosis).

Symptoms: Bulbar–dysarthria and dysphonia, dysphagia and difficulty in chewing with nasal regurgitation of fluids, recurrent chest infections and dyspnoea; limbs–weakness of a hand or the whole upper limb, with wasting that the patient has noticed, progressive foot drop;

cramps or fasciculations are common and can precede other symptoms by months.

- Dysarthria (pseudobulbar palsy: "hot potato" speech; bulbar: "Donald Duck" speech due to palatal weakness), dysphonia,
- Wheel-chair/stick,
- *Tongue:* Wasting and fasciculation (bulbar) or a stiff spastic tongue with brisk jaw jerk (pseudobulbar),
- General fasciculations,
- Wasting,
- *Tone:* Usually spastic but can be flaccid,
- Mixed upper and lower motor neurone signs (spasticity with areflexia or flaccidity with hyperreflexia),
- *Reflexes:* Absent and/or brisk,
- No sensory deficits. No extra-ocular muscle, cerebellar or extra-pyramidal involvement,
- Sphincter and cognitive state disturbance is rarely seen,
- Tell the examiner about your wish to enquire about possible difficulties in swallowing.

Differential diagnosis: MS–no sensory abnormality in MND, polyneuropathies, cervical myelopathy, motor neuropathy, cord or cauda-equina compression (causes sphincter disturbance which does not occur in MND), myasthenia gravis (weakness of the external ocular muscles does not occur in MND), diabetic amyotrophy, cervical and lumbar stenosis. A key differential diagnosis in a tertiary unit is progressive multifocal neuropathy.

Investigations: Clinical diagnosis, laboratory results are usually normal, EMG – fasciculation/denervation, fibrillation potentials and positive sharp waves, abnormal motor units of increased amplitude and potential, reflecting widespread anterior horn cell damage, NCS – usually normal, MRI – excludes the main differential diagnosis of cervical cord compression and myelopathy.

Management: Supportive, e.g. PEG feeding and NIPPV, multidisciplinary approach to care, riluzole® (glutamate antagonist) slows disease progression by an average of 3 months but does not improve function or quality of life and is costly. This has been recommended by NICE for asymptomatic patients with amyotrophic lateral sclerosis; it extends the time to mechanical ventilation in this invariably fatal disease. Quinine is used for cramps. Baclofen, dantrolene and diazepam are used for spasticity. Lactulose and isphagula husk are used for constipation. Important non-pharmacological therapy includes counselling for depression, radiotherapy to the parotid glands for excess saliva, and assisted ventilation for respiratory failure.

OLD POLIO

This man is normally wheelchair bound.

Examine his lower limbs and suggest to the examiners why.

One of the legs is short, wasted, weak and flaccid with reduced reflexes and a normal plantar response. There is no sensory defect. The disparity in the length of the limbs suggest growth impairment in the affected limb since early childhood. The complete absence of sensory and pyramidal signs point to a condition affecting only lower motor neurones. The diagnosis is old polio. Differential diagnosis includes spinal muscular atrophy, AIDP and causes of a motor neuropathy.

Examiners if pushy may ask you about post-polio syndrome.

HEREDITARY SENSORIMOTOR NEUROPATHY / CHARCOT-MARIE-TOOTH DISEASE OR PERONEAL MUSCLE ATROPHY

This gentleman complains his legs begun to look unusual over the last few years. Please examine his lower limbs neurologically.

An Extremely Common Cause

Clinical Signs

Type I: Is a severe, symmetrical wasting of distal lower limb muscles with preservation of the thigh muscle bulk (inverted champagne bottle appearance), kyphoscoliosis, pes cavus (seen also in Fredreich's ataxia), weakness of ankle dorsiflexion and toe extension, variable degree of stocking distribution sensory loss (usually mild), gait is high-stepping due to foot drop and stamping (absent proprioception), tremor in upper limbs, wasting of small muscles of the hand, palpable lateral popliteal nerve in some families only.

Presents in 1st decade with difficulty in walking, or foot deformity.

Type II: Tends to be confined to the lower limbs, wasting and weakness is less severe, reflexes are absent in the lower limbs but normal in the upper limbs, foot and spinal deformity are less common, peripheral nerves are not palpable.

Later onset, with a peak in the second decade, but many cses present in the middle or even late adult life, with weakness or wasting.

Differential diagnosis: Peripheral neuropathy, mononeuropathy, L4/5 root lesion (may cause bilateral foot drop but inversion at the ankle is obviously lost, with dermatomal sensory signs), cauda equina lesions (this must be actively considered where there are distal signs, e.g. absent ankle jerk, and there is saddle anaesthesia and sphincter involvement), and motor neurone disease (complete absence of sensory involvement).

Discussion: Types I and II are distinct. Men are more severely affected than women. The commonest HSMN types are I (demyelinating) and II (axonal), autosomal dominant inheritance. The degeneration is mainly in the motor nerves. It is sometimes also found in the dorsal roots and dorsal columns, and slight pyramidal tract degeneration is often seen. The condition usually becomes arrested in mid-life. Nerve conduction velocity is severely reduced in type I, but is either normal or slightly reduced in type II. Sural nerve biopsy demonstrates hypertrophic onion bulb changes and reduced density of myelinated fibres in type I. The reduction in conduction velocity indicates a severe demyelinated neuropathy. Orthotic appliances and sometimes surgical correction of the foot deformity or tendon transfer can affect affected individuals. Type I is most usually dominantly inherited, but sex-linked recessive forms are also encountered. Mutations in PMP22 underlie commonly type I; myelin protein Po gene mutations have been found in HSMN I and II.

FREDREICH'S ATAXIA

This person has noticed unsteadiness for as long as he can remember. Please examine his upper limbs, and anything else that you feel is appropriate.

Clinical signs: Young adult, wheelchair, pes cavus, bilateral cerebellar ataxia (ataxic handshake), pyramidal leg weakness (bilateral extensor plantars), peripheral neuropathy with muscle wasting and loss of ankle and knee jerks, posterior column signs (loss of vibration and joint position sense), cerebellar signs in the arms, nystagmus and scanning dysarthria, kyphoscoliosis, optic atrophy (30%), sensorineural deafness (10%), listen for the murmur of HOCM, ask to dip the urine (10% develop diabetes).

The oldest person to have presented to the National Hospital of Neurology in London was in his early 60's but that is unusual. Inheritance is usually autosomal recessive, onset is during teenage years, survival rarely exceeds 20 years from diagnosis, there is an association with HOCM, mild skeletal abnormality and mild dementia. It is caused by an increased number of GAA trinucleotide repeat sequences at a gene encoding the protein *frataxin* on chromosome 9.

MYOTONIC DYSTROPHY (DYSTROPHIA MYOTONICA)

This man complains of weakness in his hands. Please examine his upper limbs.

An Extremely Common Cause

Males > females, autosomal dominant, presentation in 3rd/4th decades

Symptoms: Myotonia is rarely intrusive initially, but the failure to release grip can be troublesome. Myotonia is often worse when cold or excited. Poor vision, weight loss, impotence, ptosis and increased sweating are common. Later in the course of the disease, low-output cardiac failure and hypersomnolence occurs. Stokes-Adams attacks can occur.

Clinical Signs

- Myopathic facies (long, thin, expressionless),
- Wasting of facial muscles (temporalis, masseter and sternocleidomastoids),
- Gynaecomastia,
- Altered oesophageal and bowel motility,
- Testicular atrophy,
- Slow release of hand grip,
- Percussion myotonia,
- Generalised wasting and weakness of upper limbs (distal wasting is more prominent in DM-1, proximal wasting is more prominent in DM-2),
- Bilateral ptosis,
- Frontal balding (try to avoid this term when presenting in front of the patient),
- Cataracts,
- Myotonia (difficulty in releasing grip on handshake),
- Dysarthria due to myotonia of the tongue and pharynx,
- Hyporeflexia and subsequently areflexia develop in later stages of the disease due to muscle weakness and/or diabetic-related peripheral neuropathy,
- External ophthalmoplegia (rare),
- Pacemaker,

- Cor pulmonale due to diaphragmatic weakness with subsequent hypoxaemia or heart failure,
- Testes are small and firm.

The tingling in this case may be due to a neuropathy secondary diabetes or muscle wasting from the disease itself.

Hands – "Grip my hand, now let go", "Screw up your eyes tightly shut, now open them". Wasting and weakness of distal muscles with areflexia. *Percussion myotonia:* Percuss thenar eminence and watch for voluntary thumb flexion.

Extra points: Cardiomyopathy (brady- and tachyarrhythmias), diabetes mellitus due to impaired insulin secretion (ask to dip urine), nodular thyroid enlargement, peripheral neuropathy may occur in long-standing myotonic dystrophy due to diabetes. In advanced disease, the degree of myotonia may paradoxically be less obvious.

Inheritance: A trinucleotide repeat disorder, with its mode of inheritance autosomal dominant with the locus at 19q13.2 - q13.3, onset in 20s, genetic anticipation (worsening severity of the condition and earlier age of presentation with progressive generations due to expansion of tri-nucleotide repeat sequences). Also occurs in Huntington's chorea and Fredreich's ataxia. Condition may show "anticipation" – progressively worsening signs and symptoms.

Differential diagnosis: Facioscapulohumeral dystrophy, limb-girdle dystrophy and hypothyroidism.

Investigations: CK (2-10x normal), IgG, thyroid function tests, FSH due to gonadal resistance, *ECG:* Low voltage P waves, bradycardia, first-degree block or more complex disorders. *EMG:* Demonstrate myotonic discharges evoked by movement of the electrode; myopathic potentials are recorded from weakened and wasted muscles during volitional movement. Muscle biopsy–frequent long chains of nuclei are seen in the middle of muscle fibres; these changes are seen more marked postmortem.

Management: Weakness is a major problem – no treatment, procainamide/phenytoin may help myotonia, advise against general anaesthetic, fit a pacemaker for symptomatic bradycardia.

SYRINGOMYELIA

This 40-year-old man has weak hands. Examine his upper limbs and suggest why.

Syringomyelia is caused by a progressively expanding fluid-filled syrinx within the cervical cord, typically spanning several levels. Frequently associated with Arnold-Chiari malformation and spina bifida.

- Weakness and wasting of small muscles of the hand.
- Loss of reflexes in the upper limbs.
- Dissociated sensory loss in upper limbs and chest: Loss of pain and temperature sensation (spinothalamic) and with preservation of joint position and vibration sense (dorsal columns).
- Scars from painless burns.
- Charcot joints: Elbow and shoulder.
- Pyramidal weakness in lower limbs with upgoing plantars.
- Kyphoscoliosis is common.
- Horner's syndrome. (ask if you can examine the cranial nerves for signs of syringobulbia: Loss of pain and temperature sensation on the face).
- Look for evidence of Charcot's joints at the shoulder and trophic changes in the hands.
- If the syrinx extends into brainstem (syringobulbia) there may be cerebellar signs and lower cranial nerve signs.

Investigation of choice: Spinal MRI.

BROWN-SÉQUARD SYNDROME

This 40-year-old man has weak hands. Examine his upper limbs and suggest why.

There is spastic weakness (monoplegia – one limb; hemiplegia – one arm and leg) and enhanced reflexes and loss of propioception and vibration sense on one side (ipsilateral to the lesion) and loss of pain and temperature sense on the other (contralateral to the lesion). True Brown-Sequard syndromes, with 50% hemisection, are rare. Causes are same as those described for a spastic paraparesis. Demyelination and degenerative vertebral disease are the commonest causes. Ask about evidence of decompensation – including bladder or bowel symptoms.

MUSCULAR DYSTROPHIES

This 40-year-old man has weak hands. Examine his upper limbs and suggest why.

Table 6.2: Types of muscular dystrophies.

Type	Features	IQ	Prognosis
Severe X-linked Duchenne muscular dystrophy	Presents 3rd year of life, severe proximal weakness of lower limbs, calf hypertrophy, cardiac muscles affected, onset 5th-25th year	May be low	Death towards end of second decade
Benign X-linked Becker type muscular dystrophy	Weakness and wasting of pelvic and shoulder-girdle muscles	Normal	Many survive to normal age
Facioscapu-lohumeral dystrophy associated	Often in adolescence. Facial weakness: prominent ptosis. Difficulty in closing eyes. Speech is impaired owing to difficulty in articulation of consonants.Wasting of sternomatoids, lower pectorals, triceps, biceps. Marked scapular winging. Occasionally deltoids hypertrophy to compensate.	Normal	Normal life span. The mode of inheritance is autosomal dominant, both sexes equally affected. The gene is to the long arm of chromosome 4.
Limb girdle muscular dystrophy	Onset usually in second or third decade. Weakness and wasting may begin in either shoulder or pelvic girdle muscles. Hip flexors and glutei are weak. There is early wasting of medial quadriceps and tibialis anterior. Hypertrophy of calves and/or deltoids may occur. Ankle jerks preserved. The face is never affected.	Normal	Often severely disabled by middle life with death before normal age. Autosomal recessive.

To demonstrate facial-scapulo-humeral dystrophy, if having been asked to examine the upper limbs, you should specifically demonstrate facial weakness (for example by asking the patient to scrunch up their eyes or to blow out their cheeks). It is also important to expose the trunk properly (this may involve asking the patient to take his shirt off).

CERVICAL MYELOPATHY

Patients present with chronic weakness of the lower limbs and loss of sensation; bladder or bowel disturbance can occur; sensory symptoms in the lower limb are not always present, even with clear signs; painful cervical spine even with clear signs. Clasp-knife spastic legs with preserved bulk, clonus at the ankle ± knee, weakness in a pyramidal distribution, hyperreflexia (in the lower limbs, Babinksi's sign), dorsal column (vibration and cutaneous sensation before proprioception) or spinothalamic loss, loss of abdominal reflexes. In the upper limbs – often asymmetrical reflexes, inverted reflexes of the mid-cervical reflex pattern. The signs in the upper limbs are often not marked; wasting of the small muscles does not occur unless there is a radiculopathy affecting C8 or T1.

Aetiology: Cervical spondylosis – degenerative disease is usually most pronounced in the mid-cervical region at C5/6.

Differential diagnosis: Demyelination, syringomyelia (dissociated sensory loss ± bulbar signs). Investigations: Cord needs imaging, measure B_{12}.

Management: Consult with a neurosurgeon for myelopathy at one level or multiple levels due to diffuse narrowing of the canal. Conservative management with a collar, only if surgery is unsuitable. Inverted reflexes are the extension of triceps when the biceps is tapped and finger flexion when supinator is tapped. Biceps and supinator jerks may be absent due to damage at C5/6, whereas the triceps and finger jerks are brisk because their reflex arcs lie below the level of the lesion. This is the mid-cervical reflex pattern.

Extensor Plantars and Absent Knee Jerks

This 40-year-old man has weak hands. Examine his lower limbs and suggest why.
- Fredreich's ataxia
- Subacute combined degeneration of the cord
- Motor neuron disease
- Taboparesis
- Conus medullaris lesions.

Combined upper and lower pathology, e.g. cervical spondylosis with peripheral neuropathy.

MYAESTHENIA GRAVIS

Examine this patient's cranial nerves. She has been suffering from double vision and dry eyes.

An Extremely Common Cause

Peak incidence: 4th decade, Women 2x as affected as Men.

Clinical signs: Bilateral ptosis (can be unilateral), the head may be held back, the patient looking down their nose to counteract the ptosis, complicated bilateral extra-ocular muscle palsies, expressionless face/ myaesthenic snarl (on attempting to smile), diplopia on holding the extremes of gaze, inability to read aloud or count continually (the voice becoming quiet), nasal speech, palatal weakness and poor swallow (bulbar involvement in around 10% of patients), demonstrate proximal muscle weakness in the upper limbs, particularly neck weakness on holding the head up from the pillow,and fatiguability (10% of patients) (reflexes are normal), shoulder weakness > pelvic weakness, sensation normal, bulbar weakness can lead to regurgitation of fluids, respiratory weakness, look for sternotomy scars.

Associations: Other autoimmune diseases, e.g. diabetes mellitus, rheumatoid arthritis, thyrotoxicosis and SLE, and thymomas. *Causes:* IgG anti-nicotinic acetylcholine receptor antibodies affect motor end-plate neurotransmission. Titre of antibody does not correlate with disease activity or progression. Many patients have thymic hyperplasia especially those with AChR antibodies. Thymic hyperplasia is present in 70% of patients under 40-years of age. These patients have an increased association with HLA B8 and DR3.

Exacerbating factors: Pregnancy, hypokalaemia, over-treatment, change of climate, emotion, exercise, certain drugs (e.g. aminoglycosides, penicillamine, β-blockers).

Tests: (a) Edrophonium (Tensilon®) test: An acetylcholineesterase inhibitor increases the concentration of ACh at the motor end plate and hence improves the muscle weakness. Can cause heart block and even asystole. Two syringes are prepared, 10 ml Normal saline and 10 mg edrophonium with 10 ml. Give 2 ml of each IV injection. Observe. It is positive only if edrophonium improves muscle power (b) AChR antibodies (and also striated muscle antibody) (90% specificity, 100% sensitivity). (c) Vital capacity. (d) EMG: Characteristic decrement in the evoked muscle action potential following stimulation of the motor nerve (e) CXR – mediastinal mass, (f) CT or MRI of the mediastium to look for a thymic mass.

Cholinergic crises: Salivation, lacrimation, urination, diarrhoea, gastric, emesis, small pupils. The features which distinguish myaesthenic crisis are response to edrophonium and absence of cholinergic phenomena.

Treatments: Acute (I/V immunoglobulin or plasmapharesis), chronic (acetylcholine esterase inhibitor, e.g. pyridostigmine, immunosuppression: steroids and azathioprine (the steroid-sparing agent of choice), thymectomy is beneficial even if the patient does not have a thymoma), ice on closed lid for 2 minutes will improve ptosis by at least 2 millimetres. Bone densitometry is advisable for patients commencing long-term corticosteroids. Plasma exchange can be tried in emergencies (e.g. respiratory difficulty/facility to intubate and ventilate should be available).

Lambert-Eaton myaesthenic syndrome: Diminished reflexes that become brisker after exercise, lower limb girdle weakness, associated with malignancy, e.g. small-cell lung cancer, antibodies block pre-synaptic calcium channels, EMG shows a 'second wind' phenomenon on repetitive stimulation.

WASTING OF THE SMALL MUSCLES OF THE HAND

This 56-year-old lady has noticed wasting in her hands. Please examine her upper limbs and discuss.

Remember that rheumatoid arthritis and old age are common causes of this. First establish whether the wasting and weakness is generalised or whether it is restricted to the muscles supplied by the median or ulnar nerves (test abductor pollicis brevis and interossei). NB. Combined median and ulnar nerve lesions will of course produce generalised weakness and wasting but this is rare; distal muscular atrophy is another rare peripheral cause. Test for any sensory deficit and fasciculations, and look carefully for signs of rheumatoid disease.

If the disturbance is generalised the lesion is likely to be central, i.e.

- Lesions of the cord affecting T1, e.g. Motor neurone disease, syringomyelia, spinal cord tumours.
- Lesions affecting T1 root, e.g. Neurofibroma, cervical spondylosis (relatively rare at this level), apical lung tumours.

- Lesions of the brachial plexus affecting T1, e.g. Klumpke's paralysis, cervical ribs, Pancoast tumour.
- Peripheral nerve lesions, e.g. median and ulnar nerve lesions
  You should therefore:
- Look for fasciculation in the hand and arm (prominent in motor neurone disease: if you suspect the diagnosis proceed).
- Test for loss of reflexes and spinothalamic sensation in the arm.
- Test sensation over T1 dermatome.
- Palpate for cervical ribs.
- Observe for Horner's syndrome.
- Look for a site of ulnar nerve damage at the elbow.

Cranial Nerve Disorders: A quick reminder.

The candidate should be able to examine each of the cranial nerves (in sequence), and to recognize and discuss the pattern of abnormal signs.

General inspection

Ramsay-Hunt syndrome. Herpes zoster visible in the outer ear, together with a facial palsy and/or hearing loss.

Benign intracranial hypertension: Short, obese, hairy women with papilloedema.

Acromegaly – associated visual field defects.

Graves' disease – impaired extra-ocular movements, secondary to nerve palsy.

1. "Has there be a change in the sense of smell or taste?" – suspect anterior cranial fossa floor fracture, frontal tumour or Kallman syndrome (genetic cause of anosmia and infertility). This is not likely to be appropriate for examination.
2. Visual acuity using a Snellen chart (other means include counting fingers, perception of movement, perception of light), and then exclude red-green colour blindness (Ishihara), as patients with demyelination may have obvious impairment in both. If visual acuity is impaired: Is this correctable with spectacles or a pinhole? If you think the patient is near-blind, then establish if movement and light can be detected.

Pupil Reactions

Test for afferent papillary defect, preferably using the swinging light test (greater constriction with a consensual response than a direct light response). This defect may be caused by lesions of the retina (including severe macular degeneration), optic nerve, chiasm and optic tract. It is particularly associated with optic nerve damage in multiple sclerosis. The papillary response is also known as a Marcus-Gunn pupil. When the normal eye is stimulated by a bright light, the pupil constricts and remains constricted. In contrast, the pupil of the affected eye reacts slowly, less completely and transiently, so that it may start to dilate again even while the light is shining on it – the so-called papillary escape phenomenon. The reaction is best seen if the light is rapidly alternated from one eye to the other, each stimulus lasting 2-3 seconds, with a second between. While the normal pupil constricts and stays small, the abnormal pupil dilates instead of constricting as the light falls on it.

Check the size and shape, symmetry, reaction to light – direct and consensual reaction, accommodation.

The candidate should be able to discuss Horner's syndrome, a tonic pupil and Argyll-Robertson pupil.

HORNER'S SYNDROME

Reactions to light and accommodation should be present and normal.
- Look at the ipsilateral side of the neck for scars (trauma e.g. central lines, carotid endarterectomy surgery or aneurysms) and tumours (Pancoast's tumour).
- Examine for weakness of the small muscles of the hand (T1) and for loss of sensation over the T1 dermatome.
- Test for loss of pain and temperature in the arm and face, loss of arm reflexes, bulbar palsy and nystagmus (syringomyelia/syringobulbia).
- Tell the examiner that you would like to examine the chest clinically and radiologically for evidence of a Pancoast's tumour. *Cause:* Following the sympathetic tract's anatomical course (brainstem: MS, stroke), spinal cord (syrinx), and neck (aneurysm, trauma, Pancoast's tumour). Congenital Horner's syndrome: Iris is of different colours (*heterochromia*).

TONIC (HOLMES-ADIE PUPIL)

- A unilateral dilated pupil is striking.
- Look for ptosis and test ocular movements for evidence of a IIIrd nerve palsy (the main alternative diagnosis).
- Test the response to light (very slow) and accommodation (also slow but more definite).

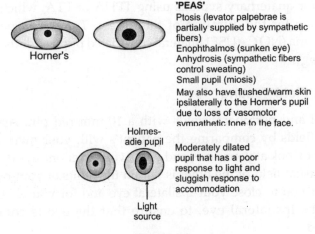

'PEAS'

Ptosis (levator palpebrae is partially supplied by sympathetic fibers)
Enophthalmos (sunken eye)
Anhydrosis (sympathetic fibers control sweating)
Small pupil (miosis)

May also have flushed/warm skin ipsilaterally to the Horner's pupil due to loss of vasomotor sympathetic tone to the face.

Holmes-adie pupil

Moderately dilated pupil that has a poor response to light and sluggish response to accommodation

Light source

Figure 6.4

- Also ask the examiner's permission to test the ankle jerks (absent or diminished ankle and knee jerks are expected).
- Mention that another cause are mydriatic eye drops.
- A Holmes: A die pupil constricts promptly to 2.5% metacoline.
- *Discussion:* A benign condition that is more common in females. Reassure the patient that nothing is wrong.

ARGYLL-ROBERTSON PUPILS

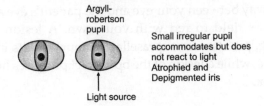

Argyll-robertson pupil

Small irregular pupil accommodates but does not react to light
Atrophied and Depigmented iris

Light source

Figure 6.5

- Pupils are small and irregular and react to accommodation but not to light.
- Look for wrinkled forehead with ptosis and absent ankle jerks, loss of joint position sense and vibration sense, positive Romberg's test and sensory ataxia, Charcot's knee joint and aortic incompetence.
- Cause is a lesion in the tectum of the midbrain.
- Usually a manifestation of quaternary syphilis, but it may also be caused by diabetes mellitus, orbital injury, hereditary neuropathies and sarcoidosis.

- Test for quaternary syphilis using TPHA or FTA, which remain positive for the duration of the illness. Treat with penicillin. Aniscoria (NO CAUSE) Bilateral constricted pupil (elderly–normal finding).

Visual Field Testing

Central and peripheral fields with a 10 mm red pin. Assess the visual fields by comparing the patient's with your own. Ask the patient to look at your nose, and while you cover one eye determine if the visual field of the other is within the limits of your own. It is best for you to close your ipsilateral eye and for you to cover the patient's ipsilateral eye, to ensure that the eye is completely covered.

Central scotoma: This is usually found using a red pin. *Hint:* If a patient complains of a hole in his visual field, it is often easier to give him the pin and ask him to place it in the hole in his vision. Causes of a central scotoma: Retrobulbar neuritis most commonly in cases of multiple sclerosis, choroidoretinitis, pressure on the optic nerve by a tumour, optic atrophy due to toxins or vitamin B_{12} deficiency.

Bilateral hemianopia and homonymous hemianopia can be found using confrontational visual field testing. When using a red pin, ask the patient to tell you when the pin is seen *as red*. Ensure the pin is midway between your eye and the patient's eye and compare the patient's field to red with your own. A lesion at the optic chiasm (e.g. pituitary or suprasellar tumour) results in bitemporal hemianopia, while a lesion of the optic tract produces homonymous hemianopia.

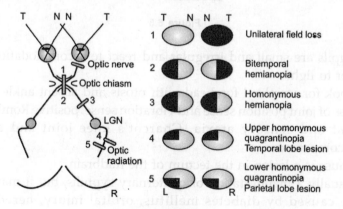

Figure 6.6

It may be relevant to map out the blind spot. Cover your left eye and tell the patient "*Could you please cover your right eye with your right hand* (pause to let them do this.) *Thank you, could you fix your gaze on the bridge of my nose again. I am going to slowly move a red pin in front of you. You will see the pin disappear and then reappear again. Please tell me when you first notice it go and then when you see it again.*" Now bring the pin slowly across your visual field midway between you and the patient. Compare the size of your blind spot with the patient's. A central scotoma occurs with defects in the retina or optic nerve.

Optic fundi: Perform fundoscopy by first looking at the anterior chamber then the lens and finally the retina itself. Is there disc cupping (glaucoma) or blurring of the otherwise clear margins (papilloedema)? Are the discs pale (optic atrophy)? [See Station 5]. Are there any retinal changes of diabetes or hypertension?

III, IV, VI 3 = oculomotor, 4 = trochlear, 6 = abducens.

Ptosis – seen with both Horner's syndrome and III nerve palsy.

Palsies and Ptosis

Causes of bilateral ptosis: Myotonic dystrophy, myaesthenia gravis, ocular myopathy, bilateral Horner's syndrome due to syringomyelia, syphilis (Argyll-Robertson pupils). Causes of a unilateral ptosis. Complete IIIrd nerve palsy (complete ptosis, pupil large, divergent strabismus, diplopia on adduction), partial IIIrd nerve palsy (partial ptosis with a large pupil on the affected side), Horner's syndrome.

Investigations of ptosis: Glucose (diabetes mellitus), ESR/CRP (mononeuritis multiplex), anti-AChR antibodies, CXR (apical malignancy/cervical rib), syphilis serology, MRI, EMG.

Exopthalmos: When gross will result in impaired ocular movements. Best assessed together by asking the patient to focus on your finger (kept about a metre away) as it moves horizontal and vertical extremes noting the full range of movement in each eye, and asking the patient if there is any 'double vision'. If the patient does see double establish which eye's movement is responsible by covering each eye in turn at the point of double vision. The eye from which the most distant image disappears when covered is the one with the impaired muscle.

Check the function of individual oculomotor nerves. Candidates should be able to make a general assessment of external ocular movements by getting the patient to fixate on an object and follow it in a H pattern. On inspection, III and VI nerve palsies may be obvious. You must quickly demonstrate which nerves are weak and the direction in which reported diplopia is maximal. In less obvious cases, you should be able to analyse the diplopia by using the cover test (when looking in the direction of action of the weak muscle, the outer image disappears on covering the affected eye). In the case of a III nerve palsy, you must state whether the lesion is complete or partial. In a complete lesion there is complete ptosis, the eye is deviated downwards and outwards with loss of upward, downward and medial movements, and a dilated unreactive pupil. It is obviously necessary to elevate the eyelid to observe the latter findings because of the ptosis. Note that in vascular lesions of the III nerve (e.g. in diabetes, arteriosclerosis or arteritis) the pupil may be spared.

You should demonstrate whether the IV nerve is intact by lifting the eyelid and asking the patient to look down: If the nerve is intact there will be intorsion of the eye. Test lateral gaze to confirm that the VI nerve is intact.

You may be asked the likely cause: Remember that the commonest causes of a pure III nerve palsy are posterior communicating artery aneurysm, diabetes, atherosclerosis and raised intracranial pressure. The latter three are also common causes of a VI nerve palsy.

Remember that the III, IV and VI nerve palsies may be affected singly or in combination as part of a cranial neuropathy due: Diabetes, polyarteritis nodosa, multiple sclerosis, sarcoidosis, basal meningitis: Tuberculous, syphilitic and carcinomatosus.

Look specifically for internuclear ophthalmoplegia (failure of adduction in one eye and nystagmus in the abducting eye) and causes (multiple sclerosis, vascular disease, tumour such as pontine glioma, inflammatory lesions of the brainstem, drugs such as phenytoin and carbamazepine). Investigations include MRI scan. The lesion is in the medial longitudinal bundle which connects the sixth nerve nucleus on one side to the third nerve nucleus on the opposite side of the brainstem. The eye will not adduct because the third nerve, and, therefore, the medial rectus have been disconnected from the lateral gaze centre and sixth nucleus of the opposite side.

Nystagmus:

Nystagmus is defined as a slow drift in one direction with a fast correction in the opposite direction.

Key signs: Lasting <2 beats on extreme gaze – normal; involuntary usually jerky eye movements; horizontal – often due to vestibular lesion – acute away from lesion/chronic towards lesion; cerebellar lesions nystagmus towards the affected size; if greater in eye that is abducted, there may be an intranuclear ophthalmoplegia suspect MS.

The direction of nystagmus is defined by the direction of the fast phase. The slow phase is the pathological component; the fast phase is the correction. Some neurologists also grade nystagmus into: Grade 1 (present in looking in one direction only), grade 2 (present with the eyes in the neutral position), and grade 3 (present on looking on either side). Ataxic nystagmus is a popular case so be sure that you can demonstrate the signs (nystagmus in the abducting eye often associated with weakness of adduction due to internuclear ophthalmoplegia). For horizontal nystamus which occurs only on looking laterally, the direction of the fast phase is away from the lesion in a peripheral lesion, but towards the lesion in a central lesion.

Tinnitus may imply Meniere's, varies with head position implying benign positional vertigo. Up and down nystagmus – midbrain or 4th ventricle lesion. *Investigations:* Appropriate to the possible cause. *Management:* As for cause.

Pendular nystagmus is symmetrical moving at the same speed in both directions. Jerk nystagmus has a fast phase in one direction with a slow phase in the other. The type of nystagmus is ascertained by this flow diagram:

Aetiology: Peripheral lesions (labyrinth/vestibular apparatus), central lesions (brainstem or cerebellar pathology).

Prolonged horizontal nystagmus on lateral gaze – commonly drugs (e.g. phenytoin, barbiturates, benzodiazepines and alcohol) and demyelinating disease.

Vertical nystagmus: Upbeat – Wernicke's encephalopathy, MS, brainstem tumours; downbeat – tumours at the foramen magnum (where a cerebellar lesion is suspected, look for other cerebellar signs).

Ataxic nystagmus is closely allied to INO.

Pendular nystagmus: No fast phase and due to congenital or retinal pathology (e.g. albinism); therefore, examine visual acuity and examine the fundus.

Investigations: Audiogram, caloric tests (peripheral VIIIth nerve function), MRI (lesions), phenytoin level, alcohol, LFTs, red cell transketolase (Wernicke's encephalopathy).

Management: Dependent on the cause.

V *Shingles:* Reactivation of latent trigeminal nucleus zoster may be associated with dysaesthesia.

The ophthalmic and maxillary divisions carry only sensory fibres, the mandibular division carries additional motor fibres. Test for jaw opening, teeth clenching and horizontal jaw translocation, along with sensation in the face (know the quintothalamic distribution). Cutaneous distribution of the three components: You should test light touch and/or pinprick in the three divisions of the V nerve (ophthalmic, mandibular and maxillary); compare one side with the other, right or left.

Jaw Jerk

Inform the examiner you would like to perform the corneal response.

Masseter ("Clench your teeth"), temporalis, ptyergoid muscles ("Open your mouth and don't let me close it").

In a cerebellopontine angle syndrome, any combination of cranial neuropathies involving the trigeminal, facial and vestibulocochlear nerve may occur. Corneal reflex loss is often the first sign, followed by facial sensory loss. Facial weakness can be late sign. There may be nystagmus. There may be sensorineural deafness. Cerebellopontine angle lesions, including acoustic neuromas and meningiomas, may cause slowly progressive hearing loss or tinnitus. Vertigo is a rare or late sign. The next step is neuroimaging. The cerebellopontine angle is the angle between the cerebellum, lateral pons, and petrous bone. Cranial nerves 5-8 emerge from it from the pons in cranio-caudal sequence.

VI. The facial muscles are served by the facial nerve. The facial nerve is almost entirely a motor nerve, supplying all of the muscles of the scalp and face except the levator palpebrae superioris.

Upper and lower motor neurone facial palsy.

"Smile", "Show me your teeth", "Blow out your cheeks like this", "Screw your eyes up tightly."

LMN facial palsy (e.g. altered taste, hyperacusis, altered lachrymation as the parasympathetic fibres in the greater superficial petrosal nerve are interrupted).

Lower motor neurone palsy has paralysis of the upper and lower face, so that the eye cannot be closed.

Unilateral facial nerve palsy: Unilateral facial droop, absent nasolabial fold and forehead creases, unilateral inability to raise the eyebrows (frontalis), unilateral inability to screw the eyes up (orbicularis oculi) and smile (orbicularis oris).

Palpate for parotid enlargement (the VII nerve may be involved in a malignant tumour).

Inspect the external auditory meatus and fauces for vesicles (*Ramsay-Hunt syndrome*) and the tympanic membrane for evidence of otitis media (a rare cause today).

Tell the examiner that you would like to ask the patient whether he has become unilaterally intolerance to high-pitched or loud sounds (hyperacusis due to paralysis of the stapedius muscle) and that you would normally test taste sensation on the anterior two-thirds of the tongue (involvement of the chorda tympani).

Look for evidence of corneal damage, conjunctivitis or lateral tarsorrhaphy.

Level of the lesion:

Pons (MS, stroke) + VIth nerve palsy and long tract signs.

Cerebello-pontine angle + V, VI, VIII, cerebellar–tumour, e.g. acoustic neuroma.

Auditory/facial canal + VIII, cholesteatoma and abscess.

Neck and face + scars and parotid mass – tumour, trauma.

Commonest cause is Bell's palsy: Rapid onset (1-2 days), HSV-1 implicated, induced swelling and compression of the nerve within the facial canal causes demyelination and temporary conduction block. Treatment: steroid and acicyclovir. Remember eye protection. 85% make a full recovery.

Other causes of a VIIth nerve palsy: Herpes zoster (Ramsay Hunt syndrome; reactivation of herpes zoster in the geniculate gangion), mononeuropathy due to diabetes, sarcoidosis or Lyme disease, tumour/trauma, MS/stroke (the long intrapontine course from the nucleus makes the nerve vulnerable), cerebellopontine angle lesion, parotid swellings, cholesteatoma (epithelial cells accumulate behind the tympanic membrane: Needs urgent appraisal by an ENT surgeon), Millard-Gubler syndrome (Vith and VIIth nerve palsy and contralateral hemiplegia).

Bilateral facial nerve palsy is very easy to miss but the patient has an expressionless face. Causes of a bilateral facial palsy: Guillain-Barre, Lyme disease, facioscapulohumeral dystrophy, dystrophia myotonica or myaesthenia gravis, Parkinson's disease (akinesia rather than weakness), bilateral Bell's palsy, sarcoidosis and myasthenia gravis.

Consider also causes of mononeuritis multiplex.

Investigations: None for Bell's palsy, EMG done at 1-2 weeks after the onset can demonstrate axonal degeneration in up to 15% of those with a total paralysis, CT brain (UMN lesions where stroke is likely), MRI (cerebellopontine angle tumour, demyelination, brainstem stroke), ultrasound (parotid tumours), serum ACE (sarcoidosis), AChR antibodies (myaesthenia gravis).

Management: Bell's palsy (corticosteroids, lateral tarsorrhaphy), Ramsay-Hunt (acicyclovir, prednisolone to reduce post-herpetic neuralgia). Stroke and tumours need investigation and treatment along standard lines.

VII. Hearing

A crude whisper is insufficient at the level of MRCP especially if the diagnosis is a cerebellopontine angle tumour. Perform Weber's and Rinne's test.

For Weber's test, sound is referred to the deaf ear in conductive deafness, and to the better ear in sensorineural deafness.

For Rinne's test. BC>AC in the deaf ear in conductive deafness, but AC>BC in both ears in sensorineural deafness.

Further features in a patient with unilateral deafness: Ipsilateral facial weakness, depressed facial sensation or a depressed corneal response

Lateral medullary syndrome (Wallenberg's syndrome) or posterior inferior cerebellar artery syndrome. There is ipsilateral Horner's syndrome (disruption of the sympathetic tract), cerebellar signs (cerebellum and its connections), palatal paralysis and diminished gag reflex (IXth and Xth nerves), decreased trigeminal pain and temperature sensation, and contralateral decreased pain and temperature sensation (spinothalamic tract). Involvement of the nucleus and tractus solitarius may cause loss of taste. Hiccups may occur.

IX. Tonsillar fossa: Gag reflex

The function of the nerve can only be assessed by a painful stimulus to the tonsillar fossa, and should not be examined.

X. Palatal sounds (e.g. EGG or RUG); the palate moves away from the side of the lesion.

To assess the patient's swallow, they must be fully conscious, able to follow commands, and be sitting upright. The instructions are to take a sip of water, swallow it, the patient says his name, and observe throughout for coughing or choking.

Palatal deviation: "Open your mouth and say aah". The candidate should be able to recognize palatal deviation, and be aware that the palate deviates to the intact side in a unilateral palatal palsy. Jugular foramen syndrome involves the 9th, 10th and 11th nerves which pass through the jugular foramen (between the lateral part of the occipital bone and the petrous portion of the temporal bones). Examination reveals sluggish movement when the patient says "aah" on the affected side. Absent gag reflex on the same side. There is flattening of the shoulder on the same side. Wasting of sternomastoid. Weakness when the patient moves his/her chin to the opposite side. Difficulty in shrugging the shoulder on the same side. Look for wasting and deviation of the tongue (12th nerve palsy), and tell the examiner you would like to look for two signs (bovine cough and husky voice).

XI. Spinal accessory nerve (sternocleidomastoid and upper fibres of trapezius).

For sternomastoids, place one hand on the patient's forehead asking the patient to push the head up off the pillow, and observe and palpate for the bulk and power of sternomastoids. For trapezius, ask the patient to shrug shoulders. Observe for asymmetry.

XII. Tongue (wasting, fasciculation of the non-protruded tongue).

Unilateral palsy (ipsilateral wasting, fasciculation and deviation to the paralysed side).

A pseudo-bulbar palsy (stiff, immobile tongue).

Communication Skills and Ethics (Station 4)

7

[The MRCP Clinical Examining Board have kindly made available sample scenarios for this Station: these may be viewed and downloaded using the following link: http://www.mrcpuk.org/PACES/Pages/PACESscenarios.aspx]

INTRODUCTION TO THE GENERAL APPROACH OF THIS STATION

Station 4 aims to assess the candidate's ability to guide and organize a consultation with a subject who may be a patient, relative or surrogate, such as a health care worker. The candidate is expected to provide emotional support, discuss further management of the case and deal with ethical and legal implications as they arise. The inclusion of this task in the PACES examination is significant, since the medical interview is considered central to clinical practice. Doctors are thought to perform around 200,000 interviews in a professional lifetime. Communication is therefore the clinician's responsibility, with multiple influences. It is an essential component of the physician role. Effective communication builds trust between the patient and the doctor, improves patient satisfaction, recall, understanding, concordance, decision-making and disease outcome.

The importance of communication was recently emphasised by the British Medical Association in an article entitled "Communication Skills education for doctors: an update" (November 2004) and the Royal Colleges of Physicians themselves, "Improving communication between doctors and patients" (Royal College of Physicians of London, 1997). All patients irrespective of race, gender and social class are entitled to good standards from their doctors. The essential tenets underlying this good practice are: professional competence, good relationships with patients and colleagues, and thinking ethically about decisions regarding patients and colleagues. In this chapter, we are obviously unable to cover all eventuality in the examination. Rather, we have used 24 scenarios to outline the fundamental principles of communication skills and ethics which cover the key areas of the values tested, including breaking bad news, confidentiality and consent, explaining diagnosis and treatments, different styles of patient response, and end-of-life decisions (Sections A-G of this chapter).

The RCP want a Registrar that they feel is competent to deal with such scenario so that the patient/family will be satisfied with the explanation they are given. It is not possible to try and prepare for all possible scenarios.

Instead, make sure you have:
- A broad knowledge of general medicine.
- Knowledge of (national or international) clinical guidelines and protocols: Useful guidelines relevant to this station are the DVLA guidelines, NICE guidelines, details about coroner referral, and BMA guidelines on DNAR.
- Intimate knowledge of acute medical management protocols for common medical emergencies.
- A management plan for all common non-acute conditions.
- Knowledge of major trials that have altered clinical practice in some way.
- An idea of any topical newspaper reports on medical subjects.

Candidates are *not* expected to have a detailed knowledge of medical jurisprudence. For overseas candidates in the UK, detailed knowledge of UK law is not required, although candidates should be aware of general legal and ethical principles that may affect the case in question.

PRINCIPLES OF COMMUNICATION SKILLS

Structure of the Consultation for the Examination

In the examination, five minutes are allowed for reading the referral letter, 14 minutes for talking to the patient, 1 minute for the candidate to collect his/her thoughts and five minutes' discussion with the examiner. Read the scenario carefully before going in, decide the important issues that you are addressing and what you should stress for the patient to take home. Make sure that you write the main points you want to discuss otherwise you may forget once you go inside that room. You are given a blank sheet of paper to scribble on. If possible, use this time to decide which words are likely to constitute medical jargon and think of equivalent words a lay person would understand. When in the room, take a short time to establish rapport, and lead/direct the interview without being too controlling. See if the chair has been left a bit further away from the patient; see if there is a barrier between you and the patient. *One of your colleagues tried to bring the chair around the table near the patient to break bad news and the examiner said, "It is alright. I know what you are trying to do. Point taken."* You are supposed to have, after the 15 minutes, a discussion of 5 minutes when they will ask you questions concerning the case and if there are any ethical dilemmas. Timing is therefore absolutely crucial to a decent performance in this Station, and time management, whilst not explicitly stated, as in real life and indeed for the clinical stations, can help to determine success. The 5 minutes spent reading the task is of critical importance.

You should be able to put patients at ease, particularly with regard to beginning an interview and enabling the patient to raise and discuss sensitive personal issues. In this station, you should be demonstrate your ability to adapt their interviewing style to accommodate different patient styles (overtalkativeness, reticence, depression, hostility, confusion), the communicative abilities of different patient groups (e.g. children, patients who understand or speak very little English, patients with learning difficulties), and the changing demands of the situation (e.g. within one consultation the candidate may be required to elicit information about a medical problem, discuss a psychosocial problem, deal with emotional distress, and provide education). Some of these issues are discussed in part E of this chapter.

Most of all, you *must* undertake the task. Do not attempt to convert the case into something that you would rather do. Each examiner also has a copy of the written instructions to the candidates, together with the written subject information and Examiners' information. Each examiner has a structured marking schedule for the case and will examine independently and without discussion. Be frank with the patient (honesty means integrity)! You are expected to have agreed a summary and plan of action with the patient/subject before closure and discussion.

The structure suggested below is based on the Cambridge-Calgary formulation. This structure can be applied to virtually all scenarios. These scenarios may be set in any branch of adult medicine that an FY2/ST1 is likely to encounter in an in-patient or outpatient setting. The semi-structured marking schemes involves sections covering initiation of the interview, appropriate exploration and planning, and exploration and problem negotiation, and conclusion of the interview, as well as the discussion of relevant issues of medical ethics and/or law. This marking scheme is given below (reproduced by kind permission of the Federation of the Royal College of Physicians).

This Station can go Easily Wrong!

The new PACES format allows candidates to receive more structured feedback on why they failed this particular station. This station is an evolution of the old viva system. The easiest way to ensure that you are given a "clear fail" in this section of the exam is by saying something that is downright dangerous medical practice, or indicates a complete lack of basic understanding about a subject.

Reasons How the Station Could go Wrong

1. *Taking the station for granted:* It is very important to see as many clinical cases as possible in the run-up to the exam – both to refine one's examination skills and to pick up key signs. Nevertheless, to ignore the communication skills and ethics station nor to devote a proportion of your time in proportion to the examination is unwise.
2. *Not showing enough empathy:* It is relatively easy to distinguish those candidates who are trying to show empathy from those who do not. It is important that the candidate is seen to demonstrate empathy in dealing with their situation. Empathy is the ability to identify or understand with another person's predicament. Synonymous words include compassion and sympathy. One useful tip in helping you develop more empathy is to try and imaging how you would feel if you or a relative were caught up in that person's situation.
3. *Using medical jargon:* Do not use medical jargon. Remember that this station is testing your ability to communicate effectively. You are not communicating effectively if the person in front of you who has no medical knowledge cannot understand what you are saying. Bear in mind that medical jargon is not necessarily limited to medical terminology but also "medical speak". By medical speak, we mean words that are not for the most part purely medical but convey a different meaning to health professionals.
4. *Misreading the scenario given to them:* Read the scenario carefully. In addition, the information contained in the scenario may be extremely important, for example, why have they made the patient a young woman (issues of contraception, pregnancy) or why have

they mentioned that the pastient is attending with their relative (issue of confidentiality).

5. *Being insensitive with patients/relatives:* This does not need any explanation.

6. *Volunteering wrong information:* Although, this station is not testing your clinical skills, it is important that the candidate does not communicate erroneous clinical information. This in itself may lead to the interview going in a completely different direction to that intended by the examiners. Examples, include making up information, not given to the candidate either from the scenario or from the actor/actress. Another error is assuming that the patient has had tests not mentioned in the scenario. For example, although in some scenarios when it says the cancer has metastasized, it is very likely that you have performed a CT to find out where it has metastasized. However, some of your colleagues suggested the patient's confusion is secondary to metastases (when the primary was lung cancer). As you well know, hypoxia or secondary infection could have caused the confusion.

SECTION 1: CONDUCT OF THE INTERVIEW

The first third of the structured marking scheme is devoted to the general conduct of the interview, in particular, an appropriate initiation followed by adequate exploration of the patient's beliefs, concerns and expectations.

Initiation

- Introduction of doctor to patient; introduction as Dr.
- Establish reason for the discussion/explain role clearly.
- Agree the purpose of the interview with the patient: Ask the patient what he/she wants or needs.
- Put the patient at ease and establish good rapport. Ways in which to develop good rapport include accepting non-judgementally what the patient says, acknowledging the legitimacy of the patient to hold their views ("I can understand that you wish to get ... checked out"). It is vital not to be too judgemental, patronising or paternalistic.
- Make appropriate eye-contact early in the interview. General principles of non-verbal communication include appropriate body-posture, proximity, touch, body movements, facial expression, eye behaviour, vocal cues, use of time, physical presence, and

environmental cues. Use non-verbal cues to demonstrate attentiveness and build the relationship. Patients and examiners alike are good at picking up non-verbal cues.

Explanation and Planning

Explanations should be tailored to the patient's preferences in terms of the amount and timing of the information provided.
- Assess the patient's level of knowledge,
- Assess the patient's concerns,
- Assess the patient's expectations and feelings.

You need to assess the patient's starting point. Discover what the patient already knows, is fearful of, and what they are hoping for, particularly when they are frightened. The rewards of obtaining an accurate picture of where the patient and their relative is coming from before giving information about prognosis or treatment options are great. Gauging how much the patient wishes to know also requires skill. Do not fall into the trap of doing most of the talking (this is a mistake that leads to failure). Remember that the actor in front of you will have been given information that would not be initially available to you and can only be gleaned by asking relevant questions. In addition to that, it is a well known fact that listening is respectful and polite. Try not to interrupt.

Beliefs

We're here to talk about X. Is that correct?
    What do you think is causing it?
    Why do you think that might be happening?
    Have you had any ideas about this yourself?
    Have you got any clues or theories?
    You've obviously given this some thought; it would help me to know what you think it might be?
    Is there anybody else you know who has this problem?

Concerns

What are you concerned that it might be?
    Is there anything particular or specific that you were uneasy about...?
    What was your worse fear or thoughts about this?
    In your darkest moments... what had been going through your mind?
    Is there anything else that you would like to talk about?

Expectations

How were you hoping I might help you with this?
What were you hoping we might be able to do for this?
What do you think might be the best plan of action?
You've obviously given this some thought, what were you thinking might be the best way of tackling this?
What sort of information do you want to know?

Feelings

How has all of this made you feel?
>   How has this left you feeling?
>   How have things seemed to you?
>   In the subsequent part of the interview, you will be expected to:

- Demonstrate empathy, response and non-judgemental attitude. Empathy is the understanding and sensitive appreciation of another person's predicament or feelings, and the communication back to the patient.
- Give the information required in simple language avoiding medical jargon, abbreviations or slang.
- Inform the patient about the options as to what can be done or should be done and what you are going to.
- Avoid patronizing the patient by talking extremely slowly or loudly, calling them *"dear"* or saying *"sure, sure"* dismissively.
- Check out non-verbal cues – this allows doctors to express **empathy** and **compassion** for the patient's position. It also gives the doctor space to enquire about further concerns and respond to them with feeling. *"I can see that you look very distressed to hear the results of the tests confirm your worst fears. I am extremely sorry (pause) you mentioned your husband is diasbled; have you any other concerns you wish to discuss now?"* or *"The last point made you look worried. Is there something more serious about the point you would like to tell me?"*
- *Encourage active listening:* Wait time, facilitate responding (encouragement, repetition, paraphrasing), and encourage non-verbal transmission.
- Facilitate questions and answer them, but avoid distressing too much.
- Prioritise problems.
- Redirect interview as necessary with sensitivity.
- Offer support in terms of concern, understanding, willingness to help, partnership and sensitivity.
Some golden rules of things of what **not** to do!

- Do not talk over the patient; if it is necessary to interrupt, do it sensitively and rarely.
- Do not get angry with the patient if they cannot remember things or do not accept your views.
- Do not use "statement" questions, such as *"You don't have diabetes?"*

SECTION 2: EXPLORATION AND PROBLEM NEGOTIATION

The next section of the marking scheme assesses the ability of the candidate to agree a clear course of action, involving achieving an appropriate diagnosis and treatment plan, and to summarise and check the patient's understanding. It is expected that the candidate within 14 minutes concludes the interview appropriately, without overrunning. A possible way in which these goals can be achieved is suggested below:

- Use an appropriate questioning style (generally open-ended to closed as the interview progresses).
- First it is a good idea to start with encouraging the patient to contribute their thoughts first and it's useful to be forewarned about potentially strong feelings against a course of action, before rather than after, it has been suggested.
  Doctor: "Before I suggest a way... I'd like to hear what you had in mind – or anything you wouldn't be keen to consider?"
  Patient: "I've heard a lot about the dangers of surgery and I'm not too keen on being reliant on drugs for the rest of my life. Is there a homeopathic remedy you can recommend?"
- Next you should share your own thoughts about management - this allows patients to understand your own reasoning as well as your difficulties and dilemmas. Enlistment is a term that conveys the initiation of the physician to do this.
  Doctor: "I can well understand your concerns about medication – but having a blood pressure of this level makes me think it is unlikely that you will be able to control it by diet and exercise alone. There might be a risk involved if you exercise vigorously in the meantime ...I think the best ways is to.... What do you think?"
  "Are these treatments acceptable to you?"
- Next, you need to provide clear and relevant information about the various approaches and options – continue by involving the patient by offering choices and making suggestions (*not directives*).
  Doctor: "There are clearly pros and cons to each of these options ... what preferences do you have?"

Patient: "Yes I agree – I'm really not sure now"

Doctor: "My suggestion is that we get an expert opinion about your gallstones…and see what this involves… what do you think?"

- Finally - actively seek and encourage their reactions, views and acceptability about what is proposed – and negotiate a mutually acceptable plan

- Doctor: "Perhaps we can start with something mild and check to see if there are any problems before going on… Is this acceptable or do you have any other ideas"

- Summarise the subject's understanding.

  "Is there anything else that you are unclear about or didn't understand?"

  "From what we have talked about today, what do you think is most important?"

  "I want to make sure, I've got everything. You are concerned about…."

- Formulate a plan of action with the patient.

- Reiterate your discussion with the patient to ensure understanding.

- Offer co-partnership and support. Overt statements such as *"we need to work on this together"* or *"I will undertake to speak to the specialist on your behalf"*, *"you will not be left to cope with this on your own … how can we go forward now?"* are examples of phrasing which may help patients and need to be underlined.

- Ask if there are any important issues not covered or if they have any further concerns that they would like you to address.

- Remember it is often appropriate to say that you would seek senior or specialist advice.

- Offer further information sources, e.g. leaflets, societies, and support groups.

- Close the interview appropriately. Offer a clear follow-up plan, set a date for a next appointment. Offering to contact relatives or carers when the patient has expressed concern about informing others about their diagnosis or prognosis is often helping. This all arises from the need to inform the patient that the interview is over.

Common questions that can be expected from the Examiners:

How do you feel that went? Did you put the patient at ease?

What could you have done differently?

Which areas if you had time would you have covered?

What and how do you the patient has taken from your consultation?

They will then discuss legal and ethical issues (see below).

SECTION 3: MEDICAL ETHICS

In dealing with your case scenario in the examination, you must be able to communicate your argument with relation to the four fundamental ethical principles. The examiner will expect you to have some understanding of these principles which underpin the practice of good medicine, and may refer to these as part of the semi-structured oral examination which follows the interview.

Beauchamp and Childress' Principles

These four principles derive from Beauchamp and Childress (1979), and are:

Autonomy: This literally means self-rule, and means in practice **respecting** and following the patient's decisions in the management of their condition. Competent patients hace the capacity to think, decide and act on the basis of such thought and decision, freely and independently. Respect for patient autonomy requires that health professionals (and others, including the patient's family) help patients to make their own decisions (e.g. by providing appropriate information), and respect to follow these decisions (even when the health professional believes the patient's decision is wrong).

Beneficence: This means promoting what is in the patient's best interests. In most situations, respect for the principle of beneficence and for the principle of respect for patient autonomy will lead to the same conclusion. The two principles conflict when a competent patient chooses a course of action that is not in his or her own best interests. However, a patient can be advised that a course of treatment in her best interests if there is evidence to do so (e.g. subcutaneous heparin in a young pregnant lady with a suspected pulmonary embolism, who is beyond the first trimester).

Non-maleficence: This means avoiding harm. The potential good and harms and their probabilities must be weighed up to decide what is in the patient's best interests. Sometimes it means that appropriate safety measures are taken to perform certain essential investigations, e.g. using an X-ray shield for a CT scan of the chest in a pregnancy lady.

Justice and sharing: Doing what is good for the population as a whole in terms of time and treatments. In real terms, this may mean distributing resources fairly in the provision of care; health professionals have to decide how much time to spend with different patients, and decisions must be made about limitations on the treatments that can be offered at various levels within a health care system.

In the following sections, general advice is given about the possible principles being tested, followed by specific examples of tasks which illustrate these principles.

We have organised these sample scenarios according to the broad category of their main focus: Breaking bad news, giving information about diagnoses and treatments, informed consent, differing patient styles and responses, the ethical issues concerning genetic counselling, confidentiality and good medical practice, and end-of-life decisions. We have provided details for the candidate, as well as a description of a possible consultation in response to that instruction. Of course, various ethical issues are brought out in these different scenarios. In the real examination, however, any scenario can be used to examine your competence at communication skills, law and ethics (e.g. advising a nursery school teacher not to attend work, even if she wants to, because of the danger of passing on an infectious disease).

EXAMPLES OF TYPES OF SCENARIOS

Breaking Bad News

A review of candidates' experiences of PACES suggests that 'breaking bad news' has been the focus of many scenarios. Bad news is any information which is likely to alter drastically the patient's view of the future, for example a diagnosis of multiple sclerosis or the news that a patient is brain-dead. It is the most potent cause of distress and, for the medical profession, if done incorrectly, an important cause of complaints and law suits. Genuine communication is characterised by attentiveness, listening and dialogue. The required skills can be learned. Health care professionals sometimes find it difficult to understand the physical, social, occupational and financial consequencves of bad news. There are gradations of bad news: subjective, dependent on individuals' life experiences, personality, spiritual beliefs, philosophical structure, perceived social supports, and emotional hardiness. A useful structure to this type of task is given below. We will use a few scenarios which you can use to consider how these principles may be put into practice.

A STRUCTURE FOR BREAKING BAD NEWS

Initiation

- Use a private setting, involve other health workers, opportunity for relatives to attend if they wish.
- Set your behaviour with correct positioning, eye contact, body language, listening skills. Some examiners are impressed if you physically move the chair near the patient, but obviously at a comfortable interpersonal space.
- Check there is privacy.
- Ask about attendees.
- Offer good eye contact and the patient comfort.
- Greet the patient, and obtain the patient's name.
- Provide a proper introduction of self and role, outline plan for the consultation.
- The clinician should first find out if anything new has happened since the last encounter. Begin with a neutral question about what is happening.

Assess beliefs before giving the bad news with appropriate signposting (signals moving to information).

- It is important to hear the patient's narrative of events to allow them to explain what has happened and where they are up to in their illness, e.g. ask *"How did it all start?"* and *"What happened next?"*
- Ask about his/her beliefs about the situation. Repeat and reflect *"So you had been worried about something like that?""Have you thought about what may be causing your symptoms?"* or *"What has been the most difficult part of the whole thing for you"*. This way you understand the patient's perspective and what they understand by their illness and therefore can avoid giving shocking information, if, for example, it is their belief that they have had curative treatment when you know that their prognosis is only a few weeks.
- Acknowledge what the patient has been told in the past.
- *"You said you wanted me to be honest and open with you. Are you the sort of person who likes to be told about his medical condition?"*.
- Ask what he/she understood about why a test was done, for example, *"Do you know why we did the biopsy?"*
- Give clear signposting/warning shot that serious information is to follow. *"I'm afraid it looks more serious than we hoped."* *"Unfortunately, the test results show ..."* Give time for the patient to think about this.

- Watch your body language particularly when breaking bad news – look at the patient and lean a bit forwards, pause and acknowledge distress, recap what has been discussed and check understanding of the key facts.
- Give the bad news simply and clearly in small pieces, without fudging, in an organised manner.
- Build the news up layer by layer.

Reaction and Prognosis

- Allow the patient time to respond. There is good evidence that most doctors interrupt the patient within 30 seconds of speaking. Encourage the patient to contribute reactions, concerns and feelings. Be prepared for the patient to have disorderly emotional responses of some kind and acknowledge them early on.
- If the patient is distressed acknowledge this e.g. *"I can see this news has really upset you. Can you bear to tell me what distresses you most about this?"*. Many patients are distressed but can be uncertain what the distress is mainly about. Giving permission to discuss concerns enables the patient to start clarifying the issues and then prioritising their concerns. This feels like a positive process to the patient and is always helpful. Avoid premature reassurance or excessive explanations which can cause dissatisfaction and frustration. Avoid the use of confusing language and jargon.
- Denial is a way of coping with fear and it should be respected as a coping strategy, especially if the patient is coping. If a patient declines further information, it should be acknowledged, but also acknowledge the discomfort of uncertainty and give permission to ask questions at a later date. Few patients adopt a stance of denial permanently, most start to ask more information once they feel more secure. Patients usually experience belief once that they are able to discuss some of their fears.
- Check understanding. *"Is this making sense?"* or *"Have I covered what you want to talk about?"*
- Repeat certain information.
- Keep pausing to allow the patient to think.
- Acknowledge the patient's concerns and feelings through attentive listening. Allowing ventilation of feelings provides a therapeutic part of the dialogue. *"How does this leave you feeling at the moment?"* is the key phrase. The aim is to help the patient try to name their feelings. Encouraging the ventilation of feelings conveys empathy. Stay calm and allow time for the person to think about their feelings.

- Discuss prognosis. If the prognosis is unclear, give a range rather than leave it entirely open, i.e. avoid saying *"No one can tell for sure"*. Be realistic and honest, but try to leave room for hope.
- Outline likely consequences in a sympathetic and empathetic manner.

Treatment

Do not rush into treatment options, if it is clear the patient/relative is not prepared for the information yet.

- Explain clearly the treatment options and outcome, with an approximate time frame.
- Ask for any other or new worries and deal with them systematically, bring the discussion to a close but offer an opportunity to speak again and elicit the help of other groups, e.g. specialist cancer nurses or societies, offer services for the future, offer transport for the patient. Be prepared for anger and denial, despair and depression. Consider the long term implications, the importance of the support network of family, friends and agencies now and in the future. Identify problems of the patient which are fixable and make a plan.
- Identify coping strategies of the patient and incorporate them. Identify other sources of support for the patient.
- Encourage feedback and check understanding.
- Leave room for hope.
- Summarise and emphasise what can be done.
- Encourage the patient to articulate his personal goals.
- Make appropriate arrangements for follow-up contact. Some examiners like the candidates to enquire what the subject will be doing in the immediate short-term (e.g. by offering if they are travelling alone to arrange a cab to go home if the news has been devestating).

This framework can be applied to the scenarios below, but we have also included some further details specific to each scenario.

BRAINSTEM DEATH AND ORGAN DONATION

Scenario 1

Problem: Breaking bad news (brainstem death and organ donation).
Subject name: Helen Roberts (sister of the patient, Charles Roberts).

You are the FY2/ST1 for ITU. Charles Roberts is a 28-year-old accountant who was admitted a week previously following a road-traffic accident. He was treated for multi-system trauma, and was being kept alive on a ventilator. The nurses have requested you to tell the sister of the patient that he has been declared brain-dead by two consultants. It is documented that he had wished his organs to be donated to medical science, in a private conversation with his parents many years' ago (obviously without having foreseen these particular tragic circumstances). Please inform his sister that Charles Roberts is brain-dead, and approach, if appropriate, the issue of organ donation.

- Introduce yourself and establish a good rapport.
- Ask if he would like anyone else there for the discussion. Assess how much emotional support the subject has in dealing with the situation.
- Acknowledge that it must have been a very difficult time for all of the family.
- Ask what the family has been told in the past, and signpost the bad news. Explain briefly the history of admission to ITU.
- Explain the patient is brain-dead simply. *"He has technically died and only the ventilator is keeping the other organs working. For all intents and purposes, Charles is dead because the parts of the brain vital in keeping someone alive are damaged beyond any possibility of recovery"*. Explain that brain cells cannot be replaced once damaged and so these cells will not recover. You can also add that if the machines were to be switched off then his heart and lings would stop. It can also be helpful to volunteer to involve a neurologist to confirm the patient is genuinely brain dead.
- Explain the next appropriate step is to stop the ventilation. Explain carefully that this is not to allow her father to die but that continuing ventilation is inappropriate if a person has already died. Explain that it is the medical team who makes the decision who makes the decision as they may think that they are giving you permission to end his life (you are not actually causing death).
- Pause for reflection and allow plenty of time for reaction. Express condolence.
- Show empathy, e.g. "I realize that this must be extremely distressing for you. I only wish that I had better news for you".
- Confirm that there is no hope of recovery.
- Give opportunity to discuss the situation with family and friends.
- According to the subject's response, consider whether a subsequent discussion regarding organ transplantation would be appropriate. If so, outline the benefits of organ donation: The shortage of hearts,

lungs, kidneys, for example, which may enable other people to live who would otherwise die. In this case, Charles Roberts, the patient, had previously suggested the notion that his organs to be put to medical science.

- Nurses in ITU often open the discussion by asking something like *"What do you think your mother/sister would have wanted in these circumstances?" "I wonder if your father/husband would have wanted his organs donated for the benefit of others"*. Remember that this is not an all-or-nothing situation–relatives, who are legal guardians of the body, may specify which are acceptable or unacceptable organs for donation.
- If there is strong emotional resistance, then you should respect and acknowledge their resistance. *"I can see you find the idea distasteful, so I won't pursue it any further"*.
- If, instead, the relatives are sympathetic to the idea, you should explore their reasons and determine whether their reasons are appropriate are realistic. *"What exactly makes you support the idea of organ donation?"*
- Offer him the opportunity to have a discussion with other members of the family; arrange to meet again in a few hours. Ask the father if there is anyone else he would like to inform. Ask if he has any questions. Ensure all staff involved in the case of the father's decision.
- Arrange a further appointment with somebody.

Mistakes candidates have made when acting out this scenario including adding information not given to them, e.g. "The CT scan shows a very large bleed" or using graphic descriptions of injuries which are unpleasant.

Definitions

The definitions of death have to some extent varied with altering technologies. The examiners may be interested in your understanding of terms such as "brainstem death". In 1979, the Medical Royal Colleges volunteered the definition that brain death represents the stage at which the patient truly becomes dead. There is no legal definition of death. Death is now accepted as meaning brainstem death or brain death. Brainstem death is a deep coma with absent respiration, with absence of hypoxia, hypothermia, hypoglycaemia, neurolomuscular blocking agents, acidosis, abnormal biochemistry and sedative drugs. Tests include fixed dilated pupils, absent corneal response and vestibulo-ocular reflex. There is no gag reflex or motor response in the cranial nerves. There is no respiratory effort on stopping the ventilator and allowing the $PaCO_2$ to rise to 6.7 kPa. The definition involves two medical practitioners; with two sets of tests; the tests are repeated at an interval that is left to clinical judgement. A persistent vegetative state (Jennett and Plum, 1972) is in patients whose brainstem function persists despite loss of cortical function; there is no behavioural evidence of awareness of self or the environment. Their quality of life is at best uncertain, and their life depends on artificial feeding. There are no reversible causes present, and at least 6 months and usually 12 months have passed since the onset. The causes are severe head injury (40%), hypoxia (40%), and others. There are about 600 new cases in the UK. There is brain damage consistent with the diagnosis. These patients breathe spontaneolusly, open and close their eyes, swallow and make facial grimaces. However, they show no behavioural evidence of awareness.

MULTIPLE SCLEROSIS

Scenario 2

Problem: Breaking bad news (multiple sclerosis).
Patient name: Sarah Lewis (aged 26).
Sarah Lewis is a 26-year-old lady who had noticed some numbness of her feet, with some difficulty in walking, and odd sensations when taking a bath in her upper limbs, a few weeks' ago. You are the FY2/ST1 in clinic for Neurology. The MRI scan organised by your Consultant demonstrates multiple peri-ventricular plaques most in keeping with a diagnosis of multiple sclerosis. Miss Lewis is a local teacher. She has attended clinic today, and would like the results of her investigation. On previous occasions, the patient has never asked what the problem might be and nobody has volunteered a differential diagnosis. Please discuss with her.

- Introduce yourself to the patient and establish good rapport. Ask if she wishes for anyone else to be present.
- Explore the patient's understanding of her symptoms and what they possibly meant, i.e. expectations/suspicions of what may be wrong.
- Ask what she understood by the tests. The patient should be given small pieces of information in a logical manner; pauses are essential and give the opportunity for questions. Patients can be given too much information in one consultation after receiving bad news. Explain that the MRI scan findings do suggest multiple sclerosis. Pause to allow this to sink in.

- Watch for her reactions, such as anger or denial. Express empathy.
- Ask what she knows about multiple sclerosis (MS). Explain that myelin is a substance that sheaths around nerves in the body for insulation. Damage to them is called 'demyelination' and the bare patches interfere with the smooth conduction of nerve impulses. Aim to reassure her that there are specialists who look after patients with multiple sclerosis and that they will help her with the best available therapy.
- *"How many attacks will I have in a year?"* Reassure her that she may have no further attacks.
- *"What happens if I have an attack?"*. Mention that there is treatment (iv methylprednisolone) for a 'sudden' attack, but that this usually requires admission for a few days.
- Tell her that there are many people with multiple sclerosis who lead very active lives. In terms of prognosis, explain that there are different forms of the disease. Tell her that patients with relapses and remissions may go on for many years without any major disability.
- Ask if she has any specific concerns; these may include her worries about future pregnancies, or her ability to hold down a particular job such as teaching.
- Tell her the causes of the condition are unknown.
- Explain that there are treatments that prevent the disease from relapsing, but that these do not affect the final outcome. β-interferon reduce the rate of relapse, but at this point is unlikely to be warranted.
- MS has no effect on fertility and does not affect pregnancy outcome (but may worsen in the puerperium period").
- Offer general advice (polyunsaturated fat may be good, and hot climate may worsen the condition").
- Reassure her that this is not hereditary.
- Tell her about the Multiple Sclerosis Society 0800 800 0800. Explain that joining such groups may allow her to come into contact with other people who have MS. It may even help her to see other people who are coping well with the condition. Other advantages of MS groups in addition to encouragement include educagtion, tips and awareness of new discoveries.
- Ask about her support mechanisms and enquire about his social circumstances including job. Arrange early follow-up to discuss this further. Say you will refer her to a specialist and tell her you will inform her GP.

- Conclude the interview appropriately, and arrange a follow-up appointment. Give her a contact number if she wants to ring you for advice.

  A note on the term 'multiple sclerosis': this is normally referred to in the clinical cases as a demyelinating disorder.

LUNG CANCER

Scenario 3

Problem: Breaking bad news (Lung cancer).
Patient name: Michael George (aged 58).
Michael George is a 58-year-old architect. He has smoked 10 cigarettes a day for the last 40-years. He was admitted a week ago with cough and shortness of breath. Investigations were normal, apart from a slightly low serum sodium, and a high resolution spiral CT scan of the chest demonstrated left-sided hilar lymphadenopathy. The Radiology report states that the appearance is most suggestive of a neoplasm of the lung. You are the FY2/ST1 for General Medicine. He is feeling much better, and would like to go back to work as soon as possible. You are to discuss with him the results of his investigations, and their possible significance.

- Introduce yourself and establish a good rapport.
- Ask the patient what he thought the symptoms meant: Possible symptoms include cough, shortness of breath, bloody sputum, chest pain, wheezing or pneumonia.
- "I've read a summary from the GP, but what have you been told?" Check what is known already. Is more information wanted? What is his concern?
- Signpost that the news is worse than may first appear (the "warning shot", Faulkner (1998)). "I've had a look at your scans, and it's not good". Ask about why the patient thought he was having tests and what they mean in the long term, despite the fact he is currently feeling very much better.
- Break the news that he has an abnormal growth of cells in the lung, a lung cancer. Explain that diagnosis of a lung cancer is normally through imaging findings (including CXR and CT), as in his case, but further details about the type of cancer can only be obtained through further investigation (e.g. induced sputum). The spread of cancer can be ascertained through further imaging (e.g. CT of the abdomen). Pulmonary function testing may be useful for determining suitability for surgery, or safety of further

investigation (such as bronchoscopy). It is very important, however, to absorb jargon.

- Ask about the beliefs about the cause. Inform him that 80% of lung cancers are related to tobacco smoke, and therefore smoking cessation is advised.
- Explain that foreseeing the likely prognosis of his condition depends upon information from these tests.
- Ask the subject if he has any questions. Explain that there will be appropriate management with the respiratory physicians and oncologists, and he will be introduced to the physicians and nurses.
- Beware of information overload (Greger, 1993) and allow denial, *"I'm going to be the first person to beat this, Doctor. You'll be proud of me!"* Give time for the news to be absorbed, and don't be afraid of silence. Allow ventilation of feelings. Stay calm.
- Arrange a further appointment with somebody in the near future. Offer availability.

Discussion

Whilst this station is primarily an assessment of communication skills, the examiners may reasonably be interested in your understanding of the basic principles of the management of lung cancer. Lobectomy and pneumonectomy are used for non-small cell carcinoma, and can prolong life, improve quality of life and relieve pain. Adenocarcinoma is the most common non-small cell cancer, when tend to develop to the periphery. They tend to metastasize to the bone, CNS, adrenal glands, liver and opposite lung. Squamous cell carcinomas tend to be located in the more central part of the lung. Small cell carcinoma is the most aggressive type of cancer and has the worst prognosis. Radiotherapy and chemotherapy is the primary treatment for small cell carcinomas. Contraindications to surgery in non-small cell lung cancer include: Metastatic carcinoma, transfer factor < 50%, severe pulmonary hypertension, uncontrolled cardiac arrhythmias, poor lung function, left laryngeal nerve palsy, malignant effusion, dysphagia, mediastinal lymph node involvement, superior vena cava obstruction, phrenic nerve palsy, rib or distant metastasis.

The examiners may wish to discuss related oncology issues, such as the importance of oncology patients entering multicentre clinical research trials. It may be useful to be aware of documents such as the "Calman-Hine" report which was produced in response to concerns about variations in treatment around the country. This report recommends that cancer services should be organised at three levels.

Primary care is seen as the focus of care; the commoner cancers will be treated in Cancer Units in local hospitals which have the expertise and facilities to support a multidisciplinary team; and the less common cancers will be treated in Cancer Centres situated in larger hospitals, which will also support Cancer Units by providing specialist services such as radiotherapy.

ALZHEIMER'S DISEASE

Scenario 4

Problem: Breaking bad news (a diagnosis of Alzheimer's disease).
Patient name: Peter Matthews (aged 64).
Peter Matthews is a 64-year-old man who presented with increasing memory difficulties. He himself reported an incident where he went to his local corner shop, but on arrival forgot what he had intended to purchase. Overall, he feels that his mood has been fine, and he reports that he has had no other difficulty. In light of this symptom, his GP arranged a CT head scan which demonstrates cerebral atrophy. Neuropsychology confirmed short-term memory problems. You are the FY2/ST1 for Neurology and General Medicine, and you are to see Peter Matthews in outpatients regarding his investigations. The multidisciplinary 'memory clinic' team have discussed Mr. Matthews, and they feel that the most diagnosis is Alzheimer's disease.

- Introduce yourself to the patient and establish good rapport. Ask if she wishes for anyone else to be present.
- Explore the patient's understanding of the condition and expectations/suspicions of what may be wrong.
- Discover what the patient understood about the tests (e.g. CT scan demonstrating cerebral atrophy). Explain that there is no single test for this particular condition, although results may be supportive of such a condition.
- Explain that the disease tends to be a slowly progressive disease, but the rate of progression can be unpredictable. The disease is characterised in its early stages by loss of memory. *"I can see how hard your memory loss has been to deal with."*
- He should aim to optimise general health, and should use cognitive aids (e.g. clear labelling diary). Current medications include donepezil, a cholinesterase inhibitor, for mild dementia. Main side effects are cholinergic. It is a case of taking things as they happen.
- Explain that lifestyle changes can be helpful (for example, locking up any rooms in the house that are not in use, locking up any drawers that contain important documents).

- The patient may wish to know whether the condition runs in families. Alzheimer's disease where there is a family link is called familial Alzheimer's disease, and is more common among younger people (under the age of 65). Research has shown that even for people with a strong family history of early onset Alzheimer's disease, only 50% of cases are caused by a genetic defect. Some cases of Alzheimer's disease in people under 65 are, however, inherited. On average, half of the children of a person with one of these rare genetic defects inherits the disease. Probably all those who inherit the genetic defect develop Alzheimer's disease at a comparatively early age.
- Tell him about the support offered by the Alzheimer's Disease Society. Mention that benefits are available to patients with Alzheimer's disease, and their carers, and these can be ascertained from the Citizen's Advice Bureau.
- Explain that daycare may be available for the patient, giving respite for the carer.
- Ask her if he has any questions. Offer an appropriate time for follow up.

TESTICULAR CANCER

Scenario 5

Problem: Breaking bad news (A diagnosis of testicular cancer).
Patient name: William Charles (aged 21).
William Charles is a 21-year-old man saw his GP because of a lump in his testes. A nurse had accidentally done a pregnancy test which was positive. However, he was unaware this had been done, and had just been told that a urine sample was needed to look for infection. A CT scan, with subsequent biopsy, arranged by his GP, demonstrates a testicular tumour. He has a girlfriend of two years, to whom he is close. You are the FY2/ST1 for General Medicine. He has attended clinic to discuss the result.

- Introduce yourself to the patient and establish good rapport. Ask if she wishes for anyone else to be present.
- Explore the history of how the patient realised that something was wrong. Once the patient's understanding of the condition has been established, it may be possible to predict if he is expecting a diagnosis of cancer. If he is aware that cancer is a possibility, the patient should be informed of the diagnosis in a clear and sympathetic manner. He may wish to see his CT scans or the histology report, which is sometimes useful.

- Explain the nature of the disease, the need for cyclical combination therapy over a period of several weeks, and its side-effects. Explain that the treatment will give him a very good outcome. If the patient has not considered cancer as a possible diagnosis, the patient should ideally be given small pieces of information at a time, working towards the diagnosis. The doctor should be relatively positive, as the outcome is usually good with chemotherapy.
- Allow the patient time to react to the diagnosis and pause.
- He may ask why the urine sample was taken. The author of this scenario would like you to consider what **ethically** you would do in this scenario.
- Explain the need for subsequent cytotoxic chemotherapy: Logistics (when and where) and side-effects (e.g. infection, alopecia, nausea and infertility).
- Explain the implications of the treatment of his condition: Cosmetic – testicular prostheses can be inserted; fertility–unaffected by previous surgery, likely to be infertile after chemotherapy, but semen can be frozen and stored; need for future monitoring of response to treatment: CT body and blood tests. He may wish to discuss these findings in light of his personal circumstances (such as his girlfriend).
- Emphasise the very good prognosis for testicular cancer: Around 90% cure. Ask the patient if he understands what has been said. Summarise the consultation and ask if he has any questions.
- Arrange medical follow-up. Arrange a point of contact with the oncology nurse specialist. Make sure that there is someone he can talk to, or someone at home with him.

HODGKIN'S DISEASE

Scenario 6

Problem: Breaking bad news (Hodgkin's disease).
Patient name: Claire Barron (aged 27).
Claire Barron aged 27 presented to her GP feeling unwell a month ago with fever and loss of appetite. A chest X-ray in the clinic showed bilateral hilar lymphadenopathy. The consultant did not discuss the diagnostic possibilities but arranged for a mediastinal biopsy (mediastinoscopy) which was performed by a thoracic surgeon 2 weeks ago. You are the FY2/ST1 for a firm that specializes in haematology and oncology. Your Consultant is away today, and Miss Barron has come back for the biopsy result. Unfortunately, this result states Hodgkin's disease as the diagnosis.

- Introduce yourself to the patient and establish good rapport. Ask if she wishes for anyone else to be present.
- Explore the patient's understanding of her symptoms and expectations/suspicions of what may be wrong.
- Ask her if she has heard of "Hodgkin's disease".
- Explain that Hodgkin's disease is a malignant proliferation of a certain type of cells which are involved in the immune system and called lymphoid cells. Prognosis depends upon sampling these in biopsy.
- The symptoms should be explained to the patient. Patients usually present with enlarged, painless nodes, and 25% have constitutional upset, e.g. fever, weight loss, night sweats, pruritus, and lethargy.
- Explain that there are doctors who specialize in this disease and that there are well-established treatments available. The tests which need to be done should be explained, including lymph node biopsy, blood tests, CT/MRI thorax, abdomen and pelvis.
- Tell her that you will refer her urgently to the clinical oncologist for further staging, which confers a treatment plan and prognosis.
- Explain the options for treatment: radiotherapy is for stages IA and IIB, chemotherapy for IIA with >3 areas involved to IVB. Complications of treatment include hypothyroidism, lung fibrosis, nausea, alopecia, infertility, infection and secondary malignancies.
- Ascertain how much the patient has taken in regarding the information.
- Avoid giving specific times regarding prognosis, and provide hope.
- Ask who is at home to support her. It is wise to inform the GP straight away for primary care support. Check that she is not driving home on her own.
- Offer an appropriate for follow-up.

Discussion

The prognosis of Hodgkin's disease depends on the histological type of disease. Lymphocyte-depleted has a poor prognosis, the others have good prognosis (nodular sclerosing, mixed cellularity, lymphocyte rich). It also depends on the staging of disease. The examiners may expect some understanding of the staging of disease. Stage I is confined to a singly lymph node region, II involves two or more regions on the same side of the diaphragm, III involves nodes on both sides of the diaphragm, and IV involves spread beyond the lymph nodes.

Recurrence of Breast Cancer

Breaking the bad news of a recurrence of breast cancer is a particular example of a 'bad news' scenario, but there are features of this scenario which reflect that palliative care is a speciality where patients can lose hope. It is therefore essential to elicit a patient's own specific fears, before addressing them.

*   Consider the understanding of illness, the expectations and concerns about the future.
*   Consider the effect of the illness physically and emotionally.
*   Provide medical reassurance (their symptoms will be identified promptly, controlled as far as possible and that they will remain comfortable).
*   Explore the social support (in terms of Doctors, Nurses, Church *etc.*)
*   Explore thoughts and fears about the future, dying, worries, plans made, plans not made.
*   Explore how the family is coping with the illness.

Scenario 7

Problem: Recurrence of breast cancer.
Patient name: Anna Fine (aged 48).
You are the FY2/ST1 on the medical ward to which Mrs. Fine, a 48-years-old lady, who was admitted a month ago with acute confusion secondary to mild hyponatraemia and severe hypercalcaemia. She was treated with intravenous fluids and pamidronate, and was then well orientated and lucid. She had a mastectomy for breast cancer 12 years ago followed by radiotherapy but no chemotherapy. She was last seen only 6 months ago in breast clinic, and reassured that everything was going well. She even underwent a mammogram at that stage, reported as "normal". She had been otherwise well on this admission, until she began to complain of increasing back and sacral pain. The House Officer requested X-rays which demonstrated changes consistent with bone metastases, confirmed on a later DEXA bone scan. Her chest X-ray also demonstrates a moderate effusion and cytology confirming malignant cells. Your task is to explain to Mrs. Fine that she has advanced metastatic cancer, and will be referred to the oncology team for further care that is likely to include chemotherapy and radiotherapy.

*   Introduce yourself to the patient and establish good rapport. Ask if she wishes for anyone else to be present.

- Explore the patient's understanding of the condition and expectations/suspicions of what may be wrong. Explore the understanding of her prognosis: She may have been convinced that she has been completely cured of cancer, but her recent admission cast may have doubt upon this.
- Explain the meaning of the tests and results (e.g. bone scan), and explain that the cancer has spread.
- Be prepared for the patient's response. She may demonstrate denial, before being angry towards the initial therapy given. The candidate should not criticise previous treatment, and even if he is not able to understand the logic of the initial therapy, he should still find some way of reassuring the patient about the appropriateness of initial therapy.
- Explain that it is difficult to predict what course the disease will take. However, prompt investigation of the cause of symptoms, and treatment for these symptoms and side-effects can be given. Inform the patient that you will comply with her wishes. Explain that you will listen to the patient's concerns and involve her in decision-making.
- Explain that her symptoms will be treated, but that the treatments have side effects, for example chemotherapy can cause nausea and vomiting, diarrhoea and constipation. The 'best treatment' may involve radiotherapy, chemotherapy or hormome therapy, either given alone or in any combination or order. Explain that the treatment will shrink the cancerous growths but it may be impossible to get rid of the cancer completely. Some patients go into complete clinical remission. The candidate should be prepared to discuss the pro's and con's of an optimistic versus a pessimistic approach in discussion.
- Outline that breast cancer treatment is carried out by different specialists who work together as a team, including psychologists, physiotherapists and also members of the appropriate religion. There are a number of sources of professional support. It is impossible to predict who will do well until the treatment is underway. The GP has responsibility for health care, and the District nurse can provide nursing care and organise for equipment. Macmillan nurses are available, who are specialists in pain and symptom control for people with cancer, and emotional and psychological support for carers. Palliative Care Teams have expertise in symptom control and support for patients and their carers. A social worker can assess what welfare benefits a patient

may be entitled to. They can arrange social services and other practical help. Explain that there are organisations such as Cancer BACUP can help, and these organisations usually have their own websites on the internet.

- Enquire further about any further expectations (for example, she may have booked a holiday abroad, in which case you would need to inform her about the possible need for assessment for a fitness to fly, and what local arrangements could be made at the place that she is flying to regarding local therapy for emergency such as cord compression).

- It is important to maintain a positive and optimistic outlook. Ask the patent if he has told other members of the family, or if he would like them to know of his decision. Ask if he has sorted things out at home. Is there any one else who would like to be contacted? Explore the patient's understanding of what refusal will entail. A good candidate should be able to agree a summary and plan of action with the subject. Summarise what has been discussed. Ask if he has any questions. Make appropriate follow-up arrangements.

- At some later date (guided by the scenario), it may be important to discuss resuscitation status.

Giving information: Explaining diagnosis, treatment and prognosis to competent patients.

Several scenarios used in this station involve simply explaining a diagnosis or treatment to competent patients. A definition of competence is provided in the next section C, and is not the focus of this section. A recent study by Kindelan and Kent (1987) in British general practice showed that patients placed the highest value on giving information about diagnosis, prognosis and causation of their condition. Doctors however greatly tend to underestimate their patients' desire for information about prognosis and causation, and overestimated their desire for information concerning treatment and drug therapy. Patients' individual information needs were not elicited.

You should explore the patient's perception of their condition and prepare them. Consider *"What have you been told about your condition?"* Find out what the patient wishes to know. Bear in mind that patients are often extremely well informed, and therefore if a patient presents with a condition that you may in actual fact know not that much about, for example alpha-thalassaemia trait, listen to the patient! You should show you are listening through body language, and encourage the patient to tell their 'story' too.

Do not forget that some scenarios will deliberately go beyond the scope of a junior doctor in a medical firm's professional experience or authority (e.g. a certain condition in a pregnant lady). In such cases, you will be expected to recognise the need to refer the matter.

Examples of suitable scenarios for this station include:

Giving Information About Diagnoses

This will not be a test of your knowledge of particular medical conditions, but rather an approach of how you impart information about these particular diagnoses. Some useful points to consider are:

1. Information must be related not only to the facts, but also the patient's ideas about the condition. *"Have you heard of this condition before?"*, *"Have you any ideas about this condition?"*, or *"What have you been told about this condition?"*
2. Use a logical sequence to explain the cause and effect of the condition in the context of the patient's symptoms (why it occurs, possible clinical problems, the likely natural history with/without treatment).
3. Be alert to beliefs, concerns and expectations. Establishing prior experience can help you understand any specific fears that may relate to it.
4. Tell one thing at a time and check the patient understands before moving onto the next.
5. Use simple language; translate any unavoidable medical terms and write them down.
6. Make your information direct. Repeat important information.
7. At the outset, show patients that you will write down the key words, use a simple diagram, and offer them aids to memory.
8. Acknowledge the possible need for further referral in diagnosis or management.
9. Encourage feedback, invite questions and check understanding. Be prepared to admit uncertainty if the patient asks you something you cannot answer.

A NEWLY DIAGNOSED DIABETIC

Scenario 8

Problem: Giving information (a new diagnosis of diabetes mellitus).
Patient name: Tim Scott (aged 19).
Tim Scott is a 19-year-old man who was referred to endocrinology outpatients after his fasting blood sugar was found to be elevated.

He had noticed some transient blurring of vision, which has subsequently thought to be due to osmotic changes in the lens as a result of blood sugar problems. His glucose tolerance test supported the diagnosis of diabetes mellitus. Please discuss with him.

- Introduce yourself to the patient and establish rapport. Establish the patient's understanding of his symptoms and their implication (e.g. *"You say that you have been passing water frequently, and felt thirsty. Have you had any thoughts about what these symptoms might be due to?"*), and expectations.
- Ask the patient whether he has had any experience of diabetes in other people (e.g. his father may have had diabetes and developed complications from that), and respond empathetically.
- Explain to the patient the basic mechanisms underlying the diabetes mellitus. You should then ask the patient if he would like any other information (e.g. *"Would you like to know about the tests I would like to do to confirm the diagnosis and the stage of your diabetes?"*).
- Explain the aims of treatment – to reduce the risk of complications: macrovascular (IHD, cerebrovascular and peripheral vascular disease) and microvascular (nephropathy, retinopathy and neuropathy). All of these can be reduced with optimal glycaemic control, but other important risk factors are smoking, alcohol excess, hypertension, hyperlipidaemia, and obesity.
- Emphasise the need for lifelong treatment.
- Explain the multidisciplinary approach: Diabetic specialist nurse, dietitician, chiropodist, ophthalmologist, and need for teamwork.
- Outline possible treatments: emphasise that dietary modification is a most important aspect of treatment, combined with exercise.
- Discuss the possibility of oral medication, if this is unsuccessful.
- Discuss the possibility of insulin therapy in the future. Address other risk factors, i.e. hypertension, hyperlipidaemia, smoking. Emphasise the need for compliance and regular review. Introduce him to the diabetic team.
- Point the patient in the direction of further information about diabetes. Arrange patient education sessions. State clearly that he will require follow-up for review of his diabetes to detect and treat any complications.
- It is important that you check the patient's understanding by asking, *"Can you now tell me what you understand about what I have explained to you in terms of the tests needed, the extent to which we should be able to control your illness, and the likely treatment?"*
- Arrange appropriate follow-up with the multidisciplinary team.

THYROTOXICOSIS

Scenario 9

Problem: Giving information (a new diagnosis of thyrotoxicosis)
Patient name: Annabel Smith (aged 29)
Annabel Smith is a 29-year-old lady who has lost 2 kg over the last few months, despite a good appetite and intake of food. She has become somewhat irritable at work, and slightly tremulous in both her hands which she thought was due to her anxiety. Blood tests confirms that she is hyperthyroid. Examination, apart from the tremor, is normal. Her pulse is 90, regular. You are the FY2/ST1 for Endocrinology. She has returned to clinic for the results of her blood tests.

- Introduce yourself and establish rapport.
- Explore her knowledge of the symptoms, and what they possibly meant. Ask what she understood by the need for the blood test. Explain the results of the blood test.
- Explain the nature of an overactive thyroid and the pathological consequences of an untreated disease. This might focus on current symptoms. When considering loss of weight, confirm that this weight is lost despite a good appetite and eating vast amounts. Advise about some of the manifestations of thyrotoxicosis can take, e.g. skin (warm and sweaty due to vasodilatation), cardiovascular (tachycardia, with increased cardiac output due to increased peripheral oxygen utilisation and increased cardiac contractility, atrial fibrillation, mitral valve prolapse), ocular, gastrointestinal (weight loss due to increased basal metabolic rare, increased gut motility with associated diarrhoea and malabsorption), locomotor, neurological (emotional lability, insomnia, irritability, anxiety, proximal muscle weakness, tremor) and reproductive system.
- If a smoker, the patient is at greater risk of eye disease, and so therefore should be asked if there is any noticeable bulging of the eyes or double vision. Discuss the treatment options.
- Explain that her symptoms will resolve with treatment, but may take months to resolve completely. For medical therapy, warn of the potential side-effects, especially agranulocytosis. Thus, must be given both verbally and in writing. Establish her last menstrual period, wishes for pregnancy and if she has any children.
- Establish the need for regular review.
- Point the patient in the direction of further information about thyroid disease. Arrange patient education sessions.

- It is important again that you check the patient's understanding by asking, *"Can you now tell me what you understand about what I have explained to you in terms of the tests needed, the extent to which we should be able to control your illness, and the likely treatment?"*.

Giving Information About Treatments

Encouraging a patient to adopt a treatment requires that the patient understands the risks and benefits of that treatment, and it is necessary before consent for a treatment can be acquired. For any procedure, treatment or operation, the doctor needs to explain the nature of the procedure. The doctor must exercise sensitivity to patient's fears, and it is a legal requirement to inform the patient of risks, benefits and alternative treatments which demonstrate both good practice and avoidance of negligence. Doctors may be faced with litigation when patients understand the benefits of the treatment, but do not understand the risks of the procedures that they are undergoing. The duty of the doctor is to provide this information frankly to the patient. The nature by which consent is obtained is not only fundamental to the doctor/patient relationship, but is also a key way to which patient autonomy is respected. In order to obtain consent, the doctor discloses information to a patient who is legally competent. A sensible approach in which to do this is suggested below:

1. Explain the reasons for considering the treatment (Is the treatment critical, essential, elective or discretionary).
2. Give the patient a chance to react to the need for treatment.
3. Consider whether there are any likely benefits of treatment according to currently accepted medical practice, but be aware of overwhelming patients with outcomes of studies.
4. Explain what the treatment will need for the patient in terms of the frequency of dosing, the duration of therapy, any special instructions, how long the treatment will take.
5. Any requirement for any specific monitoring, e.g. blood monitoring.
6. The common, as well as uncommon, side effects and any discomfort of treatment.
7. Suggest any alternative to treatment. You should be offering suport, i.e. making supportive statements but also giving practical advice such as details of counselling services and appropriate literature.
8. How soon knowledge about the effects of the proposed intervention will be made available.

9. Give ample opportunity for questions.

10. Keep it short and simple.

11. Finally seek consent. Remember that you are explaining the reason for a treatment and not telling your patient that they must have it. Following your explanation, you should seek informed consent to proceed.

12. For negotiating a management plan, clarify the task, explore concerns and explanations, keep to a framework, share management options *"It might help if..."*, *"I wonder if..."* etc.

13. Show respect for the patient's autonomy; do not behave coercively.

14. Invite the patient to ask any questions.

Studies have consistently shown that between 10 and 90% of patients prescribed drugs by their doctors (with an average of 50%) do not take their medication at all or take it incorrectly. Walton et al (1980) estimated the cost of wasted drugs per year in the UK is of the order of £300 million. In the scenario, you should specifically ask how the patient is with regard to symptoms. Ask any patient who appears not to be compliant with his medical regimen whether he has not been taking his medication, and, if so, enquire why, e.g. side-effects, forgetfulness, inability to get hold of the tablets, poor information about how to get the tablets, the purpose of taking the mediction, unpleasant side-effects. Consider alternative simplified drug regimens. Consider arranging with the health visitor and your Consultant directly observed therapy where ingestion of every dose is witnessed. Patient recall is increased by categorisation, signposting, summarising, repetition, clarity and use of diagrams (Ley, 1988).

HORMONE REPLACEMENT THERAPY (HRT)

Scenario 10

Problem: Commencing treatment (hormone replacement therapy)

Patient name: Laura Wood (aged 57)

Laura Wood is a 57-year-old lady who has been experiencing the symptoms of the menopause. She has read about HRT, and has considered it as a treatment for her troubling symptoms. You are the FY2/ST1 for General Medicine. Please discuss with her HRT as an option, and advise accordingly.

• Introduce yourself to the patient.

• Establish the patient's perception of her symptoms.

• Explain the concept of HRT and explore the patient's beliefs and concerns about it. Establish then the patients's expectations.

- Explain the potential benefits: HRT is an effective means of controlling the vasomotor and genital symptoms associated with the menopause. It prevents osteoporosis. There is a possible decrease in the risk of ischaemic heart disease, but the evidence is unlear. It decreases the risk of uterine carcinoma and possibly colonic carcinoma.
- Explain the likely course of treatment, and related issues. Current recommendations are to stop HRT after 5-10 years of treatment, although the increased risk of breast cancer attributable to HRT is not thought to begin until around 50 years of age. Oestrogen-only HRT tablets or patches may be used in hysterectomized patients, but preparations associated with progesterone should otherwise be used to limit endometrial hyperplasia and the risk of endometrial malignancy. Amenorrhoea need not be awaited before starting HRT. Cyclical (sequential) hormone regimens are generally used in perimenopausal women and continuous combined regimens in postmenopausal women. Continuous combined treatment is associated with a high risk of irregular bleeding in perimenopausal women but should not cause induced bleeding in postmenopausal women. Postmenopausal bleeding generally necessitates investigation to exclude endometrial malignancy.
- Describe briefly the evidence concerning the risks associated with hormone replacement therapy. HRT increases the relative risk of venous thromboembolism, but again the absolute risk is low, and possibly offset by the favourable effects of HRT on lipid profiles and potential cardiovascular benefit. Studies are inconclusive as to whether HRT induces (or even increases) cardiovascular risk. There is no current evidence to support the use of HRT in either the primary or secondary prevention of coronary heart disease, and no evidence that HRT reduces stroke risk. A systematic review and meta-analysis has suggested that HRT may have a role in reducing dementia and cognitive decline. HRT does not cause weight gain. Discuss alternatives to HRT, e.g. clonidine for hot flushes, evening primrose oil, topical oestrogens.
- Explain the need for annual mammograms and self-examination. Explain that HRT will result in her continuing to have regular withdrawal bleeds that she may find troublesome. Ultimately the decision is the patient's, and she needs to weigh up the theoretical risks and inconvenience against her troublesome symptoms. Ensure that she understands all the issues. Finally ask if she has any questions.

WARFARIN

Scenario 11

Problem: Commencing treatment (warfarin)

Patient name: Jennifer Salmon (aged 34)

Jennifer Salmon is a 34-year-old lady who has recently undergo a mitral valve replacement. She was diagnosed both clinically and echocardiographically with severe mitral stenosis. She is about to be discharged having undergone the replacement, but your Consultant would like you to discuss with her the need for anticoagulation with warfarin. She has made it known to the senior CCU nurses that she and her husband had been wishing to try for a family by the end of the year. You are the FY2/ST1 for Cardiology. Please discuss with her the need for warfarin treatment, and any concerns she may have.

- Introduce yourself and establish rapport. Explore the patient's perception of her condition, and what she has been told about it in the past. Ask about her beliefs, concerns and expectations of her valve replacement.
- Ascertain what she knows about aspects of the treatment plan, including knowledge of warfarin.
- Some people only have heard of warfarin in the context of "rat poison". Explain that blood clots normally form to stop bleeding that has occurred as a result of injury to the tissues. Explain that the clotting process is complicated, but sometimes a blood clot can form abnormally within blood vessels and dislodge such that blood supply to a vital organ such as the heart, brain or lungs is impeded (thromboembolism).
- State that 'loading' with warfarin is necessary, and explain what this involves.
- Consider the need for treatment and the precautions needed. It is used for abnormal blood clots in conditions with increased risk (e.g. prosthetic heart valves, atrial fibrillation), and prevention of PE's and DVT'S. Consider all the drug history and lifestyle factors that would impact upon taking warfarin, i.e. the patient should be warned to take extra care when participating in physical activities because minor injury can result in bleeding. Also, warfarin inhibits vitamin K, therefore eating large amounts of green vegetables can reduce the effect of warfarin and should be avoided. Large amounts of alcohol can also increase the effect of warfarin.
- The candidate should be able to give adequate information to the patient about how to take the treatment and what precautions to

observe, in terms suitable for a patient to understand. If there is any bruising, bleeding, dark stools, dark urine, or fever, then a Doctor should be seen.

- Warn about common side effects including easy bruising, rash, jaundice, alopecia, skin necrosis, liver disorders, pancreatitis and nause and vomiting. OCP and rifampicin can reduce the effect of warfarin.
- The need to monitor the INR should be explained, as too much anti-coagulation can adversely increase the risk of bleeding. If there are any problems with ongoing bleeding, the patient should seek medical attention immediately. Warfarin is the long-term anticoagulant of choice in non-pregnant patients, but its great disadvantage in pregnancy is that it freely crosses the placental barrier because of its low molecular weight and can harm the fetus.
- Explain the need to carry an anticoagulation book, and the need to tell the dentist/other doctors about treatment.
- Ask for any further questions, and make appropriate follow-up arrangements.

Discussion

The anticoagulant effect of warfarin is mediated by inhibition of the vitamin K-dependent gamma-carboxylation of coagulation factors II, VII, IX and X and proteins C and S. The laboratory test most commonly used to measure the effects of warfarin is the prothromnin time. Loading is necessary because, in the first few days, factor VII is depressed, but five days are needed before factors II, IX and X are suppressed.

Adverse fetal effects from warfarin may result from the teratogenicity of the drug and its propensity to cause bleeding in the fetus. Warfarin should also not be used in pregnancy, peptic ulcer or uncontrolled high blood pressure. Difficult decisions arise when patients are on long-term warfarin therapy because of prosthetic valves or recurrent pulmonary embolism become pregant. Any changeover to low molecular weight heparins (LMWH) must be carried out with care and under the multidisciplinary care of the obstetrician and the haematologist. Warfarin crosses the placenta with a risk of placental or fetal haemorrhage. Warfarin therapy is contraindicated in the first trimester because of its association with fetal epiphyseal haemorrhage. In the second and third trimesters, warfarin may cause fetal atrophy, microcephaly, optic atrophy, spasticity, and mental retardation. However, warfarin is safe during breastfeeding. In the initial treatment of a DVT, LMWH which does not cross the placenta may be administered subcutaneously according to body weight. LMWH is not contraindicated in breast-feeding women.

STATINS

Scenario 12

Problem: Commencing treatment (a statin)
Patient name: Luke Dunn (aged 48)
Luke Dunn is a 48-year-old who, despite a good BMI, has a consistently high cholesterol. He had an uncomplicated myocardial infarction 4 years' ago, but made an excellent recovery. Recent investigations showed: plasma cholesterol 7.2 mmol/l, LDL-cholesterol 4.9 mmol/l, HDL-cholesterol 1.1 mmol/l and triglycerides 1.4 mmol/l. He is a life-long non-smoker, and his diet has been good. Despite dietary advice, his cholesterol remained high. You are the FY2/ST1 for General Medicine in clinic. Please discuss with him the possibility of commencing the statin simvastatin.

- Introduce yourself and establish rapport.
- Explore his knowledge of his condition, and the relevance of cholesterol. Explore briefly relevant risk factors: i.e. cardiovascular history, diabetes history, hypertension history, family history of ischaemic heart disease, alcohol, smoking, dietary and exercise history, concerns of patient.
- Explain the need for reducing cholesterol in terms of the future, e.g. heart attacks, stroke. There is 'bad' cholesterol (LDL) and 'good' cholesterol (HDL). Simvastatin decreases the production of LDL cholesterol (and total cholesterol) by competitively blocking the action of the enzyme in the liver that is responsible for its synthesis (HMG-CoA reductase).
- Explain that, as the body produces most cholesterol at night, statins are generally more effective at night.
- Explain the likely benefits of the therapy (cause regression of coronary atheromatous plaques, may ameliorate peripheral vascular as well as coronary artery disease, slightly reduce the risk of stroke), and explain what the treatment will mean for the patient in terms of frequency of dosing, the duration of therapy, any special instructions (e.g. the tablet should be taken with meals), any requirements for blood monitoring.
- Advise that excessive amounts of alcohol should not be taken, and grapefruit juice should ideally be avoided in excess because it can increase the amount of medicine in the blood.

- The patient should see the doctor if there is pain or tenderness in the muscles, particularly if accompanied by symptoms of generally feeling unwell. Blood tests should be monitored before treatment (e.g. LFTs), and during it. It should be used with caution in the elderly and in patients with hypothyroidism, or history of liver disease. It should not be used in pregnancy.
- Explain the side effects which are common or serious, and explain how the side effects weigh up against the benefits. These side effects are abdominal pain, constipation, flatulence, headache, dizziness, pins and needles, indigestion, nausea and vomiting, anaemia, liver disorders, hair loss and muscle disorders.
- Common medications that increase side effects are amiodarone, verapamil, diltiazem, itraconazole, and erythromycin. Explain what should be done when a side effect occurs.
- Give ample opportunity to react to the information, and ask for questions. Seek consent to proceed. Explain that other health professionals may be involved, such as dietitians. Arrange appropriate further information if necessary, and follow-up.

STEROIDS

Scenario 13

Problem: Commencing treatment (steroids for rheumatoid disease)
Patient name: Sarah Collins (aged 37)
You are the Rheumatology FY2/ST1 in clinic in outpatients. You have just discussed the case of Mrs. Collins, a 37-year-old woman, with your consultant who feels that she should start steroids. She has had rheumatoid disease for three years. So far, her main symptoms have been stiff hands, and she required NSAIDs to control her symptoms. However, over the last few months, she has worsening disease, and your team decision is that she should start prednisolone 30 mg od to control her symptoms. Please discuss with her.

- Polite introduction and establish rapport.
- Establish the patient's understanding of her disease and the need for steroids.
- Try to get some feel of the impact of the disease on her life, including the use of her hands (eating, washing) and other aspects of a routine functional assessment (for example, managing stairs, using a telephone, cooking, shopping).
- Explain that corticosteroids are hormones produced naturally by the adrenal glands which have important functions including the

control of inflammatory responses. Explain that prednisolone is a synthetic corticosteroid that is used to increase inflammation in various diseases.

- Explain the need for steroids to prevent attacks and the consequences of poorly controlled disease. Explain that steroids should be taken after food. A steroid card will be needed if prednisolone taken for more than 3 weeks, which contains details of prescriber, the type of steroid, dose taken and duration of treatment. There will also be a need for medic alert bracelet and a hydrocortisone pack (for parenteral self-administration if she's unable to take oral medication). If there is any illness, trauma or surgery, the steroid dose may need to be temporarily increased.

- A good candidate should be able to explore the impact of disease on the patient's daily activities and quality of life, and explain the need for further treatment and advantages of using steroids.

- Warn that the steroids should also not stopped suddenly, as long-term use suppresses the natural production of steroids by the adrenal glands. She should therefore not miss a dose. There may be increased susceptibility to infections.

- Common side-effects are difficulty in sleeping, depression, skin thinning, weight gain, irregular menstrual cycle, osteoporosis, diabetes, acne, increased susceptibility to infection, high blood pressure.

- Your role in discussing the adverse effects should not be confined to reeling off a long list of adverse effects but rather to have a balanced discussion. Remember you are automatically making (or should be making) risk-benefit calculations in your everyday jobs when considering investigations and treatments.

- She may mention *weight gain*. You can say, "Yes, these steroids can cause weight gain and they do this not only by causing the retention of fluid but also by increasing appetite. So knowing this you can plan ahead and try to eat more sensibly with smaller portion sizes (although offer her a dietitian appointment to help her plan the strategy more effectively). She could also exercise more frequently. By saying this, you are offering back some control of the situation.

- She might have heard that steroids will *thin her bones*. Again explain that this is a possibility but that as a young person she is likely to have strong bones to begin with. Reassure her that you will be ordering a (DEXA) scan that will monitor her "bone strength". Explain that there are effective treatments she can take that will prevent bone loss and that exercise can also help.

- "What about the *blood pressure* doctor?". Steroids tend to cause retention of water and this may cause an increase in blood pressure. Reassure that regular measurements of blood pressure can be taken, and that treatments are available to counter the rise in blood pressure.
- "What about the *blood sugar* doctor?". Corticosteroids do not precipitate high blood glucose (say "sugar" instead of glucose) in everyone who takes the tablets. Some people are more susceptible especially if there is a family history of diabetes and if they are overweight. Again, there are effective ways of monitoring for this and treating if ncessary.
- State that these will be minimised by ensuring her dose is tailored to her condition. Osteoporosis can be minimised by concomitant bisphosphonate therapy. The effects of steroids are reduced by antiepileptics, rifampicin, barbiturates and aminoglutethimide. When taken with NSAIDs, there is an increased effect of adverse effects on the gut. Ensure that the patient understands what has been said and ask if she has any questions.
- It is very important to ask the occupation of the patient in certain situations. If you are not given this information, it is a good idea to ask. If the person has never had chickenpox, close personal contact should be avoided. If exposed, the patient should see his/her doctor urgently, as these diseases can be threatening. This would be especially important if, for example, she was working as a nanny.
- Summarise what has been discussed. Arrange appropriate follow-up.

SURGICAL TREATMENTS FOR MEDICAL DISORDERS

Benefit and risk of a CABG in a patient with triple vessel disease.

Scenario 14

Problem: Proposing treatment (coronary artery bypass graft)
Patient name: Andrew Foster (aged 53)
Andrew Foster, a 53-year-old man, was admitted with his third episode of chest pain at rest this year. This pain was cardiac sounding in history, and the ECG demonstrated dynamic changes. His troponin was elevated 12 hours after the onset of the pain. A coronary angiogram was arranged on this admission, which demonstrated

multiple narrowings in the coronary circulation. He had hoped that these vessels would be amenable to stenting, but the Cardiology Consultant on review of the angiogram data feels that he ought to be referred to Cardiac Surgery. You are the FY2/ST1 for Cardiology. Please discuss the possibility of coronary artery bypass grafting as an option for him.

- Introduce yourself and establish good rapport.
- Establish the patient's beliefs and concerns of understanding the disease, its severity and likely expectations. Ask about smoking behaviour, but avoid being judgemental about his smoking.
- Explain the results of the recent angiogram. Establish the patient's understanding and expectations of possible treatment options. Explain the need for the procedure, e.g. none of the vessels are amenable to stenting.
- Explain that coronary artery bypass graft (CABG) surgery, sometimes just called bypass, is the procedure that enables a blocked area of the coronary artery to be bypassed so that blood flow is not hindered. During bypass surgery, a healthy artery or vein is taken from the leg, arm or chest and transferred to the outside of the heart. The new healthy artery or vein then carries the oxygenated blood around the blockage in the coronary artery. Explain why CABG surgery is performed, i.e. to relieve symptoms of coronary artery disease, reduce the possibility of more heart problems, and to prolong life.
- As with seeking consent for any procedure, explain explicitly that there are complications and risks associated with CABG procedures. Complications associated with coronary artery bypass grafting may include stroke, damage to the aorta, the potential damaging effect of emboli, bleeding, vein graft occlusion or stenosis, arrhythmias, acute myocardial infarction, angina, or death. After the procedure, the patient spends 5-7 days in hospital. After a day in the ICU, the patient normally moves to a hospital wound, and the incision heals. Recovery from any surgery varies for each patient. Most patients start feeling better within 4-6 weeks. It is important in the post-operative phase to follow doctor's instructions and to report any problems (abnormal pain, signs of infection) immediately.
- Arrange for the patient to meet the surgical team, and arrange appropriate follow-up.

RENAL TRANSPLANT

Scenario 15

Problem: Proposing treatment (renal transplant)
Patient name: Elaine Cook (aged 58)

Elaine Cook is a 58-year-old lady who has polycystic kidney disease. Four years ago, she commenced continuous ambulatory peritoneal dialysis, but her renal function has remained poor. She now has end-stage renal failure, and requires further support. Haemodialysis has previously failed. You are the renal SHO. Mrs. Cook would like to discuss with you the possibility of a renal transplant, and what practicalities will be involved.

- Introduce yourself to the patient and establish rapport.
- Explain the patient's understanding of the condition requiring renal transplant. A candidate should be able to explain to the patient that the kidneys are not working and why. They should be able to explain the significance of this and what would happen if left untreated. This should be done in an empathetic manner in terms the patient would be able to understand, avoiding technical terms.
- The candidate should be able to ascertain the current level of functioning and quality of life of the patient in a sensitive way, to determine the appropriateness of dialysis (See Station 1 for a description of types of dialysis).
- Discuss the reasons for not coping with other renal replacement therapy, e.g. CAPD.
- Explore the patient's expectations of CAPD and transplantation. Explain that he has endstage renal failure and requires support. If he is not managing CAPD, renal transplantation is the only alternative, as haemodialysis has previously failed.
- Explain the practicalities of obtaining a transplant: Cadaveric vs. live donor, the waiting list is long, the length of wait for transplant depends on finding an acceptable HLA match, explain the complications of transplant, i.e. short-term (surgical risks), medium term (immunosupression and risk of rejection) and long-term (immunosuppression – secondary malignancy and infection; recurrent renal failure – 5-year graft survival).
- Ensure the patient understands what has been said. Ask if he has any questions. Arrange a follow-up.

Lifestyle Adjustments

To illustrate two discussions of lifestyle, scenarios 17 and 18 tackle the issues of smoking cessation and lifestyle adjustments following a MI respectively.

SMOKING CESSATION

Scenario 16

Problem: Smoking cessation

Patient name: Ken Wood (aged 59)

Ken Wood is a 59-year-old bar manager who has been smoking 10 cigarettes a day for the last 20 years. His previous medical history is otherwise unremarkable. His wife has mentioned to you that he would like to give up smoking, and he has attended clinic today to discuss this with you. You are the FY2/ST1 for General Medicine.

- Introduce yourself and establish rapport.
- Explore his knowledge of the effects of smoking on health. Ask about current smoking status. Explain that smoking cessation reduces the risk of many diseases, including stroke, coronary artery disease, peripheral vascular disease, COPD, cancers of the lung, mouth, throat, larynx, oesophagus, pancreas, bladder, and peptic ulcer disease (and in women ca of cervix and complications of pregnancy).
- Explain also the risk of smoking to others; that adults are at risk of developing heart and lung disease from passive smoking.
- Emphasise that there are social and cosmetic benefits from stopping smoking.
- Ask whether she has been given any "quitting smoking" leaflets.
- Explain symptoms of nicotine withdrawal (such as tremor and nausea). Inform about the benefits of stopping smoking. Involve family and friends. Nicorette products and 'zyban' (buproprion) may help to avoid these withdrawal symptoms, but consider contraindications include hepatic cirrhosis, seizure, CNS tumours, EtOH withdrawal, benzodiazepine withdrawal.
- Advise the patient to aim to stop completely rather than cut down. Ask your patient if he/she really wants to stop smoking and if he/she would be prepared to stop now or within the next few weeks.
- Say that it may be useful to get rid of all ashtrays, lighters and cigarette holders *etc.*
- Find out whether previous attempts have been made, and what measures helped/hindered.
- Discuss ways of assisting, including setting a date and stopping completely, enlisting the help of family and friends, enlisting the help of health promotion services, and amfebutamone.
- Watch out for relapse. Amfebutamone is a possible medication. Advise the patient that he has access to specialist counsellors and/

or psychotherapists. Make appropriate follow-up arrangements.
Lifestyle adjustments after an uncomplicated acute myocardial infarction

Scenario 17

Problem: Lifestyle adjustments after an uncomplicated acute MI
Patient name: Chris Goddard (aged 48)
Chris Goddard is a 48-year-old computer programmer who has just sustained an uncomplicated anterior myocardial infarct. He was successfully thrombolysed, with complete resolution of his ST changes. You are the FY2/ST1 for Cardiology. He smokes about four cigarettes a day, and drinks around ten pints of beer a week. He is about to be discharged. He has been happily married for 15 years. He is keen to discuss with you the lifestyle adjustments that will be necessary. Please discuss with him, and advise accordingly.

- Introduce yourself and establish rapport.
- Explore his knowledge of the term "heart attack". Explain in simple language what a heart attack is, i.e. it is caused by a blockage of a blood vessel that supplies blood to the heart, but reassure him that he has the correct and best treatment available and that he is on the road back to health. Reassure him that many people do well after a heart attack and that the reason for the tablets is to offer some prevention from a second attack.
- A patient's specific concerns can be overlooked when giving advice after a myocardial infarction (e.g. a flight to somewhere abroad in a month's time), because there are usually standard areas that are usually discussed. Patients do not always voice their concerns.
- Explain the need for tablets. Explain that he should change his lifestyle, and tackle exercise, smoking and weight. Activity may be restricted by an overprotective spouse. Returning to work depends on the type of work and completeness of recovery. With less physical jobs, 4-6 weeks off work is advisable. With physical jobs, defer the return to work until after stress testing. Anxiety is common. Most exercise programmes recommend at least three types of aerobic exercise (e.g. brisk walking, jogging, swimming, aerobics classes). Point out that regular exercise has benefits for preventing further heart attacks and encourage him to go for walks.
- Speak that you will speak to the cardiac rehabilitation nurse who will arrange rehabilitation programmes. Offer pamphlets from the rehabilitation team and the British Heart Foundation.

- Say that he should not drive for a month and that he can have sexual intercourse only after increasing his activity level, say to going up briskly two flights of stairs. Explain the need for moderate amounts of alcohol at maximum (e.g. around 21 units/week), as heavy drinking can increase the patient's weight and 'weaken' the heart muscle.
- Ask if he has any questions. Offer appropriate follow-up.

INFORMED CONSENT

This section takes further some of the issues discussed in the previous last section, namely, one aspect of medical practice is the approach a doctor takes to obtain consent from a patient regarding investigation and treatment for a given condition. Consent is only valid when the individual is competent (or in legal terms has "capacity"). A patient is not incompetent because they act against their best wishes. For consent to treatment to be valid, the patient must be legally competent to give consent, the patient must have sufficient information to make a choice, consent must be given freely.

A competent patient can refuse any, even life-saving, treatment. For example, in the case of Jehovah's witnesses, you may ask to explain the benefits of blood transfusion, but you should allow the patient to explain religious beliefs with respect. The use of components such as albumin, immunoglobulins and haemophilia preparations may be allowed on an individual basis. For normal blood transfusions, non-haemolytic febrile transfusion reactions may occur, acute haemolytic transfusion reactions, bacterial and viral contamination, wrong blood group, iron overload, and circulatory overload (see "Better Blood Transfusion", 1998). Capacity is not a global term but is specific to each decision, i.e. a patient may be competent to make a will but at the same time incompetent to consent to treatment. A clinician does not have to prove beyond all reasonable doubt that a patient has capacity, only that the balance of probability favours capacity. The critical stages in assessing capacity are: Comprehension and retention of information needed to make a decision, ability to believe the information, ability to weigh the information, consider the degree and severity of risk to the patient, the risk to benefit ratio of the treatment, the patient's mental state, and ability make the decision. Patients under 16 years of age can consent to treatment if they are deemed 'Gillick competent', i.e. are deemed mature enough to understand the implications of their actions.

A patient has a right therefore to refuse treatment ordinarily, but not where there is an issue of public health. Section 37 of the Public Health Act magistrates orders to allow compulsory treatment olf a patient with notifiable disease. This is almost never needed if appropriate negotiation with the patient is undertaken.

CONSENT AND THE LAW

This PACES station is **not** intended as a test of medicolegal issues, but obviously candidates need to be roughly aware of them. The main issues candidates are expected to know about are expressed consent (consent either oral or in writing), statutory requirements (where law requires particular consent for particular treatment), and implied consent. At present, consent forms are used if a patient is exposed to any invasive procedure. After providing the patient with adequate information about the procedure, as well as risks and benefits, doctors should document what has been said on the consent form. The patient then reads the consent form with the doctor and signs accordingly. The consent form provides a mechanism to ensure that consent is obtained, and also to communicate the fact to other members of the health team. Consent forms are not, themselves, absolute proof that valid consent was obtained to the treatment specified on the form. These tasks may be delegated to a person who is suitably trained and qualified, with appropriate knowledge.

From a legal point of view, lack of consent engages two key aspects:
- *Battery/assault:* Non-fatal offences against the person. A procedure or treatment that is performed without consent.
- *Negligence:* Harm caused by a doctor acting outside accepted medical opinion or practice (the Bolam principle). If a patient does not receive certain relevant information when consented for a procedure, a doctor may be found negligent. It is advisable to tell the patient of all potential serious complications and those with an incidence of at least 1%.

Situations Where Consent is not Possible

A doctor, by acting in the patient's best interests, can treat a patient against their will under common law. The "*doctrine of necessity*", which underpins the treatment of patients lacking capacity, is made up of the necessity to act and the action being in the best interests of the patient, where a patient is unable to give the necessary consent required for treatment. If relatives are available for discussion, they should be informed rather than opinions canvassed. It is advisable that they remain well informed. The patient has the right to be free from discrimination, have privacy, have confidentiality of personal health information with information disclosed only to the nominated next of kin, liberty (i.e. free from interventions that inhibit liberty), and continue dignity (according to social and cultural views). Legally, when consent is not available and there is no advanced directive, the responsibility for emergency operations rests with the consultant in charge particularly if the team believes this is in the patient's best interests.

An advance directive is that a person can anticipate losing the mental capacity to decide or communication how she wishes to be treated by drawing up a formal advance statement of her values and preferences or by naming a person who can be consulted. Whilst advance directives may not always be legally binding or unambiguous, it will be increasingly unwise to ignore these directives, and they can be helpful to clinicians. If there is disagreement, a second opinion can be arranged. Views about the patient's preferences given by a third party who may have more knowledge of the patient should be taken into account. There are different types of advance directive.

If mental impairment is suspected, a psychiatrist may be consulted to make the diagnosis. Medical staff may be required to make decisions which are deemed to be in the best interests of the patient.

Be aware of the meaning of the following specific terms used in relation to consent:

- Proxy consent: A relative cannot consent on behalf of an incompetent patient.
- Implied consent: By going to hospital a patient should expect a nurse to take their blood pressure and therefore consent for this procedure should not necessarily be sought.
- Emergency consent: Where consent cannot be obtained, medical treatment can be provided to anyone who needs it.
- Advanced directives or living wills: a patient makes a choice on their future medical care before they become incompetent. A doctor that treats a patient in the face of an advanced directive could be liable in battery.
- Power of attorney: A patient nominates a person (usually a relative) whilst competent to make decisions on their behalf if they were to become incompetent. However, this does not include medical

management decisions. With an increasingly elderly population, there is growing need for people to delegate control of financial and legal affairs to others close to them. A power of attorney is a legal document enabling this to be done, allowing, for instance, someone to sign cheques and letters on another's behalf if he or she were going abroad for some time; or if you became seriously ill, or were mentally incapacitated, business and personal interests could be looked after.

- Ward of court: A doctor may apply to a judge to make medical decisions on behalf of the patient. This is advisable if it is not clear what the correct course of management should be and there is opposition from colleagues or relatives against the intended treatment.

MENTAL HEALTH ACT

The **Mental Health Act** [1983] (but please note **Mental Health Act** [2007]) can be used to treat psychiatric illness in non-consenting patients. This may be useful in patients who present with deliberate self-harm either due to a temporary or permanent illness. Factors suggesting suicidal intent include act in isolation, precautions to avoid discovery, preparation made in anticipation of death, active preparation for the event, leaving a suicide note; consider the events preceding the act, concomitant psychiatric illness, personal and family history, coping resources and the risk of suicide (male, < 19, > 45, separate, living alone, chronic physical health, problems with alcohol and drugs, psychiatric disorder including depression, schizophrenia and alcoholism). They can be detained/restrained for varying periods, depending on the clause of the Act, and can be given treatment, but only for their mental illness, which is deemed in the best interests for themselves or the public.

Section 5(2): Emergency Doctor's Holding Power

Applied by one physician or an *inpatient* to enable a psychiatric assessment to be made. 72 hours duration. Good practice to convert this to a Section 2.

Section 2: Admission for Assessment Order

Applied by two written medical recommendations (usually a psychiatrist and a GP) and an aproved social worker or relative, on a patient *in the community*. 28 days duration. May be converted to a Section 3. The patient has a right of appeal to a tribunal within 14 days of detention.

Section 3: Admission for Treatment Order

Applied as in a Section 2 on a patient already diagnosed with a mental disorder. 3 months duration and then reviewed.

Section 4: Emergency Admission to Hospital Order

Applied by one doctor (usually a GP) and an approved social worker or relative. Urgent necessity is demonstrable. May be converted to a Section 2 or 3.

MENTAL CAPACITY ACT [2005]

This is an Act of the UK that came into force in April 2007. It applies to everyone over the age of 16 in England and Wales. Its primary purpose is to provide a legal framework for acting and making decisions on behalf of individuals who lack the capacity to make particular decisions for themselves The five principles are outlined in the Section 1 of the Act. It aims to protect people who lack capacity to make particular decisions, but also to maximise their ability to make decisions, or to participate in decision-making, as far as they are able to do so.

1. A person must be assumed to have capacity unless it is established that they lack capacity.
2. A person is not to be treated as unable to make a decision unless all practicable steps to help him to do so have been taken without success.
3. A person is not to be treated as unable to make a decision merely because he makes an unwise decision.
4. An act done, or decision made, under this Act for or on behalf of a person who lacks capacity must be done, or made, in his best interests.
5. Before the act is done, or the decision is made, regard must be had to whether the purpose for which it is needed can be as effectively achieved in a way that is less restrictive of the person's rights and freedom of action.

Please note that this Act was amended by the **Mental Health Act [2007]** in July 2007.

Examples of common 'consent' scenarios:

ACQUIRING CONSENT FOR AUTOPSY

Scenario 18

Problem: Acquiring consent for autopsy

Relative name: Winnifred Thomas, wife of the patient Edward Thomas (aged 84)

Edward Thomas, 84, was admitted yesterday with acute confusion. He was tachypnoeic with a respiratory rate of 30/minute, and cyanosed. His urea was 13 mmol/l, but his C-reactive protein was < 8 g/l. He was admitted to ITU, where an initial chest X-ray was unremarkable. At 2 am this morning, he died suddenly. He had been thought to have been suffering from a pneumonia, but this cause of death was not certain. You are the ITU SHO. Your objective is to inform his wife of his sudden death, and to acquire consent for an autopsy if appropriate.

The principles of the breaking of bad news are outlined above.

- Ensure that you will not be disturbed. In real life, you will also ensure that you are appropriately dressed (e.g. not in blood-stained theatre clothes).
- Introduce yourself to the patient and establish rapport. Ask her if she would like anyone else present at this point.
- You must break the news about her father's death early on. You must provide the necessary background for the grave news, e.g. the seriousness of the pneumonia, the expectation of her father's illness. Explain that attempts were made to contact her, but he deteriorated suddenly and resuscitation was attempted. Avoid making assumptions about the direct causes of any incident (e.g. a drink-driver going off a road into the river) if there is a risk of being judgmental. Mention that the death was swift and painless. Avoid euphemisms for the death. Be prepared for the emotional response, and be prepared to repeat information patiently.
- Tell her how sorry you and all the staff who have looked after him are.
- Check if the relative has come alone or is with others – if possible, know who they are at least in general (the family).
- If the relative would like to go on, explain that the doctors looking after her father would like to know exactly what caused the sudden deterioration. This can be done by performing a postmortem examination. Ask if she knows if the patient himself had any known objection towards a post mortem before his illness.

- The relatives need a general understanding of the procedure. The pathologist first carries out an external examination of the body, before proceeding to an internal examination. Reassure her that the body will not be disfigured.
- Explain that she will be asked to sign a consent form.
- Tell her that she can obtain the results of the post mortem as the results are sent to thhe consultant looking after her father, and she can arrange an appointment with him to have the findings explained. Explain that the body can be viewed by relatives after the post mortem if necessary.
- Ask if she has any questions. Ask if she would like to contact someone. Ascertain how much emotional support the subject has in dealing with the bereavement.
- If agreed, the medical certificate is issued before the post-mortem so that the funeral arrangements can be made. Express condolence and appreciate that the subject has maintained a major loss.
- Allow the subject to speak and ask questions which should be answered with sensitivity and empathy. Make follow-up arrangements to speak to her or other members of the family again. Offer to put them in touch with the transplant coordinator once the family members have been consulted before reaching a decision. Arrange immediate follow-up, e.g. further meetings with a Doctor, including a GP.

Discussion

Organ and tissue retention at hospital postmortem examinations is currently an issue attracting much public attention and is subject to independent enquiries. Postmortems are introduced as a way of discovering the cause of deterioration and are carried out by a histopathologist according to standards set by the Royal College of Pathologists, and may be full or limited in nature; if something suspicious is found, consider objection to retaining of organ part for educational or research purposes which can be kept indefinitely, or disposed of in a legal and proper manner if the relatives change their mind. Autopsies are useful where the cause of death is unclear, where the disease is rare and an autopsy can shed new light on the disease, and where information may shed light on other family members who suffer from the condition. Coroners' post mortems are required for sudden unexplained death, deaths from an operation, suspicion of unnatural cause of death (e.g. violence, neglect, drug poisoning). An autopsy should not delay funeral arrangements, and relatives can view the body afterwards. Finally, it is now widely accepted that specific consent is required for organ/tissue retention. This issue is an area of intense debate and leglislation is likely to be forthcoming.

The **Human Tissue Act** [1961] does not mention the requirement for relatives of the deceased to consent to postmortem examination. A donor card is sufficient legal authority to proceed; however, it is good practice to assess the relatives' wishes and few centres would proceed if the relatives did not assent to organ donation. Contraindications are infections such as HIV, prion disease, metastatic tumours, severe atherosclerosis. Time delays involved prior to the certification of death and the release of the body.

Regarding live organ donations, a donation may be obtained from a non-genetically related person provided no payment is expected. The **Human Organ Transplants Act** [1989] restricts transplants between persons who are not genetically related. All proposals are referred to Unrelated Live Transplant Regulatory Authority (ULTRA). Living donor kidney transplantation is only considered if the risk to the donor is low, the donor is fully informed, the consent is fully and freely given, the donor can withdraw his consent anytime before the operation, the offer of the organ is voluntary, and the transplant procedure has a good chance of success. To sell an organ is **illegal** (under s.16(1)). Please note that the UK currently does not operate a system of presumed consent, where consent is assumed unless notification is given otherwise. This is in contrast to some jurisdictions.

CONSENT FOR A HIV TEST

This is a relatively common examination scenario. We will therefore attempt to consider the component parts of this discussion carefully.

Scenario 19

Problem: Acquiring consent for a HIV test
Patient name: Hannah Jones (aged 22)

Hannah Jones is a 22-year-old journalist who has a sore throat and a rash. You have a clinical suspicion of HIV seroconversion. She has recently returned from a trip abroad to SE Asia.

Discuss this possibility with her, and counsel her regarding an HIV test.

A suggested plan for this consultation is:
- Introduce yourself and try to establish a good rapport. The patient must be aware that confidentiality will be respected.

- Ask how the patient feels and explain that you are now in a position to be able to tell her what the cause of the problem is.
- A good candidate should consider a brief history of the current illness as an introduction to the issue, and explore risk factors for HIV infection so as to go onto sensitively introduce HIV infection as a possible diagnosis. Ask her if she has been prone to infection in the past.
- The risk factors for HIV include current state of health, sexual orientation, sexual behaviour (e.g. numbers of partners, type of intercourse, use of condoms), partners, ethnic background (HIV-2 is common in parts of Africa), history of sexually transmitted disease, sexual behaviour whilst overseas, history of drug abuse (has she shared needles either now or previously), history of blood or blood product transfusion here or overseas, or organ donation. Review HIV risk reduction measures.
- Discover the patient's knowledge about HIV, how it is transmitted and its prognosis. Avoid being judgemental. Review the natural history of HIV infection.
- Distinguish between anonymous and confidential testing, availability of rapid-home-testing kits, and lab-send away from home kit.
- The candidate should be able to discuss the implications of a positive test including who to tell and implications for employment. Include that you can test for HIV infection, and not for AIDS. The window period between infection and seroconversion is normally no more than three months during which a false negative result may be obtained. The course is usually transmission, primary HIV infection, seroconversion, the asymptomatic period when lymphocyte counts fall and then AIDS.
- State explicitly that the test is for HIV antibodies, and it involves talking a small amount of venous blood, tell the patient when the result will be vailable, and tell the patient that the result will be given verbally, ideally by you. The tests are ELISA and Western Blot. Strict protection of client confidentiality must be maintained for all persons offered and receiving HIV counselling services.
- Explain that HIV is lifelong infection. Without treatment, there is a relatively short life expectance due to immune suppression. New drugs have revolutised the treatment with a marked improvement in life expectancy. HAART treatment can now prolong life of sufferers for up to 30 years. New treatments are being researched all the time.

- When applying for a mortgage, the patient may be asked whether she have had an HIV test. If the test is positive, the patient will be strongly encouraged to give consent for his GP and dentist to be notified and the result will then be permanently be in his GP records. The patient may be asked about his HIV status at employment medicals, although they are not legally obliged to divulge information. If positive, the patient's partner(s) should be informed. Say that you will not divulge details of the HIV test (even if the test was negative) to any insurance company without the patient's consent.
- You should assess the patient's ability to cope with the implications of a positive test and prepare them for it. Some implications of a positive test are: It would need to be repeated to confirm its positivity; it would give the patient greater uncertainty albeit of an unpleasant nature; there might be social discrimination and adverse psychological reaction; the patient would be offered continued medical support including anti-retroviral therapy and follow-up including prophylaxis of opportunistic infections including appropriate vaccinations; it should motivate the patient to practise risk minimization (decrease the number of partners, condoms and spermicide, detoxification regarding i/v drugs, use sterile needles, do not share razors or toothbrushes).
- If the test is positive then all insurance policies taken out prior to this will be honoured, although he may find difficulty in taking out future policies; all prior policies will be honoured. There are specialist companies for mortgages (and group-employment schemes and opt-outs).
- If the test is positive, it has to be considered that she may be at risk of other transmitted viruses. For example, Hepatitis B and hepatitis D which requires co-infection with Hepatitis B to replicate successfully.
- Ask who else needs to be told the result. Assess the personal and social support, and advise the patient where to obtain information about other services.
- If negative, the possibility of a false negative has to be considered, it might give the patient reassurance, and the patient will still have to behave responsibility to minimise her risk of HIV. Explain about seroconversion but dispel the false beliefs about immunity.
- Having weighed up the pro's and con's, the patient should be encouraged to make a decision, and appropriate follow-up made.

(This question has featured in a number of different guises, including oesophageal candidiasis, and hypoxia and abnormal CXR).

Discussion: **Causes of a false negative ELISA (0.2%)** Multiple pregnancies, blood transfusions, liver disease, parenteral substance abuse, haemodialysis, hepatitis B vaccination, rabies, influenza.
Causes of a false negative Western Blot (0.00001%)
Clerical error, contaminated sample, misinterpretation of results.

JEHOVAH'S WITNESS

Scenario 20

Problem: Jehovah's witness requiring blood transfusion
Patient name: Kirsty Fox (aged 42)
Kirsty Fox is a 53-year-old church volunteer. She presented with a history of tiredness, palpitations, raised blood pressure 180/110 mmHg. CT of the abdomen revealed that she has a large phaeochromocytoma on the right side adjacent to the aorta. She is about to undergo an operative procedure to remove the phaeochromocytoma. She has a past medical history of having three TIA's within the last year. However, in view of the position of the tumour, there is a high risk that the patient may bleed, making blood transfusion a critical matter.

- Jehovah's witnesses refuse to take any blood or blood products, they refuse any blood to be reintroduced to their body. They regard this as a sin.
- This patient needs the operation. There is a high risk that the patient will bleed. And if the patient continues to refuse the surgeons may have the right to cancel the procedure, if he/she feels the risk is more than the benefit. So you are left with a dilemma, if he/she feels the risk is more than the benefit. So you are left with a dilemma that you need to convince the patient of the necessity for the blood.
- It is difficult if you know little about their beliefs. *"Tell me a little more about your faith"*. Your best option is first to build a rapport and find out how much the patient knows about the condition.
- Their confidentiality is paramount; it is up to them, if they take blood and does not inform the church. Explain the options: EPO but the patient is hypertensive. Another possibility is re-introducing one's own blood (amount-limited and the period to save it in the fridge is also limited). Offer her the option of discussing this with the elders of the Church.

- Bring to her attention the watchtower policy. *"When it comes to fractions of any of the primary components, each Christian, after careful and prayerful meditation, must conscientiously decide for himself"*. Refer to the Bloodless Surgery Centre (the Watch Tower Society has lists).
- Be aware of patients' refusal or childrens' consent – best interests principle/only one parent's consent required.

ETHICAL ISSUES REGARDING GENETIC COUNSELLING

Consent is clearly crucial in situations regarding genetic counselling. This type of task poses particular problems.

The principles of genetic counselling whatever the condition

The subject should be encouraged to select a companion for the stages of the testing process: The pretest stage, the taking of the test, the delivery of the results and the post-test stage. The tests performed are:

Carrier-testing: Usually for AR/XLR conditions to base reproductive decisions. Give information regarding reliability of test, implications of carrier status. Children are advised to delay this until old enough to make personal decision.

Predictive testing: Presymptomatic tests: Usually for complete penetrance AD conditions, e.g. HD. If no useful treatment, the value of testing is questionable. This has profound implications regarding insurance, etc.

Predisposition testing: Increased risk, not certain of disease (e.g. BRCA for breast cancer, APO for Alzheimer's disease).

The aim of genetic screening is to identify people who might benefit from the new medications, help genetic researchers understand the disease better and so lead to improved treatment, and help people plan for the future. However, the disadvantages are that a genetic defect cannot be repaired. Neither prevention or cure is possible. The test may not accurately predict who will develop the disease; testing positive does not necessarily mean that a person will definitely develop the disease and testing negative does not guarantee they will not. There could also be an effect of a positive test on buying property, getting insurance and financial planning for the future. Alternatives the applicant can consider are not to take the test for the time being, to deposit DNA for research, and to deposit DNA for possible future use by family and self. Discuss how the diagnosis relates to others, e.g. mother: social aspects, legal aspects. Counsellors and multidisciplinary team (such as a geneticist, neurologist, social worker, psychiatrist, or medical ethicist) are important. Consider socioeconomic consequences on potential employment, social security, data security *etc.* Reassure the patient that there will be time to decide if he is unsure about proceeding and that at the next appointment you will provide information about addresses of support services. Say that you could refer him to a regional genetic centre if he wishes to go ahead with the testing.

Discussion

The subject must choose freely to be tested and must not be coerced by anyone. Extreme care should be exercised when testing would provide information about another person who has not requested the test. This issue arises when an offspring with a 25% risk requests testing with full knowledge that his or her parent does not want to know his or her own status. Ownership of the test result remains with the subject who requested the test.

HUNTINGTON'S DISEASE AND GENETIC COUNSELLING: EXPLAINING A TEST RESULT

Scenario 21

Problem: Explaining a test result (genetic test for Huntington's disease).
Patient name: Anne Wood (aged 37).
Anne Wood, aged 37, has attended clinic following the recent diagnosis of her mother with Huntington's disease five years' ago, which followed a 2 years history of psychiatric disturbance and choreiform movements. She agreed to have a genetic test for Huntington's disease. You are the FY2/ST1 for Neurology. She has returned to clinic to discuss with you the results of the test.

- Introduce yourself to the patient and establish rapport. Ask if she would like someone with her.
- Establish the patient's beliefs about the disease (Huntington's disease), her concerns and expectations. She must be aware of the seriousness of the condition and its untreatable nature. If she is not fully aware, the doctor should discuss the nature of the disease at length with her, including its inherited nature. Before moving on, ask if she has any questions about the disease.
- Explore why she has decided to have the test now. Explain that the test is positive.

- At this point wait for the patient's reaction.
- If the patient is not emotionally well prepared, listen and answer questions. The patient may not wish to talk about siblings or children at this point although she may already be aware of the inherited nature of the disease.
- If the patient is well prepared, ask if she has thought about telling other members of her family, the implications of inheritance and who may or may not be affected.
- Discuss support groups. Ensure that the patient has adequate emotional support at home.
- Summarise the discussion. Ask if she has any questions. Arrange follow-up.

DIFFERING PATIENT RESPONSES

In real life, we have to acknowledge that people, in response to certain situations, all tend to react differently. This is reflected in the description of the station provided by the Royal Colleges of Physicians in Station 4. Candidates are expected to react to these different patient responses appropriately. In real terms, in the exam, do not allow the actors to wind you up – you need to show that you can keep calm even when stressed. Consider the following examples:

1. If the patient is angry, acknowledge the anger and plight. Listen without interruption. Avoid being defensive. Check how intense the anger is. Keep calm and do not raise voice. Empathize. Advise of complaints procedure. Offer to meet later.
2. If the patient is depressed, ask her to tell you more about "feeling low" and the extent of it (severity, frequency, comparison with how the patient feels normally). Direct questions may be aimed at particular symptoms, for example, sleep, concentration, loss of interest, loss of energy, loss of appetite, loss of weight.
3. If the patient is confused, check their orientation according to time, place and date, and assess their short-term memory by giving them a name and address to remember and check their recall immediately. Assess whether they are having any abnormal experiences (e.g. misinterpretations, hallucinations), and whether there is any evidence for false beliefs such as delusions. Give the patient a clear explanation of their confusional state, and to reassure them that this is why they are having a confusional state. It is important to explain that every effort will be made to determine the cause of the confusion.

4. If communicating cross-culturally, ask him if there is anything special about his culture (e.g. sense of family) or religion that might be affecting him. Show acceptance of this cultural or religious dimension, and explore the patient's views. Avoid the danger of stereotypying in cross-cultural communication, by accepting that each person has their own particular view of culture or religion. Express solutions and involve other agencies if possible.

5. If communicating through an interpreter, address both the patient and the interpreter, and communicate simply in "chunks". Be aware of some problems involved with using interpreters (e.g. incorrect transmission or misunderstanding of information, avoidance of delicate topics, domination of the patient by the interpreter).

6. When talking to someone who is over-talkative, avoid interrupting too much because the more you interrupt the more your patient will tend to have to say; 'steer' the patient by selectively reflecting, paraphrasing and summarising aspects of the narrative, avoid resorting to closed questions until you have developed some sort of rapport, and, most of all, remain calm and courteous.

A MEDICAL MISTAKE AND AN ANGRY PATIENT

Scenario 22

Problem: Medical mistake (omission of a gentamicin level)
Patient name: George Ellis (aged 48)

George Ellis is a 46-year-old man who was commenced on ciprofloxacin and gentamicin on this admission for an acute exacerbation of bronchiectasis, but who has previously been admitted on multiple occasions with infective exacerbations of bronchiectasis. His previous medical history included multiple respiratory infections as a child. The drug chart indicated that he was supposed to have a gentamicin level on the 3rd dose, but this was accidentally omitted. He has found out about the error. This is the first time such a mistake has happened. He had been told yesterday that his renal function was normal. You are the FY2/ST1 for Respiratory Medicine. He would like to discuss the problem with you.

- Introduce yourself to the patient and establish rapport. Explain involvement in the case.
- Tell the patient that there has been a problem with one of the drugs. Explain the concept of a therapeutic range and the need to monitor levels.
- Explain what happened and how.

- Apologise for the error. Emphasise openness and truthfulness.
- Allow the patient to voice anger. Empathise and give legitimacy to the patient's feelings. Show your empathy verbally and non-verbally.
- Say that you are disappointed.
- Explain the side-effects of the drug (e.g. problems with deteriorating kidney function), and that therefore appropriate monitoring will be necessary (for example, blood tests).
- Explain the steps that you have taken to determine the cause and to prevent it from happening again. Explain the need for continuing medical care.
- Deal with emotions before facts; put the emotions into words and offer them back to the patient. Seek to understand the emotions. Be clear what the patient is feeling and identify the source of these feelings.
- Encourage the patient to elaborate on the background of his emotions. Avoid disagreement.
- Explain the possibility of further action for him to take in the future, e.g. formal complaint, and identify constructive actions that you and the patient can take.
- State that you will discuss the mistake openly with your consultant, an adverse incident form will be completed, and that the conversation will be documented in the medical notes.
- Ask the patient for any further worries.

The conditions for negligence are that the doctor owes a *duty of care*, that the doctor was in breach of the appropriate *standard of care* imposed by the law, and that the breach in the duty of care *caused* harm in question.

Bolam v Friern Hospital Management Committee [1957] is the English case that lays down the typical rule for assessing the appropriate standard of reasonable care in negligence cases involving doctors. The Bolam test provides that where the defendant has represented him or herself as having more than average skills and abilities, this test expects standards which must be consistent with a reasonable body of medical opinion (*De Frietas v O'Brien* [1995] which suggests that this can be as low as 11 in 1,000 doctors). It is intuitive, and the common law position, that this standard of care must not be palpably wrong (*Bolitho v City and Hackney Health Authority* [1997]), although the law does allow for different, nut valid, possible management decisions.

CONFIDENTIALITY AND GOOD CLINICAL PRACTICE

Under common law, doctors are obliged to maintain confidentiality, and MRCP(UK) candidates are expected to respect that confidentiality forms the core of any doctor/patient relationship. In terms of ethical principles, confidentiality therefore supports the principle of respect for patient autonomy, a principle that emphasises the patient's right to have control over his own life. The fundamental concept of medical confidentiality is that patients have a right to expect that information about them will be held in confidence by their doctors. Without assurances about confidentiality, patients may be reluctant to give doctors the information that they need to provide good care. The doctor must also respect requests by patients that information should not be disclosed to third parties, except in specific circumstances, where the health or safety of others would otherwise be at serious risk. The issue of when it is lawful, and when it is not lawful, for a doctor to breach confidentiality is often a question of balancing public interests, and of balancing private and public interests. The General Medical Council provides professional guidelines on the issue of confidentiality for practising doctors. Whilst these do not have the force of the law, they are taken seriously by the courts.

OBLIGATIONS FOR DOCTORS TO BREACH MEDICAL CONFIDENTIALITY

The GMC(UK) states that patients have a right to expect that doctors will not disclose any personal information which they learn during the course of their professional duties unless they give permission. Indeed, several acts of Parliament allow access of patients to material kept about them (the Data Protection Act, the Freedom to Health Records Act (1990) and the Freedom of Information Act (2005)). When a doctor is responsible for confidential information, it is the duty of the doctor to ensure that the information is effectively protected against improper disclosure when it is received, transmitted, stored or disposed. When patients give consent to disclosure of information about themselves, you must ensure that they understand what is being disclosed, the reasons for disclosure, and the likely consequences. You must also ensure that patients are informed whenever information about them is likely to be disclosed to others involved in their health care (sharing information with other members of the healthcare team is not generally viewed by the law as breaching confidentiality), and that they have the opportunity to withhold permission. Confidential information must be disclosed in the following situations. If confidential information is disclosed, the doctor should release only as much information as is necessary for that purpose.

- When legally required by a court order
- In a communicable disease notification, and the reporting of births, deaths, abortions and work-related accidents (Public Health Control of Diseases Act 1984; Abortion Act 1967; Births and Deaths Registration Act 1953). This is a statutory duty.
- Identification of patient undergoing *in vitro* fertility treatment with donated gametes (The Human Fertilisation and Embryology Act, 1990).
- Identification of donors and recipients for transplanted organs – Human Organ Transplants Act 1989.
- Drug addiction (Misuse of Drugs Act, 1973).
- In cases of national security, such as terrorism or major crime prevention or solution (Prevention of Terrorism Act, 1989).
- Police on request – name and address (but not clinical details) of driver of vehicle who is alleged to be guilty of an offence under the Road Traffic Act, 1988.

Confidential information may be disclosed at a doctor's discretion:
- When a 3rd party is risk of harm, for example, at risk of contracting a serious infectious disease,
- When it is in the public interest, e.g. patient with seizures known to be driving illegally,
- Through sharing information with the health care team
- Other than for treatment only with express consent (e.g. lawyers, Insurance companies).

In terms of public interest, the doctor is advised to disclose information promptly to an appropriate person or authority. Examples of this include a situation where a medical colleague who is also a patient is placing the patient at risk as a result of illness or another medical condition.

No information that might identify a patient examined or treated for any sexually transmitted disease should be provided to a third party, except for in a few specific situations where that third party may be in a situation of contracting a life-threatening disease, such as HIV infection. Furthermore, doctors should not write reports or disclose any confidential information which may be requested by insurance companies or employers without the patients' prior written consent.

Even after a patient has died, the obligation to keep the information confidential remains. If an insurance company seeks information about a deceased patient to decide whether or not to make a payment under a life insurance policy, information should not be released without the prior consent of the patient's executor, or a close relative, without being fully informed of the consequences of disclosure.

Possible consequences of breach of confidentiality are loss of trust, disciplinary action by the GMC, civil legal action, and investigation of serious professional misconduct by the General Medical Council.

Disclosure of information and public versus private information.

A Road Taffic Offence

In road traffic offences, the doctor must breach confidentiality and provide the police constable with the name and address of the patient (*Road Traffic Act* [1988]). The doctor must explain that he cannot without the patient's consent divulge any other information which can be used to prevent minor crime, or help convinction in minor crime. Most crimes against properties are onsidered to be minor crimes now. Details should not include clinical details. You are duty bound by a duty of confidentiality not to give any clinical information without the consent of the patient. Most crimes against properties are considered to be minor crimes now. Similarly, the doctor cannot breach confidentiality to prevent minor harm to another individual.

Fitness to Drive

The DVLA is legally responsible for deciding if a person is medically unfit to drive. They need to know when holders of a driving licence have a condition which may now in the future affect their safety as a driver. The following situations illustrate the steps taken in discussing this with patients. The ethical areas in the fitness to drive scenarios are respecting confidentiality, recognising the need to inform others when a patient refuses to take responsibility, recognising that failing to act may put others at risk, and recognising that a doctor's duty may involve doing something to which the patient has not consented.

EPILEPSY

Scenario 23

Problem: Epilepsy and DVLA
Patient name: Terri Warner (aged 21)

Terri Warner is a 21-year-old night club dancer who was admitted yesterday with a second tonic-clonic seizure. She had a similar seizure a month previously. Both seizures occurred whilst at work, in the presence of strobe lighting. She had been working the "night shift", and had felt relatively tired on both occasions. She has undergone a MRI which is normal, and an EEG demonstrated abnormal activity in relation to light stimuli. Her only medication is the oral contraceptive pill. She normally drives to work. Please discuss with her the results of her investigations. She is keen to carry on driving, especially "off road" driving, a competitive sport which is not governed by the DVLA.

- Introduce yourself, explain your role clearly, and agree the purpose of the interview.
- Explain epilepsy in a way that a layperson would understand. "A seizure is a sudden, unpredictable attack of electrical activity of the brain resulting in shaking of part of the body (or all four limbs). It may cause you to lose consciousness. Epilepsy is a term we use when somebody is having seizures".
- Establish the patient's level of knowledge of precipitating factors, including alcohol and recreational drugs, lifestyle and late nights. Inform her that alcohol will lower the fit threshold, and the medication given to avoid further fits may not work properly.
- Avoid swimming, bathing alone, cooking alone with gas cookers, heights. Ask about understanding of medication: Important issues are compliance and pill-failure, and continue anti-epileptic medication with folate cover during pregnancy.
- Ask about her occupation. Remember that with every epilepsy scenario, it is very important that you ask what the person's occupation is since their medical condition may prevent them from safely carrying out their job.
- Ask about driving and state how this would affect the person's life and job. Make sure that the patient understands that the condition may impair his ability to drive.
- Provide information about the law in relation to epilepsy. A patient can drive (on and off drugs) when they have been free of fits for 12 months, provided that they do not have continued high likelihood of seizures (e.g. a known brain tumour). If he/she has purely nocturnal (sleep) seizures he can drive, provided this pattern has been established for 3 years. Advise the patient about his responsibilities to himself and other drivers.
- The onus is on her to report the condition to the DVLA. The patient must be aware that you have the right to inform the DVLA if you

think that the patient is going to continue to drive despite careful consideration of the position. Mention lack of insurance cover if they drive and safety issues. Remain calm in the face of mild aggressive and emotional behaviour by the patient.

- If the patient refuses to accept the diagnosis or the effect of the condition on driving, you can suggest that the driver seeks a second opinion. You should advise that the patient should not drive until the second opinion has been obtained.

- Notice that she is a young woman of childbearing age. You need to tell her that certain anti-epileptics can make the oral contraceptive pill less effective and that a doubling or even tripling of the dose of oestrogen may be required. It is important to also inform her that pregnancy can ina percentage of women result in fetal teratogenic side effects. Explain that the risk is around 7% compared to 3% for the "normal" population and that there are ways of minimizing the risk, e.g. taking folic acid, using one instead of two anti-epileptics and possibly using the newer agents.

- Inform about the British Epilepsy Society. Agree a plan by the end of the interview. Advise her about the need to inform her partner. Arrange for appropriate follow-up.

The framework for the interview is likely to include: respect of the patient's autonomy (i.e. the capacity of the patient to make deliberated or reasoned decisions for himself and to act on the basis of these decisions), disclosure of confidential information (i.e. it is in the best interest of the public if this information is handed to the relevant authorities).

Table 7.1: Summary table of the DVLA and common medical disorders. For further information, please see consult www.dvla.org.uk for current guidelines.

Disease	Private vehicle license	HGV
Epilepsy	1 year fit free	Fit free, off medication
MI	1 month	3 months. Symptom-free. Completes 9 minutes Bruce-treadmill test
Stroke	1 month	Banned
IDDM	Notify DVLA	Banned

Public Health

A patient may refuse treatment ordinarily, but Section 37 of the Public Health Act, 1984, magistrates orders to allow compulsory treatment of a patient with notifiable disease. This is almost never needed if appropriate negotiation with the patient is undertaken, which is a good thing as it is very difficult to work.

Compulsory Treatment of TB

The *Public Health Act (Control of disease)* [1984] states that, in exceptional circumstances where a person with TB of the respiratory tract poses serious risk of infection to others, a CDC and Respiratory Physician can enform compulsory admission of the patient.

Needlestick Injury

If you or another health care worker has suffered a needlestick injury or other occupational exposure to blood or body fluids and you consider it necessary to test the patient for a serious communicable disease, the patient's consent should be obtained before the test is undertaken. If the patient is unconscious when the injury occurs consent should be sought once the patient has regained full consciousness. If appropriate, the injured person can take prophylactic treatment until consent has been obtained and the test result is known. If the patient refuses testing, is unable to give or withhold consent because of mental illness or disability, or does not regain full consciousness within 48 hours, you should reconsider the severity of risk to yourself, or another injured health care worker, or to others. You should not arrange testing against the patient's wishes or without consent other than in exceptional circumstances, for example where you have good reason to think that the patient may have a condition such as HIV for which prophylactic treatment is available. In such cases you may test an existing blood sample, taken for other purposes, but you should consult an experienced colleague first. It is possible that a decision to test an existing blood without consent could be challenged in the courts, or be the subject of a complaint to your employer or the GMC. You must therefore be prepared to justify your decision. If you decide to test without consent, you must inform the patient of your decision at the earliest opportunity. In such cases confidentiality is paramount: Only the patient and those who have been exposed to infection may be told about the test and its result. In these exceptional circumstances neither the fact that test has been undertaken, nor its result, should be entered in the patient's personal medical record without the patient's consent. If the patient dies you may test for a serious communicable disease if you have good reason to think that the patient may have been infected, and a health care worker has been exposed to the patient's blood or other body fluid. You should usually seek the agreement of a relative before testing. If the test shows the patient was a carrier of the virus, you should follow the guidance in paragraphs 21 - 23 of this booklet on giving information to patients' close contacts.

END OF LIFE DECISIONS

This chapter concludes with the area in medical ethics that raises probably the most strong and diverse views: Those concerned with end-of-life decisions. Indeed, topics such as euthanasia, do not resuscitate orders, and even advance directives (living wills) concern many outside the medical profession.

Who Makes End of Life Decisions?

Doctors, patients and families may face the question of how actively life-sustaining treatments should be pursued. In making these decisions, there should be respect for the patient autonomy, knowledge about the limitation of the treatment and promotion of the patient's best interests. Patients are deemed to act autonomously if they act with intent, with understanding and without controlling influences. Patients of this calibre may refuse life-prolonging treatment. If the patient knew all the relevant facts, there is reason to limit life-prolonging treatment. If the desires are regarding treatment, then it needs to be clear whether the decision was formed with an adequate understanding of alternatives and their consequences, and that these decisions were made when the patient was competent, and formed without coercion. If this is the case, there is no reason to limit life-prolonging treatment. In some situations, the opposite scenario may arise when a patient requests life-prolonging treatment which may prove harmful or futile. If the patient has made this decision, having been fully advised, there is no reason to satisfy the request.

Doctrine of Double Effect

The principle of double effect permits an act which is foreseen to have both good and bad effects. This doctrine distinguishes actions that are intended to harm versus those where harm is foreseen but not intended. Frequently, doctors set out to relieve pain and suffering but see that life may be shortened. Foreseeing is not necessarily the same as intending. This is in keeping with duties of a doctor. Consider, for example, patients dying from cancer. These patients are often given heightened dosages of opiates to relieve pain by their medical care teams who willhave foreseen that these actions may shorten the patient's life by their effects on respiratory depression. Although it would be morally wrong to inject morphine into the patient's blood stream with the intent of hastening death, it may not be necessarily wrong to inject it if the foreseeable consequences of it were to hasten death if the doctor's intention was to relieve pain.

Euthanasia and Assisted Suicide

Euthanasia is intentional killing, i.e. murder under English law, and therefore illegal. Assisted suicide, i.e. helping someone take their own life, is a criminal offence.

Arguments for: Respecting a patient's autonomy over their body, beneficence (i.e. mercy killing may prevent suffering), suicide is legal but unavailable to the disabled.

Arguments against: Good palliative care obviates the need for euthanasia, risk of manipulation / coercion/ exploitation of the vulnerable, undesirable practices when constraints on killing are loosened.

Physician-assisted suicide is where the physician provides the patient with the means to commit suicide.

Euthanasia and assisted-suicide are illegal.

Best Interests

Options for treatment or investigations are contemplated by the Medical Team which are clinically indicated are in line with the patient's expressed preferences, and the patient's background (cultural, religious or employment), or the patient's preferences given by a 3rd partner.

Advance Directives

Advance directives are not covered by legislation. In cases of conflict with other legal provisions, advance statements are superseded by existing stature. A person can anticipate losing the mental capacity to decide or communicate how much he or she wishes to be treated by drawing up a formal advance statement of her values and preferences or by naming a person who can be consulted. These are statements usually written and formally witnessed made by a person when they are fully competent about the medical care he/she does or does not want to receive should they become incompetent in the future. It will be increasingly unwise to ignore these directives, and they can be helpful to clinicians. Advanced consent is not legally binding, e.g. to be kept alive as reasonably possible using whatever forms of treatment are available. Advanced refusal is legally binding if adult and competent when made, the decision was informed, circumstances have arisen which were envisaged, and the patient was not unduly influenced.

Withholding Medical Treatment

The primary goal of medicine is to benefit the patient's health with minimal harm, and this should be explained to those close to them so that they can understand why treatment is given, and why a decision to withhold or withdraw life-prolonging treatment may be considered. Balance should be in favour of treatment if there is doubt. On the other hand, treatment may prolong suffering and there is no absolute ethical or legal right to a treatment that may prolong suffering. When a patient lacks capacity to make decisions and there is uncertainty about the appropriateness of treatment, treatment that may be of some benefit should be started until clearer assessment can be made. This is particularly important in emergencies, when more time is needed for detailed assessment. Although, it may be emotionally easier to withhold treatment, rather than to withdraw that which has already been started, there are no legal or necessarily moral distinctions between the two. The BMA considers that where a particular treatment is no longer benefitting the patient, continuing to provide it would not be in the patient's best interests and maybe morally wrong. Greater emphasis on the reasons for providing treatment including artificial nutrition and hydration, rather than the justification for withholding treatment, may challenge this perceived difference (British Medical Association, Withholding and withdrawing life-prolonging medical treatment: guidance for decision-making, 1999).

Whilst the nature of the withdrawal of medical treatment will depend on the particular context, we hope that the possible structure to this difficult area below is a useful guide:

* Introduce yourself and establish rapport.
* In withholding treatment, you may start by suggesting you wish to share some thoughts on the next step if the outlook is poor.
* Explain that the team feels that continuing active treatment will not achieve the desired result and introduce the concept of withdrawing active treatment. This does not mean the same as withdrawal of all treatment. Explain that, rather, the emphasis will change from treatment with the aim of cure or prolongation of life to that of the relief of symptoms and for the promotion of

the patient's comfort and dignity. The quality of care will remain the same.

- In explaining this situation, it can be helpful to go back over the past history and place the severity in historical context. Ask if any members of the family have had views on this, or whether the patient had views on this when well.
- Explain that the patient is not in pain and well sedated. Explain that if the family allows the withdrawal of treatment, he may deteriorate quickly and die soon after.
- Point out politely that the final decision of withdrawal of treatment does not reside with the family but the ITU staff. Explain how the withdrawal will be undertaken.
- Explain that a decision is not needed right away, and ask about any queries.

The case of *Burke v GMC* [2005] suggests that artificial nutrition and hydration (ANH) cannot be withdrawn without a court order, in other words ANH rights may reside with the patient. ANH should not be withdrawn where there is doubt/disagreement about the patient's capacity, where a lack of consensus amongst doctors regarding prognosis or best interests, where the patient when competent may have wanted ANH to continue, where the patient resists/disputes the withdrawal of ANH, and where close others feel that ANH withdrawal is not in the patient's best interests.

Do-not-attempt Resuscitate (DNAR) Order

English law does not require doctors to prescribe futile treatments, even if requested so by the patient. Therefore a DNR order is an example of limiting treatment that is futile. Cardiopulmonary arrest is the most crucial of all medical emergencies. Local Trusts have their own regional guidelines usually authored by a Resuscitation Committee and ratified by the Executive Board.

The BMA, RCN and UK Resuscitation Council (1999) state that a DNAR order is appropriate:

a. Where CPR is unlikely to be successful.
b. CPR is not in accord with the recorded sustained wishes of the patient if mentally competent.
c. CPR is not in accord with a valid advanced directive.
d. CPR is likely to be followed by the length and quality of life not in the best interest of the patient. Expected benefits are outweighed by the burdens, e.g. life-burdened by severe uncontrollable pain, permanent lack of awareness, or total dependency.

Possible definitions of futility include: the likelihood of the patient regaining consciousness following resuscitation is less than 1%, the likelihood of the patient being in hospital following resuscitation is less than 10%, or the patient will love only for a few weeks because of another untreatable terminal illness. The resuscitation decision is made by appropriate health professionals and not by the patient's relative, but her cooperation is valued; address all concerns of the relative. This decision should be made after appropriate consultation and consideration of all aspects of the patient's conditioning. Emphasise the need for self esteem, dignity and comfort. Ask if other members of the family need to be involved, and consider their spiritual beliefs.

Doctors should make a decision as to whether to inform the patient of the decision. It may be inhumane and distressing to raise issues of this nature with terminally ill patients. However, ideally the patient should be fully informed of any discussions about care and decisions regarding resuscitation. The order should be conveyed to all members of the multi-disciplinary team, and reviewed in light of changes in the patient's condition. A DNAR order can sometimes be made without consulting a patient if there is no likelihood that resuscitation would be successful (futility), or if the patient is not able to make such a decision (unconscious or not competent to do so), or if the patient's quality of life is extremely poor.

DNAR

Scenario 24

Problem: Do-not-attempt-resuscitate order (DNAR)
Patient name: Tony Graham (aged 62)
Tony Graham, aged 62, was admitted with a stroke. Following management of this stroke, a palliative stent was inserted for his underlying disease, carcinoma of the head of the pancreas, but it is known that he has a very poor prognosis given that he now has metastases in the liver. He was discussed in your multidisciplinary team meeting this morning, and the Consultant signed a form to state that, in the event of a cardiopulmonary arrest, a resuscitation attempt should not be made. He has never discussed this issue with your team. You are the FY2/ST1 for General Medicine. Your Consultant would like you to discuss this resuscitation status with him.

Setting: A quiet office to ensure a lack of interruptions.

Pacing: Allow yourself enough time.

Opening: Introduce yourself and establish good rapport. Call yourself Doctor. Ask how to address the patient.

Give a warning shot. *"I have something important to discuss with you".*

- Establish the patient's understanding of the underlying condition and reason for admission. Emphasise that he on maximum medical therapy which will continue, including "strong" antibiotics for the chest infection and medications to relieve any distressing or suffering.
- Ask an open question about how his symptoms have been recently. Good listening skills prepare for the most difficult part of the interview.
- What does he think will happen on the future?
- Explain there will be a decline in his function, i.e. a grave prognosis, and the reasons for this. *"Somebody with a condition as bad as yours may suddenly take a turn for the worst."*
- Respond to emotions. *"I see that you are distressed by the situation. I find it very hard to confront you with painful facts like this".*
- *"If we were to restart your heart, we might prolong a situation which you find intolerable. We would hate to do the wrong thing for you. If your heart were to stop beating, would you want us to restart it for you?"*
- If he feels strongly that he would like every medical attempt made to prolong his life, this should be respected.
- Ask what he/she feels about this. Promise support from doctors and nurses. Agree treatments to relieve symptoms.
- If he does not wish to be resuscitated, you could say something like, *"I can see how distressing it is for you to face up to how ill you are. I can see that it's a hard decision for you, but you said that life is so bad that you wouldn't want your heart to be restarted. Have I understood you correctly?"*
- If he does not wish to be resuscited, you could explain to him that death is not a failure, and that the decision has been taken to let nature to take its course.
- Explain that the patient should be left comfortable with the aim of preserving dignity and self-esteem.
- Explain that a side-room will be organised for privacy. Ask if there are any other members of the family who need to be involved.
- Finally, address any other concerns of the patient.
- Say when you will meet again.

In most circumstances, a patient should be involved in a DNAR decision. It should be borne in mind that for every patient there comes a time when death is inevitable and cardiac or respiratory function will fail. It is essential therefore to determine for each patient whether CPR is appropriate. A DNAR order should only be given after full consultation with the patient and the medical team. Where a patient is seriously ill, decisions about CPR should be ideally made in advance. The current guidelines are that if the patient is not competent to take part in the decision, consider discussing the issue with family to help make the judgement. If the length and quality of life after resuscitation is likely to be worthwhile, do not consider a DNAR order; else DNAR. The DNAR order should be reviewed and documented at a frequency appropriate to the patient's condition. The most senior available member of the medical team is normally responsible for entering the DNAR decision, and the reasons for it.

Medicolegal Aspects of Care of the Elderly

Although the law applies to everyone, there are certain aspects which become particularly associated with the needs of elderly persons.

Testamentary Capacity

The law requires that a person making a will has a 'sound disposing mind'. Doctors are often asked to assess a patient prior to making a Will. It is important that accurate records are taken and kept of the assessment in order that your decisions can be justified by contemporaneous note keeping.

In addition to establishing and documenting the absence of cognitive impairment it is necessary to specifically assess the following:

Does the patient understand the nature of the act of making a Will and its effects?

Does the patient know the nature and extent of his/her property?

Does the patient know which persons have a claim upon his/her property?

Can he/she form a judgement on the strength of the claims made by these people on his/her property?

Has the patient expressed him/herself clearly and without ambiguity (this need not necessarily be in writing as nods and gestures can be allowed)?

Section 47

Section 47 **National Assistance Act** [1948] gave the Medical Officer of Health the power to apply to a Magistrate for the **compulsory** removal of persons who:are suffering from grave chronic disease or being aged, infirm or physically incapacitated, are living in insanitary conditions **AND** are unable to devote to themselves and are not receiving from other persons proper care and attention.

The Section 47 Act is not commonly used with only around 250 cases admitted per annum in the whole of the UK. It is good practice that Geriatricians be involved and it is probably better that patients compulsory detained are initially admitted to hospital where they can be given the full benefit of a medical assessment.

Power of Attorney

This is a legal document which gives total control of a persons financial affairs to someone else. It must be made by a mentally competent person but ceases to be valid once the patient loses the mental capacity to withdraw it. This is only really of any use for physically incapacitated patients who wish their attorney to deal with their affairs.

Enduring Power of Attorney

This is a document taken out by a person when they have mental capacity, which will continue if it is subsequently lost. This is the preferred method for elderly persons to safeguard their financial affairs and property. It does not relate to decisions regarding medical treatment.

Once it is decided that mental capacity is lost the Enduring Power of Attorney must be registered with the Court of Protection. This usually requires that the document is accompanied by a doctors opinion that the patient has now lost the mental capacity to make decisions. The patient concerned is notified and if they disagree and feel that they have not yet lost their mental capacity they may challenge the decision so providing some safeguard. It is wise that two attorneys are established, one person being a family member (usually a grown-up child) and the other to be the representative from a legal firm.

Court of Protection

This is an Office of the Supreme Court of Judicature under the direction of a master, deputy master and assistant masters. The Court's primary function is to safeguard the financial interests of a patient by providing for his/her maintenance and that of his/her family dependants and management of his/her propert, and the Public Trustee is a specific person to whom these powers are delegated. It can take months to grant receivership which is usually granted to either a firm of solicitors or to a relative, but the Court itself has to oversee all the expenditure which it must also approve. This is really the only mechanism of controlling the financial affairs of a mentally incompetent patient if no Enduring Power of Attorney has been produced. This is extremely expensive and is not to be recommended if it can be avoided.

The family solicitor will usually arrange for the patient to be examined by a doctor who will determine whether or not the patient is capable or incapable of managing and administering his/her property and affairs by virtue of mental disorder. The patient is usually served with notice of proposed proceedings so they may protest if they feel they have not yet lost their powers. The doctor may choose to recommend that the service of notice is dispenses with if either the patient is incapable of understanding it or that service would be injurious to health or for any other reason.

The Court of Protection is usually receptive to providing things which will improve the quality of life of a patient. For example, they may well fund a holiday for both themselves and their carer and may be in a position to approve purchase of a vehicle, if funds permit, in order to allow for trips out, etc.

CONCLUSION

We hope that the scenarios above help to illustrate some of the key principles underlying the communication skills and ethics which are being tested. The key mistake to avoid is to think you must have a script ready for every discussion before you attend the examination. All consultations are different, and relying on a pre-prepared formula may be dangerous if you are seen to not respond to the patient's needs. Practice with somebody this station in advance of the examination, and consider whether the principles you apply for the examination are being appropriately applied in real life. It is intended that people who pass this station in the examination are performing well in their day-to-day careers.

REFERENCES

Communication skills for Doctors. Peter Maguire. Arnold (Hodder Headline Group) (2000).

Ethics and Communication Skills. Medicine 2000; Vol 28:10.

Royal College of Physicians. Clinical guidelines for candidates: the PACES examination (2001).

PRACTICE QUESTIONS

1. Mr. Giles, a 55-year-old man, is due to be reviewed in clinic as a follow-up patient. He has been diagnosed as having type II respiratory failure, in the presence of chronic obstructive pulmonary disease. Pulmonary function tests have shown:
   FEV1 is 0.95 pre b-agonist (predicted value 3.5 l)
   FEV1 is 1.29 post b-agonist.
   He has gross ankle oedema. At present, he is on salbutamol and atrovent mdi inhalers. Please discuss future potential management strategies and Mr Giles' understanding of his disease process with him.

2. Mr. Johnson is a 46-year-old man who has undergone investigations for a six-month history of pain and stiffness in his joints, predominantly affecting the small joints of his hands, wrists and ankles. The blood tests have revealed the following:
   Normal FBC, normal biochemical profile other than mildly elevated liver function tests and significantly elevated ESR and CRP.
   The rheumatoid factor is positive at 1 in 320.
   X-ray of the hands have revealed early erosions.
   He does enjoy regular pints of beer with his friends at his local pub. He has returned for his follow-up appointment. Please inform him of the diagnosis and the potential of management strategies. You would ideally like to start him on methotrexate.

3. Miss Salt is a 19-year-old lady who was diagnosed as an insulin-dependent diabetic six years' ago. She is due to be discharged following a five-day in-patient stay after her third recent episode of diabetic ketoacidosis. You are seeing her prior to her discharge. Please advise her regarding her diabetic control.

4. The son/daughter of a 74-year-old woman with severe rheumatoid arthritis has demanded to "see a doctor now" and you have complied with this request. The patient was admitted four weeks ago with a UTI but has become weaker and less mobile. She has bed-sores and today swabs have revealed MRSA.

5. Please respond to the referral letter below.
   Re: Jane Francis
   (aged 32)
   Dear Doctor,
   I would be very grateful if you could see Mrs. Francis urgently. She has attended with a itchy skin rash on her elbows, and I wonder whether she could be started on suitable treatment for

this. She lives with her two children aged 6 and 4, who have also developed some itchy lesions. She has been trying to maintain a diet compatible with her diagnosis of coeliac disease. She seems anxious.

Yours sincerely,

6. You are a registrar. This patient has been diagnosed with acute renal failure, the creatinine is climbing despite appropriate treatment, and he/she is likely to need to commence haemodialysis tomorrow. He/she has a past history of nephrectomy for renal cell cancer treated at another hospital; you know few details about this, but the patient looks well and has been leading a relatively normal life until he/she became acutely ill three days prior to admission. However, his wife reports that he has also had diabetes for 10 years, treated with oral hypoglycaemic agents. The patient is in a high-care ward on a cardiac monitor with central line. You have come to explain about the need for dialysis.

7. You have just been phoned by the Nuclear Medicine department to say that a V/Q scan on a 35-year-old woman gives a high probability of pulmonary embolism. Your task is to explain the prognosis, and the need for treatment with warfarin. You should give the patient appropriate information to take this drug safely.

8. Mr. Peters has had open tuberculosis. He has a young family who have all received a course of chemoprophylaxis. He, to date, has fully-sensitive mycobacteria on sputum culture. He admits to being non-compliant with therapy. This is the second time that he has had to recommence treatment. Discuss the importance of completion of treatment with Mr. Peters and how this can be achieved.

9. John Harvey is a 65-year-old lorry driver who was discharged last week following a myocardial infarction. He has been found to be in atrial fibrillation (a new finding since his MI), but does not appear symptomatic with him. Please advise him about his concerns.

10. A 35-year-old cyclist is referred to you, with recurrent syncope of unknown cause. He loses consciousness without warning for 30s. He is advised not to cycle in public roads, but refuses to agree to this as he cycles as a city courier-delivery service for his job. Counsel him regarding his cycling. What legal restraints are available to prevent him from cycling?

11. You are the medical FY2/ST1 on call. You are asked to come urgently to the A&E department where Mrs. Brown has presented with 24 hours of haemoptysis and a two-month history of cough, purulent sputum and weight loss. Urgent staining of the sputum has revealed plentiful Mycobacteria (Ziehl-Nielsen staining). The A&E FY2/ST1 says that previous notes of the patient had been found and that a diagnosis of rifampicin and isoniazid resistant tuberculosis and been made 18 months previously. The patient had taken treatment for three months in an isolation unit in hospital before going home. She had been lost to follow-up and discontinued treatment after discharge. The patient is not keen to be admitted as she did not enjoy isolation and would prefer to be at home, looking after her disabled husband. Your task is to discuss with the patient:
    • The need for further investigation (including contributory underlying factors)
    • The need for treatment
    • The need for admission
    • What can be done for the household contacts?

12. Mr. Brown is a 61-year-old man who was fit and healthy until one year ago now has end-stage cardiac failure. He is not a candidate for heart transplantation because due to his age and degree of renal failure. He was admitted routinely by yourself to optimise his cardiac failure therapy but his condition has deteriorated over the weekend as your team forgot to decrease the dose of his diuretics. His renal failure worsened. The ITU team have reviewed him and refused an HDU or ITU bed due to his terminal condition. The family has requested a meeting with you, and the senior nurse looking after the patient feels a decision on resuscitation should be raised.

13. A 59-year-old man, Mr. Patel, has severe congestive cardiac failure. He has idiopathic dilated cardiomyopathy. The strict upper age group for heart transplantation is 60 years. He recently turned 62, and has developed insulin-dependent diabetes mellitus. He has been on the waiting list for three years. His cardiac function has deteriorated. He is keen to discuss the possibility of heart transplantation.

14. The son/daughter of a patient with a slowly progressive primary brain tumour has asked to discuss discharge plans. The patient has been in hospital for three weeks, can only transfer with the help of two people, and is intermittently confused. 24-hour

nursing assessment suggests that discharge home would only be possible with an acre package comprising two carers three times a day. Carers are in short supply and this is not feasible. Nursing-home placement is the only option.

15. A normally fit 74-year-old has suffered a dense right-sided stroke and is unconscious. You have arranged to see a spouse to discuss decision-making about intravenous hydration and whether or not to institute enteral nutrition.

16. An endoscopy is carried out on Mr. Hopkins, a 37-year-old gentleman who has presented with weight loss and epigastric discomfort. Endoscopy has revealed severe oesophageal candidiasis. The risk of immunosuppression had not been considered when he was initially reviewed. You are to review Mr. Hopkins during his follow-up clinical appointment. Please inform him of the findings of the gastroscopy and discuss the further potential management plans with the patient.

17. You are the FY2/ST1 in the Genitourinary clinic. Mr. Jones is a Consultant Surgeon in your local hospital. His wife is diagnosed as HIV positive. She does not wish her husband to be told. She is, however, concerned about the risks of his job to other people. She wants to know if Mr. Jones should be asked not to operate on patients this afternoon. Please counsel her.

18. A 30 year old man has presented with CMV colitis. He has returned to clinic for the results of a HIV test that is positive. He is married and his wife is expecting her first child. Explain the news to the man, discuss telling his wife, discuss the possible risks to the child, and introduce the idea of a multidisciplinary team approach.

19. This in-patient who is in his/her 40s presented with a short history of jaundice. ERCP has diagnosed a carcinoma of the head of the pancreas. You have come to him/her to explain the diagnosis and possible treatment options.

20. Mr. Evans is a 42-year-old man who has admitted following an episode of haematemesis and melaena. He was treated with variceal sclerosis during endoscopy and required four units of blood transfusion during acute admission. He is now no longer encephalopathic and has been haemodynamically stable for the past 48 hours. This gentleman's liver disease has been diagnosed to be purely related to his heavy alcohol consumption. Please advise him as you feel appropriate.

21. You have just gastroscoped this patient with symptomatic acid reflux and found a hiatus hernia with oesophagitis. You now have got to see the patient to explain the results of the gastroscopy and outline the treatment options – medication, surgery.

22. Mr. Jones is a 25-year-old pharmaceutical representative. He has been referred to you by his general practitioner. Mr. Jones was involved in a road-traffic accident whilst on holiday in Spain. He suffered head injuries from which he made a full recovery. However, 6 hours' post trauma, and on the way to the local hospital, he had a grand mal seizure. This was treated by the paramedics with lorazepam. He was discharged from the hospital on carbamazepine. He has not returned back to work yet, though it has been 3 months since the incident. He feels cognitively impaired and low in mood. He has asked to see you because he has been told he cannot drive for 3 years, and is unsure how he can regain his life back.

23. Complaints about your house officer have been made by the nursing staff. Sometimes rude, short-tempered, he/she is causing moderate friction on the ward. You need to try and sort things out.

24. You are the medical FY2/ST1 on-call and asked by the A&E staff to attend a patient who has presented with a hypoglycaemic attack. He has had some intravenous dextrose, and is now awake and orientated. This is the first hypoglycaemic episode which required hospital treatment. Your task is to convince Mr. Watkins of the need to revoke his driving licence and persuade him to inform the DVLA.

25. You are seeing the daughter of a 87-year-old lady who is ill following an extensive CVA. You wish to discuss her management, particularly nutrition, but the family seem unkeen on any further treatment. The patient has written a will with an advance directive asking to be resuscitated if required.

26. You are the SHO on the ward. You have been asked to see the son of a patient of yours, Mr. Irvine. He lives a long distance from his father and sees him only 2-3 times per year. Mr. Irvine is an elderly man with metastatic carcinoma of the lung. He is admitted with an acute episode of breathlessness and a large pleural effusion which has confirmed malignant cytology. He is very cachectic and very frail. He lives alone since his wife died 4 years ago. He claims that he has had enough and feels too unwell to undergo any further treatment. You feel that he is competent

to make this decision. Your task is to discuss Mr. Irvine's prognosis and decide with his son:

- The idea of further investigation
- Any proposed treatment
- The likely prognosis and resuscitation status.

27. You are the medical FY2/ST1 doing a ward round. You have been told by the Nurses that the wife of one of your patients would like to speak to you before you review her husband. He has severe Chronic Obstructive Pulmonary Disease and has been admitted with an infective exacerbation. He is on home nebulisers, home oxygen and is housebound due to a combination of his lung disease and depression. On the ward, he is receiving intravenous antibiotics and an aminophylline infusion as well as his regular nebulisers and oxygen. Mrs Smith does not want her husband to be resuscitated in the event of a cardiac arrest. Mrs Smith is depressed, tired and fed up with her husband's illness. She feels that whilst she would like to continue to care for him, she also cannot watch him suffer any more. She would like to discuss his resuscitation status with you, but does not want him to know, as it would upset him. She feels that he should not be resuscitated but would like this decision to be made without her husband. Your task is to explain that whilst resuscitation is likely to be futile, Mr Smith must be involved in all decisions regarding his care and that will include discussions about his resuscitation.

8 *Focussed Clinical Problem (Station 5)*

[The authors recommend that, particularly for this chapter, you consult a good quality atlas of clinical medical images.]

In the old examination, there were about five minutes allocated for each of the "minors". These correspond to short cases of the old MRCP format. The second half of this chapter includes descriptions of the skin, endocrine, locomotor, and eyes cases which can now appear in any of the four preceding stations. However, as of May 2009, the Station 5 has now changed such that it now contains a focussed clinical problem. This is because the part of the old examination was seen as artificial, and the new format of the assessment is a better reflection of what a Registrar in higher specialist training, or a Consultant, would have to do in real life given the time limits of genuine clinical practice.

PART 1: THE NEW FORMAT OF THE EXAMINATION

You will be assessed on your ability to demonstrate each of the seven clinical skills described below. Each Station tests a fixed combination of these skills. The main categories of the assessment include: Physical examination, identifying the physical signs, clinical communication, differential diagnosis, clinical judgment, managing patient's concerns, and maintaining patients' welfare (Please see the MRCP website: http://www.mrcpuk.org/PACES/Pages/PACESChanges.aspx).

There will now be two 10-minute encounters at this Station rather than the current structure in which candidates see four patients for 5 minutes each.

The encounters will each take the form of a "Brief Clinical Consultation" in which the patient presents with a single clinical problem or symptom of the sort encountered in day-to-day practice in the wards, receiving unit or outpatient clinic. You will be required to undertake a brief focussed history and brief targeted examination in the 8 minutes available with the patient, before discussing findings and diagnosis with the examiner for 2 minutes.

It is not necessary for you to undertake a full, comprehensive history (as required in Station 2) or a thorough, systematic examination (as required in Stations 1 and 3) in these encounters but to demonstrate a focussed and integrated clinical problem solving approach.

All the scenarios will be structured to ensure that a capable candidate can undertake the task within the time available. Real or simulated patients may appear in these encounters. The four disciplines currently represented at Station 5 will not always be represented in the examination, but clinical problems relating to those disciplines (dermatology, ophthalmology, endocrinology, and rheumatology; see **PART 2** of this chapter) will frequently appear at Stations 2, 4 or 5, so candidates must continue to be prepared to assess patients whose problems primarily relate to these systems. Patients with problems relating to disciplines or areas less clearly represented in the current examination, for example, acute medicine and elderly medicine, may now also be encountered. The structure of all other Stations, and the overall duration and timings of the examination remain unchanged.

The pass mark will be defined by a formal standard setting process that will also take close account of the current PACES pass standard. It is intended that the overall standard of the examination will remain the same; that is, the examination overall will be no harder or easier to pass.

Development of This Station

There were a number of significant problems with the "old" MRCP PACES Station 5. The clinical cases are presented most commonly as 'spot diagnoses' and do not assess the candidate on the competencies described in the curriculum for General (Internal) Medicine (Acute), which is the aim of PACES. The "old" Station 5 had been shown, in fact, to contribute the least to the discrimination between candidates' performance in the examination overall.

In real life, the key competencies of a doctor are the ability to take the history and interpret it, the ability to examine a patient and appreciate the clinical signs, and the ability to communicate with a patient appropriately and respond to concerns raised. These skills are tested separately at Stations 1 to 4 in PACES but they are not assessed in an integrated fashion as used every day in clinical practice.

The "new" Station 5 has been subject to rigorous pilots with feedback from current examiners. From the candidate's point of view, time management in this Station is vital, in demonstrating a competent response to what is a potentially complicated series of problems within a patient. The methods of history taking and communication described in full in the other chapters will enable one to acquire these skills. Also, the approach to identifying and analyzing physical signs will enable one to be proficient in this Station. A correct examination should be focussed to allow to formulate a detailed lists of likely conditions that may occur, and the lists of differential diagnosis in the preceding chapters will help.

Marking Scheme

Most of all, the candidate will need to demonstrate a pragmatic approach in the following areas:

a. Diagnosis, investigations and management will help one be proficient at clinical judgment;

   In practice, the doctor would be expected to make recommendations for further investigations to determine the initial diagnosis and subsequent managent, and act on the results for the benefit of the patient. Here, it is worth stressing that the function of the consultation is to address the problems of the patient, not any underlying diagnosis.

b. Addressing patient's anxieties and concerns will enable one to be proficient at managing patients' concerns.

   This could involve responding to mood clues, exploring the patient's health beliefs.

c. Clinical skills, investigation and management ("an action plan") will enable one to address and maintain patient welfare.

   The welfare of patients is at center of medical care, either at the level of delivering "technical" welfare (e.g. prescribing painkillers to an elderly lady with rheumatoid disease) or delivering "social" welfare (e.g. arranging for volunteers to attend an elderly lady who is housebound with rheumatoid disease). Such social interventions may include pastoral support and providing practical and financial advice to improve quality of life. The critical aspect to note with regard to this (and similarly for Station 5) is to know when exactly to call for specialist assistance, and how to do so. The balance between the provision of these types of welfare varies enormously between specialties, between personalities and consulting styles, and between views of the role of doctors.

The case is supported by papers similar to those used at Stations 2 and 4. Thus, the candidate is introduced to the case by a very short note:

'This: 76-year-old attended this morning for day surgery on her cataracts. and she mentioned that she had noticed swelling of joints in her hands. Your task is to assess the problem by means of a relevant history and a focussed physical examination.You should then advise the patient of your probable diagnosis, and your plan for investigation or treatment as appropriate.'

The patient has a short narrative giving 'agreed' history detailing her complaints and the information she would like from the candidate's consultation with her. The examiner will observe the history-taking, the examination, and the communication with the patient. The examiner would not be able to assess whether the candidate had accurately identified any physical signs that may be present, and might also have difficulty appreciating the differential diagnosis in the candidate's mind from observation of the encounter. For this reason, the only interaction between candidate and examiner is when the candidate is requested by the examiner to report the clinical findings and give the differential diagnosis.

The "new" Station 5 is supposed to mirror everyday clinical practice – the 'Brief Clinical Consultation' – whereby a junior physician is asked to see a patient in the ward or in the clinic who raises a particular problem.

PART 2: REVISION NOTES ON SKIN, LOCOMOTOR, ENDOCRINE AND EYES

Please note that the history of any of these disorders could be assessed as part of the History Taking Station (Station 2), and the examination of any of these disorders could be a part of any of the Clinical stations (Stations 1 and 2).

SKIN

Please look at the skin here (a certain part of the body) and discuss your findings.

Description

All pigmented lesions should be defined by size (Increasing or not), site, shape, presence of satellite lesions, bleeding, pruritus, pigmentation, associated lymphadenopathy, and features of systemic upset (history of drugs/medications, allergies, contacts with similar rash).

A few important definitions.

Macules: A flat, circumscribed area of discoloration; if >1 cm this is termed a patch.

Papules: A circumscribed elevation of the skin < 1 cm in diameter.

Plaques: A raised flat-topped lesion > 1 cm.

Bullae: A fluid-filled lesion (blister) > 1 cm.

Vesicles: A circumscribed fluid-filled elevation less than 5 mm in diameter.

Pustule: A pus-filled lesion.

Wheal: A raised compressible area of dermal oedema.

Scale: Flakes arising from abnormal stratum corneum.

Crust: Dried serum, pus or blood.

Telengectasia: Permanently dilated, visible small vessels.

NEUROFIBROMATOSIS

Multiple neurofibromata, café-au-lait spots (normal person may have up to five), axillary freckling, Lisch nodules (melanocytic harmartomas of the iris). Neurofibroma are soft or firm mobile subcutaneous lumps or nodule around peripheral nerves.

  Extra points: Hypertension (associated with renal artery stenosis and phaeochromocytoma), fine crackles (honeycomb lumb and fibrosis), neuropathy with enlarged palpable nerves.

Inheritance is Autosomal Dominant

Two non-allelic inheritable forms. Type I is classical peripheral form (associated with chromosome 17; there may be an association with other tumours of the CNS such as optic glioma, meningioma, glioblastoma, and, rarely, phaeochromocytoma; also iris harmartomas), type II is central and presents with juvenile cataracts, bilateral acoustic neuromas, meningiomas and gliomas and sensori-neural deafness rather than skin lesions (autosomal dominant, associated with chromosome 22).

Associations: Pheochromocytoma (2%) and renal artery stenosis (2%).

Complications: Epilepsy, sarcomatous change (5%), scoliosis (5%), mental retardation (10%). Spinal nerve root formation can lead to cord compression. CNS fibromas can lead to stenosis/compression of the Sylvian aqueduct and give rise to hydrocephalus.

Investigations: Genetic screening, 24-hour urinary catecholamines, MAG-3 scan for renal artery stenosis, MRI brain/spine (type I), MRI cerebellopontine angle, auditory testing (type II).

Management: Condition is autosomal dominant and therefore genetic counselling; surgery where appropriate.

Complications: Acoustic neuroma, Vth nerve neuroma, cord compression, sensory loss and Charcot's joints, lung cysts, intracranial tumours, associated with phaeochromocytoma (need to check BP), nodules on iris and hamartoma of the retina.

ECZEMA

Eczema is an inflammatory skin disorder with characteristic histology and clinical features, that include itching, redness, scaling and a papulovesicular rash. Eczema can be divided into two broad groups: Exogenous and endogenous.

Erythematous, lichenified patches of skin.

Predominantly flexural.

Scaling.

Fissures (painful), especially hands and feet.

Excoriations (a shallow abrasion due to scratching).

Secondary bacterial infection.

Differential diagnosis: Exogenous (primary irritant dermatitis and allergic contact dermatitis) and endogenous (**atopic** – a characteristic dermatitic eruption associated with a personal or family history of atopy, the age of onset being between 2 and 6 months, with males more affected than females, tends to be chronic but tends to improve during childhood; **discoid** (nummular) – well-demarcated patches on the trunk and limbs; **pompholyx** – itchy vesicles on palms and soles, **seborrhoeic dermatitis** – red, scaly rash caused by *Pityrosporum ovale*, occurring on the scalp, face and upper trunk and more common in young adults and HIV patients, gravitational, asteatotic).

History and examination are sufficient for diagnosis. Investigations: History of atopy, e.g. asthma, hayfever and allergy; patch-testing (useful in establishing potential allergic contact) and prick testing.

Complications: Secondary infection and erythroderma.

Treatment: Avoid irritants, exacerbating factors and precipitants; regular emollients, tar bandages, wet wraps, antibiotic ointment for minor infections; topical steroids; anti-histamines for pruritus; antibiotics for secondary infection; u/v (UVB or PUVA) light therapy. Also consider topic tacrolimus, pimecrolimus (recent NICE review available).

VITILIGO

Key signs are depigmented lesions.

Investigations: None although Wood's light will highlight but not fluoresce like a fungal lesion. Consider other autoimmune problems such as thyroid/pernicious anaemia.

Management: Usually cosmetic, camouflage–Red Cross run a service.

Phototherapy, topical steroid and tacrolimus have been tried with some benefit but seldom really good results.

Sun protection.

PSORIASIS

A genetically determined, inflammatory and proliferative disorder of the skin, occurring in 1-2% of the UK population.

Aetiology unknown. Association with HLA Cw6, B13 and B17 in skin disease and B27 in psoriatic arthropathy.

More common in 2nd and 6th decades, with females generally developing psoriasis at a younger age than males.

Numerous symmetrical well-demarcated/sharply-defined salmon pink/red plaques of varying sizes with silvery white scaling surfaces. The plaques are most prominent on extensor surfaces (elbows, knees)/scalp and hairline/behind the ears/at the umbilicus. Extent of severity of plaque psoriasis, presence of variant psoriasis, presence of arthropathy.

Koebner's phenomenon: Localised at the site of trauma (other causes include lichen planus, vitiligo, viral warts, molluscum contagiosum).

Auspitz's sign: Punctuate bleeding spots on scraping the scales. (Other associations are lichen planus, viral warts, vitiligo and sarcoid). Note the character of the lesions (scales, thickness, erythema, pustulation), the extent of cover, the degree of itching, and complications such as joint involvement. Skin staining from treatment.

Types: Pustular-palmoplantar pustukosis variant, yellow/brown sterile pustules and erythema affects palms and soles.

Erythodermic psoriasis: Severe systemic upset with fever, raised WBC, inflammatory markers and dehydration; confluent areas affecting most of the skin surface.

Flexural psoriasis: Affects axillae, submammary areas and natal cleft. Often smooth, red and glazed looking.

Guttate: An acute eruption of multiple "drop-like" lesions on trunk and limbs following a streptococcal infection.

Palmo-plantar pustular psoriasis.

Nail psoriasis: Include keratin thickening; loss of minute plugs of normal keratin results in characteristic pitting and sometimes the thickened, dystrophic nail separates from its nail bed; subungual hyperkeratosis, destruction of the nail plate, discolouration of the nail plates and oncholysis. Other causes of oncholysis (often with discoloured, thickened, hyperkeratotic but brittle dystrophic nails) include fungal infection, trauma, dermatitis, peripheral vascular disease, thyrotoxicosis.

Chronic plaque: Well-defined disc like plaques covered by white scale classically affecting elbows, knees and scalp.

Associations with psoriasis: Gout, arthropathy, malabsorption (Crohn's and ulcerative colitis).

Factors which exacerbate psoriasis: Trauma (Kobner phenomenon), infection (including HIV), endocrine (psoriasis generally tends to improve during pregnancy and deteriorate during the post-partum period), drugs (β-blockers, lithium, antimalarials and the withdrawal of oral steroids can exacerbate psoriasis), alcohol, stress (severe physical or psychological stress).

Investigations: Most patients do not require any investigations. Skin biopsy can be used to detect psoriafirom papillomatosis, acanthosis, hyperkeratosis and parakeratosis, with intradermal collections of neutrophils.

Treatment: A careful explanation of the disease process and the likely necessity for long-term treatment should always be given. The type of psoriasis and severity influences the choice of treatment. It is usual to use topical agents as the first-line treatment.

Topical (emollients such as oil/soap emollients and moisturisers control scale), calcipotriol ointment (vitamin D_3 analogues), coal tar (smell, stains brown), dithranol (stains purple and burns normal skin, usually effective), topical retinoids such as tazarotene, hydrocortisone.

For widespread or severe disease, further treatment options include:

Systemic: Cytotoxics (methotrexate and ciclosporin: Methotreate is used in widespread plaque, acute generalized pustular and erythrodermic psoriasis, and psoriatic arthropathy as short-term or maintenance treatment; retinoids are effective particularly in acral or generalized pustular psoriasis), retinoids (acitretin, safe and teratogenic)

Phototherapy: UVB narrowband (311-313 nm) is now replacing broadband UVB (290–320 nm) (for chronic plaque and guttate psoriasis), psoralen + UVA (PUVA).

Other biological agents (promising new treatments but as yet not licensed for psoriasis include etanercept and eflalizumab, presently under review by NICE): Efalizumab humanized monoclonal antibody – blocks T cell activation/migration; alefacept – recombinant fusion protein which interferes with activation/proliferation of T cells; etanercept – human fusion protein of the TNF receptor which acts as a TNF? inhibitor; infliximab – monoclonal antibody which binds TNFa.

Complications: Psoriatic arthropathy 10% (five forms: DIP involvement, large joint mono/oligoarthritis, seronegative, sacroilitis, arthritis mutilans), erythroderma.

Guttate psoriasis: Associated with streptococcal throat infection, resolves in 3 months.

PURPURA

These fall largely into two groups.
Vessel disorders.
Platelet disorders.
Observe the distribution of the lesions, e.g. senile purpura/steroids often affect backs of hands and forearms. Henoch-Schonlein purpura classically appears over lower limbs and buttocks. Scurvy over lower limbs/backs of thighs with perifollicular haemorrhages plus corkscrew hairs; look for woollen gums.

Inspect palate for petechial haemorrhages, gums for ulceration and haemorrhage (suggests neutropenia and thrombocytopaenia), conjunctivae and fundi for haemorrhages (fundal haemorrhages only in severe thrombocytopaenia).

Look for evidence of cause: Cushingoid (steroid), Rheumatoid, SLE, infective endocarditis, Chronic liver disease, Ehler-Danlos syndrome.

If a vasculitic cause is suspected, it is important to look for renal involvement; you should therefore offer to dipstix the urine.

DERMATITIS HERPETIFORMIS

Look for characteristic distribution on extensor surface of elbows, knees and on occiput, interscapular and gluteal regions. These are symmetrical, highly itchy vesicles or urticarial plaques on the trunk and extensor surfaces, buttocks and occasionally the face and scalp, and is associated with gluten-sensitive enteropathy (coeliac disease). Dapsone is the treatment of choice.

KAPOSI'S SARCOMA

There may be solitary or numerous reddy-purple, and bluish-brown macules, plaques and nodules. These may occur on the skin and mucosa.

Sites commonly affected: Skin, feet, mouth, stomach, lungs.

Lesions can be painful.

Systemic disease may cause abdominal pain or haemoptysis.

Endemic in African males, peripheral involvement.

In HIV +ve patients, distribution may be widespread.

Lymphatic obstruction leading to chronic oedema and cellulitis of lower limbs.

Also seen in elderly Jewish or Meditteraneam males, with indolent course on distal extremities, and in immunodeficient patients, including transplant patients.

Investigations: Biopsy and PCR for HHV-8, CD4 and viral load, endoscopy and bronchoscopy if symptomatic.

Treatment: Radiotherapy often useful for patients with oedema, interferon alpha, chemotherapy.

BUTTERFLY RASH

There is a butterfly malar rash. Look for/consider causes:

1. *Systemic lupus erythematosus:* There are raised or flat patches of malar erythema, sparing nasolabial folds. Other areas such as the forehead and neck and often unaffected. There may be marked photosensitivity. There may be mouth ulcers, Oral ulceration, Scarring alopecia, Anaemia. Vasculitic changes in the hands. Raynaud's phenomenon. Jaccoud's arthropathy (mimics rheumatoid arthritis but due to tendon contractures not joint destruction).

Typical arthropathy involves MCP and PIP joints, ulnar deviation of the joints, sublaxation of the PIP joints. *Elsewhere:* Purpura due to thrombocytopenia, livedo reticularis, pyoderma gangrenosum, peripheral oedema. *Extra points:* Respiratory (pleural effusion, pleural rub, fibrosing alveolitis), neurological (focal neurology, chorea, ataxia), eyes (Sjogren's), renovascular (hypertension, proteinuria).

Diagnostic investigation: ANA, anti-dsDNA.

Disease activity: Elevated ESR but normal CRP, elevated immunoglobulins, reduced complement, urine microscopy (glomerulonephritis). FBC, APTT, anti-cardiolipin antibodies if APTT prolonged.

Treatment: Mild disease (topical corticosteroids, hydroxychloroquine), moderate disease (prednisolone, azathioprine), severe disease (methylprednisolone, cyclophosphamide, azathioprine). Specific photoprotection advice includes using skin creams or makeup, and avoidance of sun at the middle of the day.

2. *Discoid lupus erythematosus:* DLE is a skin limited disease with well defined erythematous papules or plaques on light exposed areas including the head, neck, hands and arms. The lesions are scaling and hyperkeratosis of hair follicles gives these scales a dotted 'nutmeg' appearance. If you were to remove the scales and inspect their undersurface, you would see spicules projecting from them.

3. *Acne rosacea:* There is an erythematous, 'acneiform' popular eruption on the flush areas of the face or facial convexities – cheeks. The erythema is marked, with prominent dilated blood vessels (telenhectasia). There are pustules within the eruption. Rosacea may not spare the nasolabial folds and its pustules are characteristic. The rash of SLE and DLE spares the nasolabial folds and pustules are not a feature. Scarring, follicular plugging and scarring are features of DLE but not rosacea. Acne rosacea tends to affect females more than males, with precipitating factors including heat, sun, alcohol, spicy foods, emotion/embarrassment, and steroids. There is episodic flushing with erythema, telengectasia and papules/pastules in the earlier stages. Later there is sebaceous hyperplasia, but seborrhoea and comedones are not a feature. Rosacea is usually symmetrical. Steroids should not be used. They are not effective in the long term and tend to cause skin addiction and rebound flares. Avoidance of precipitating factors is seldom helpful except for the use of sunscreens. Topical treatments included

metronidazole or erythromycin gel, with an emollient. Systemic treatments include oral tetracycline, minocycline, and doxycycline. Isotretinoin is usually beneficial. Rhinophyma occurs in later cases. [NB. Acne vulgaris causes comedones without telengectasia, and its distribution is generally wide. It is a chronic inflammatory disorder of the pilosebaceous structure, characterized by comedones (non-infmaled lesions), erythematous papules, pustules and nodules (inflamed lesions), and scarring. Scarring tends to be hypertrophic and keloid (trunk) or 'ice pick'.]

4. *Lupus pernio:* These are purple/red/violaceous plaques on the nose, cheeks and earlobes with telengiectasia over and around the plaques. The plaques have a yellowish translucency. They tend to flatten with time. Lupus pernio and lupus vulgaris are not pustular.

5. *Lupus vulgaris:* This is the skin manifestation of tuberculosis and is rare in the UK. The lesion has an 'apple jelly' consistency when a translucent slide is rested upon it.

6. *Dermatomyositis:* There is a heliotrope rash around the eyelids. It may also affect the malar region, limb extensors, knuckles and trunk. Gottron's papules may be present on the dorsum of the hands (notably metacarpophalangeal joints and interphalangeal joints), and occasionally elsewhere. Nailfold erythema due to dilated capillaries is often present, and the cuticles may be ragged.

7. *Seborrhoeic dermatitis*

BULLOUS DISORDERS

Pemphigus: Lesions in mouth common. Autoantibodies against desmosomes which bridge adjacent epidermal cells. Bullae tend to break easily and even rubbing of normal skin causes sloughing of the epidermis (Nikolsky sign). Widespread crusting and erosions. Bullous eruption on the trunk and flexor surfaces. Treat with steroids and immunomodulatory drugs.

Pemphigoid: Mucosal ulceration rare. Autoantibodies present at the dermo-epidermal border. Tense bullae present with erythematous plaques. Many burst, leaving red, exuding, tender patches. Tends to affect the elderly. Treat with steroids.

ERYTHEMA NODOSUM

[See also painful shins under the *History taking* chapter (Chapter 4).]
   Key signs are flat, red, tender, nodular large lesions on the shins, associated with fever and arthralgia.

Signs of a cause, e.g. red, sore throat or systemic manifestations of sarcoidosis. *Investigations:* History, may be due to sarcoid, check ACE and CXR, TB.

Causes of erythema nodosum include streptococcus, salmonella or campylobacter gastroenteritis; sarcoidosis; tuberculosis; oral contraceptive pill, sulphonamides, tetracyclines, penicillin; ulcerative colitis, Crohn's disease; lymphoma/malignancy; viral/chlamydial infection; pregnancy.

Management: Often self-resolving, treat sarcoid if required, or remove cause. Other skin manifestations of sarcoidosis: *Nodules and plaques* (red/brown seen particularly around the face, nose, ears and neck. Demonstrates Koebner's phenomenon) and *lupus pernio* (bluish/brown plaque with central small papules commonly affecting the nose).

PYODERMA GANGRENOSUM

This may begin as a nodular erythema or a sterile pustule, but develops often into large areas of painful, necrotic ulceration. There are large necrotic ulcers with ragged bluish-red overhanging edges together with areas containing erythematous plaques with pustules. They are situated on the legs. The appearances are suggestive of pyoderma gangrenosum. The patient may have Crohn's disease or ulcerative colitis.

Other causes: Gastrointestinal (ulcerative colitis, Crohn's disease), rheumatological (rheumatoid disease, ankylosing spondylitis), liver (chronic active hepatitis, primary biliary cirrhosis, sclerosing cholangitis), haematological (lymphoproliferative and myeloproliferative disorders), others (diabetes mellitus, thyroid disease, sarcoidosis, Wegener's disease).

It is frequently an indicator of severity of the disease. Systemic steroids often help. The adjunctive use of minocycline may reduce corticosteroid requirements. Other causes of leg ulcers include venous ulceration, ischaemic arterial ulceration, diabetes mellitus, vasculitis, infection, Charcot's joints, tumour, haematological (sickle cell, thalassaemia, pnh), neurological (diabetes, tabes dorsalis, leprosy, syringomyelia).

LEG OEDEMA

In bilateral oedema look for:
• Signs of right heart failure, especially raised jugular venous pressure.

- Involvement of the face/periorbital tissues suggesting nephrotic syndrome.
- Signs of chronic liver disease (hypoalbuminaemia may occur, look for leuconychia).
- Palpate inguinal nodes for enlargement; malignant infiltration may occur causing secondary lymphoedema.
- Comment on the desirability of abdominal, rectal and vaginal examination to exclude malignancy.
  In unilateral oedema look for:
  Other signs of deep vein thrombosis.
- Measure the calf with a tape measure.
- Consider ruptured Baker's cyst, especially in a patient with osteoarthritis or rheumatoid arthritis. Ultrasound, arthrography and/or venography may be necessary to distinguish between the two conditions.
- Look for varicose veins, venous eczema and ulceration.

NECROBIOSIS LIPOIDICA DIABETICORUM

A common 'spot' case.
  Associated with diabetes in about 75% of cases.
  Histology: Collagen degeneration with surrounding epithelioid and giant cells.
  Well-demarcated plaques with waxy-yellow centre and red-brown edges, coalescing oval plaques on the shins. The lesions have a shiny atrophic surface and may ulcerate. Prominent skin blood vessels.

Treatment: Topical steroid and support bandaging. Tight glycaemic control does not help, but this should be tried. Steroids administered cautiously may help. The histology varies, some containing large amounts of lipid.

OTHER DIABETIC CHANGES

Cheirarthropathy: Tight waxy skin that limits finger extension.

Granuloma annulare: Flesh-coloured papules in annular configurations on the dorsum of the fingers. These are pale or flesh-coloured papule coalescing in rings of usually 1-3 cm diameter, especially on the backs of the hands and fingers. Blanching by pressure reveals a characteristic beaded ring of white dermal patches. It is sometimes associated with diabetes especially when the lesions are generalized and atypical.

LIPIDS

Details, cardiovascular history, diabetes history, hypertension history, family history of ischaemic heart disease, alcohol, smoking, dietary and exercise history, concerns of patient. Need to minimize risk factors related to the above, multidisciplinary team including dietitian, statins. Proteinuria and hypertension 24-hour urinary collection, ACE-inhibitor, angiotensin-II receptor antagonist.

Hypercholesterolaemia: Tendon xanthomata, xanthelasma and corneal arcus.

Hypertriglyceridaemia: Eruptive xanthomata and lipaemia retinalis

Secondary hypercholesterolaemia: Hypothyroidism, nephrotic syndrome, alcohol, cholestasis.

Extensor tendon xanthomata: Classically occur in the extensor surfaces and may become more obvious when the patient clenches his fist. Look also for xanthomata in the Achilles tendons and patellar tendons. Look for xanthelasmata and corneal arcus. Aetiologiy is ischaemic heart disease. Remember than tendon xanthomata are classically found in Type IIA lipoproteinaemia: This may be primary (familial hypercholesterolaemia), or secondary (seen in jaundice). Investigations are cholesterol (markedly elevated), HDL, LDL and triglycerides, family history.

   Eruptive xanthomata are multiple red or yellow vesicles which are found on extensor surfaces: Back, buttocks, elbows, knees. These are not usually associated with tendon xanthomata or xanthelasmata. Ask if you may inspect the fundi for lipaemia retinalis (found in severe hyperlipidaemia, which is associated with diabetes mellitus and obesity). Symptoms may be of diabetes, pancreatitis and ischaemic heart disease. It also occurs in Types I and V lipoproteinaemia. Findings are raised triglycerides, cholesterol may be normal. Plasma appears lipaemic. HBA1c.

   Palmar xanthomata are rare xanthomata which are orange or yellow discolourations of the palmar and digital creases being most distinctive. Look also for 'tubo-eruptive xanthomata' characteristically found over the knees and elbows. Check the eyelids for xanthelasmata, which are also associated.

Xanthelasmata: Never forget the importance of inspection. Look for the corneal arcus, which often coexists with xanthelasmata and is typically most pronounced at the 12 and 6 o'clock poitions (in contrast to corneal calcification which tends to be maximal at the 3 and 9 o'clock positions). Look for tendon xanthomas in the hands and Achilles tendons. Check the palms for xanthomata and tell the examiner you would like to take the patient's blood pressure and test the urine for glucose (hypertension and diabetes mellitus being associated with Type IIB lipoproteinaemia). Remember that xanthelasmata and corneal arcus may occur in normal people, type IIA lipoproteinaemia, type IIB lipoproteinaemia, type III lipoproteinaemia. Associations of xanthelasmata also include hypothyroidism, nephrotic syndrome and chronic obstructive jaundice.

PRETIBIAL MYXOEDEMA

Key signs: Elevated symmetrical skin lesions over the anterolateral aspects of shin.

Coarse: Purplish red

Raised with well-defined serpiginous margins.

Skin is shiny and has an orange-skin appearance. Hairs in the affected areas are coarse and lesions are tender.

Remember to check for thyroid acropachy.

Skin in the superficial area is infiltrated with mucopolysaccharide. Biopsy scars then to develop keloid.

The latent interval between treatment for hyperthyroidism and onset of pretibial myxoedema varies from 4 to 31 months with a mean time 1 year.

SYSTEMIC SCLEROSIS

An Extremely Common Cause

Female: Male ratio = 4:1, usual age of presentation is 40.

Key signs: Pinched cheeks, microstomia, telengectasia, look at fingers, ask if you can check for Raynaud's swallowing. Calcinosis, Raynaud's Phenomenon (white to blue to red), oesophageal involvement, sclerodactyly and telegectasia. *Morphoea* (focal/generalized patches of sclerotic skin which does not progress to systemic involvement; characterised by thickened, waxy plaques on the trunk or limbs), *en coup de sabre* (scar down central forehead).

Other organ involvement: Renal failure 20% may be associated with accelerated hypertension responsive to ACE inhibitors, heart (pericardial effusion), musculoskeletal, intestine (rarely hypomotility with a dilated second part of the duodenum leads to bacterial overgrowth). Pulmonary hypertension may develop independent of parenchymal changes. Interstitial fibrosis (fine, bibasal crackles).

Definition: Limited is distribution limited to hands, feet and face, tight thick skin, microstomia, CREST syndrome, slow progression (years); diffuse is widespread cutaneous and early visceral involvement, rapid progression (months).

Investigations: Skin biopsy, autoantibodies (ANF positive in 90%, 80% limited anti-centromere, 70% diffuse anti-Scl 70 antibody which has an increased association with pulmonary fibrosis), renal function (and dipstix the urine, urine microscopy for casts, and consider renal biopsy), pulmonary function, oesophageal motility, blood pressure, echocardiogram and ECG primarily to assess pulmonary artery pressures and presence of pericardial effusions. Antibody to U3 ribonucleoprotein may also occur, present mainly in parients with diffuse disease and overlap syndromes.

Management: Supportive, topical camouflage creams, Raynaud's therapy (gloves, hand-warmers, calcium channel blockers, ACE inhibitors, prostacyclin infusion for severe), dependent on systemic involvement (*Renal:* Hypertensive control; *Malabsorption:* Low-residue diets, nutritional supplements; oesophageal symptoms-proton pump inhibitors and prokinetic drugs). General–education, counselling, family support. Contractures – exercises and lubricants.

The 5 years cumulative survival is 35-75%. Adverse factors are increasing age, male sex, extent of skin, heart and renal involvement. Hypertensive renal crises are an important cause of morbidity being a 30% 10 years survival while pulmonary involvement has a 50% survival.

LEG ULCERS

Venous: Painless ulcers, gaiter area.

Stigmata of venous hypertension: Varicose veins or scars from vein stripping, oedema, lipodermatosclerosis, varicose eczema, *atrophie blanche.*

Cause: Abdominal/pelvic mass.

Investigation: Doppler ultrasound of the venous system.

Treatment: Remove exudates and slough with regular cleaning with tapwater or saline, apply liquid paraffin/white soft paraffin, treat surrounding venous eczema, four-layer compression bandaging, vein surgery. If infected, take swabs, but do not use topical antibiotics as they can be sensitizers (e.g. neomycin).

Arterial: Painful, distal extremities and pressure points, trophic changes: Hairless and paper-thin shiny skin, cold with poor capillary refill, absent distal pulses.

Cause: Check for atrial fibrillation or cardiac murmur.

Investigation: Ankle-Brachial Pressure Index (0.8–1.2 is normal, <0.8 implies arterial insufficiency), arteriography.

Many patients have contact dermatitits to previous topical treatments.

Treatment: Angioplasty, vascular reconstruction, amputation

Neuropathic: Painless, pressure areas, e.g. under metatarsal heads, peripheral neuropathy.

Cause: Look for diabetic signs, Charcot's ulcer, diabetes mellitus, tabes dorsalis, syringomyelia.

Complications: Infection, malignant change (Marjolin's ulcer).

Othere causes: Vasculitic, neoplastic, infectious, haematological, tropical.

PIGMENTARY CHANGES

Hyperpigmentation

Causes of hyperpigmentation include:
- Genetic (Peutz-Jehgers syndrome; xeroderma pigmentosum; Albright's syndrome).
- Metabolic (cirrhosis, haemochromatosis, porphyria, renal failure).
- Drugs (oral contraceptive pill, minocycline, amiodarone).
- Endocrine (Addison's disease, Cushing's syndrome, Nelson's syndrome, pregnancy).
- Nutritional (malabsorption, carcinomatosis, Kwashiokor, pellagra).
- Post-inflammatory (lichen planus, eczema, secondary syphilis and cutaneous amyloid).

Hypopigmentation

Causes of hypopigmentation include:
- Genetic (albinism, phenylketonuria, tuberous sclerosis).
- Chemical (chloroquine).
- Infections (pityriasis versicolor).
- Endocrine (hypopituitarism).
- Autoimmune (vitiligo).
- Post-inflammatory (eczema, psorias, lupus erythematosus).

ALOPECIA

Distribution: Look for hair loss on the body and signs of anaemia, thyroid disease, autoimmune or skin disease. Check for features of androgen excess in females e.g. acne, hirsutism, virilization. Don't forget to look at the nails too (e.g. lichen planus, alopecia areata, Beau's line in telogen effluvium).

Table 8.1: Types of alopecia

Scarring (usually patchy)	Discoid lupus erythematosus Lichen planus Cicatrial pemphigoid Sarcoidosis Tumours, e.g. BCC Burns Radiation Infections including fungal kerion Traction (late changes)
Non-scarring and patchy	Androgenetic alopecia Alopecia areata Tinea capitis Traction (in early stages) Secondary syphilis
Non-scarring and generalized	Iron deficiency Telogen and androgen effluvium Drugs Alopecia totalis Endocrine, e.g. thyroid disease Hypopituitarism Malnutrition SLE Chronic disease

Alopecia areata may resolve with no treatment or may fail to resolve with maimum treatment. Topical or locally injected steroids may be used; short systemic course have poor evidence of sustained benefit.

ACANTHOSIS NIGRICANS

Brown 'velvet-like' skin change commonly found in the axillae.
Associations: Obesity, cultural, type II diabetes mellitus, acromegaly, malignancy, e.g. gastric carcinoma and lymphoma.

PSEUDOXANTHOMA ELASTICUM

"Plucked chicken skin" appearance: Loose skin folds especially at the neck and axillae, with yellow pseudoxanthomatous plaques. Hyperextensive joints.

Extra points: Blue sclerae, reduced visual acuity, hypothyroidism, miscarriages, retinal angioid streaks and macular degeneration.

Cardiovascular: Blood pressure 50% are hypertensive, mitral valve prolapse, CVA and/or CCF from atherosclerosis, peripheral vascular disease.

Discussion: Inheritance: Autosomal dominant or recessive, degenerative elastic fibres in skin, blood vessels and eye, premature coronary artery disease.

TUBEROUS SCLEROSIS

There is a papular, salmon-coloured eruption on the centre of the face, especially the nasolabial folds. These angiomatous glistening papules and their configuration have the appearance of adenoma sebaceum (look for periungual fibromata and shagreen patches). There may be a history of epilepsy and mental deficiency which together with adenoma sebaceum make up tuberous sclerosis. Other organs affected are the cerebral hemispheres (multiple hamartomata or tubers), renal hamartoma in 2/3 of paients, retinal hamartoma which appear yellow, cardiac hamartoma, and cystic lung disease.

EHLER-DANLOS SYNDROME

Early scarring, 'fish mouth' scars especially on the knees. No skin folds.

Fragile skin: Multiple ecchymoses.

Hyperextensible skin: Able to tent up skin when pulled (avoid doing this)
   Joint hypermobility and dislocation.

Extra points: Mitral valve prolapse, abdominal scars (aneurismal rupture and dissection, bowel perforation and bleeding).

Discussion: Autosomal dominant, defect in collagen increasing skin elasticity, no premature coronary artery disease.

HEREDITARY HAEMORRHAGIC TELANGECTASIA/ OSLER-WEBER-RENDU

Small, flattened multiple telengectasia on the face, lips and buccal mucosa.

Anaemia: Gastrointestinal bleeding.

There may be clubbing due to aneurysms/AV malformations in the lung.

Examine the respiratory system, particularly for cyanosis and a chest bruit, and a pulmonary vascular abnormality/shunt. Their presence can result in complications such as pulmonary haemorrhage; they may be sufficiently large or numerous to cause shunting (right to left) with resultant hyoxia, and, additionally, they may be involved in paradoxical embolic events.

Discussion: Autosomal dominant, increased risk of gastrointestinal haemorrhage, epistaxis and haemoptysis.

Vascular malformations: Pulmonary shunts, intracranial aneurysms (subarachnoid haemorrhage).

EXFOLIATIVE DERMATITIS

Exfoliative dermatitis may occur in response to drug therapy, systemic disease or an idiopathic entity. Common causes are systemic disease (lymphoma, leukaemia, multiple myeloma, carcinoma of the lung, prostate, colon and thyroid, immunodeficiency, Hodgkin's disease), cutaneous diseases such as psoriasis, seborrhoeic dermatitis, atopic dermatitis, Mycosis fungoides and lichen planus, and drugs such as codeine, captopril, antimicrobials such as cephalosporins, and barbiturates. Laboratory studies include serum albumin, ESR, and investigation of cardiac, renal and intestinal failure. General measures are to withdraw implicated medications and identify underlying infection and/or disease, protect the patient from the development of hypothermia, advise local moisturizing ointments, advise high-protein diet with folic acid supplementation since protein losses can be high, and urgent dermatological referral. Complications include hypothermia, superinfection, dehydration and heart failure.

SKIN MALIGNANCY

Basal cell carcinoma: Usually on the face/trunk, sun-exposed areas, pearly nodule with rolled edge, superficial telengectasia, ulceration in advanced lesions, local invasion and distant metastasis, other lesions.

Natural history: Slowly grow over a few months, local invasion only, rarely metastasize.

Treatment: Curettage/cryotherapy if superficial, surgical excision ± radiotherapy.

Squamous cell carcinoma: Sun-exposed areas (+ lips + mouth), actinic keratoses (pre-malignant, red-scaly patches), varied appearance (keratotic nodule, polypoid mass, cutaneous ulcer), local invasion and distant metastasis, other lesions.

Management: Biopsy suspicious lesions, surgery ± radiotherapy, 5% metastasize.

Malignant melanoma: Clinical risk factors (light hair, blue eyes), asymmetrical, border irregularity, color (black – often irregular pigmentation), diameter > 6 mm. Local invasion and distant metastasis, other lesions.

Management: Excision, staged on Breslow thickness (maximal depth of tumour invasion into dermis), < 1.5 mm = 90% 5-year survival, > 3.5 mm = 40% 5-year survival.

POLYMYOSITIS AND DERMATOMYOSITIS

Heliotrope rash around the eyes. Gottren's papules on the MCP joints.
    Proximal muscle weakness and wasting with muscle tenderness.
    Diffuse calcification within the muscles.
    40% of patients have primary disease with unknown aetiology.
    Associated with malignancy in 10-25% of cases, especially lung and ovary.
    Look for clubbing, Horner's syndrome, lymphadenopathy or hepatomegaly.
    It is associated with other autoimmune disorders in 10% of cases, e.g. rheumatoid arthritis, SLE.
    Juvenile forms are associated with contractures and calcification of muscle.

Symptoms: Muscle pain and weakness, dysphagia and symptoms of the cause.

Investigations: CK, aldolase, LDH, EMG – small polyphasic potentials, spontaneous; muscle biopsy – inflammatory cell infiltrates with muscle necrosis; tumour markers, e.g. CA125, CEA.

Autoimmune profile (ANA weakly positive in 60-70%, anti-Jo-1 is specific).

Respiratory Function Tests

Treatment: Supportive, physiotherapy, exercise, immunosuppressants (high-dose steroids and azathioprine if steroid-unresponsive, 20% of patients recover fully).

Consider malignancy, if male > 45 years of age; absent autoantibodies; poor response to treatment.

LIVEDO RETICULARIS

There tends to present as an arborescent pattern of reddish-blue erythema (or pigmentary change), and may be associated with antiphospholipid antibody syndrome, collagen vascular disease–especially polyarteritis nodosa, cryoglobulinaemia or a hyperviscosity syndrome. APAS is a hypercoaguable condition leading to both venous and arterial occlusions. Lupus anticoagulant and anticardiolipin antibodies are the serological markers. DVT, transient ischaemic attack, cerebrovascular attack, migraine, epilepsy and recurrent abortions may all be manifestations. APAS is also being recognised as a primary condition.

LICHEN PLANUS

This presents as an itchy, violaceous, flat-topped, polygonal, popular rash with white lines on the surface called Wickham's striae. Other affected sites include mucous membranes, genitalia, palms, soles, scalp and nails. On the buccal mucosa, it causes a white lace-like pattern. Causes of white lesions in the oral mucosa include: Leucoplakia, chronic candidiasis, and chemical burns.

LOCOMOTOR

Examine the joints of (a certain part of the body) and discuss with the examiners.

GENERAL LOCOMOTOR SCREENING "GALS"

Joint appearance: Swelling, deformity, restricted movement.

Muscle wasting: Global and localised wasting, specific muscles or groups.

Function with relation to activities of daily living.

Look, feel, move algorithm.

Inflammatory arthritis compared to non-inflammatory arthritis.

A specific system, often used in 'short cases' is GALS: Gait (look for any symmetry, deformity in leg length, spinal curvature, arm swing), Arms, Legs, Spine (see below).

Ask with some screening questions:

Have you any pain or stiffness in your arms, legs or back?

Can you walk up and down stairs without difficulties?

Can you dress yourself in everyday clothes without any help?

Gait

You may be asked to describe the gait of a patient with hip pathology. The two main types are *antalgic* and the *Trendelenburg* gait.

Table 8.2: Differences between an antalgic gait and a Trendelenburg gait

	Antalgic gait	Trendelenburg gait
Cause	Painful hip	Inefficient hip abduction
Weight-bearing/stance phase opposite side		Shortened Pelvis droops on the
Direction to which body leans whilst weight-bearing	Towards affected side	Towards unaffected side

You may be asked to describe the mechanism of the Trendelenburg gait. Normally, when standing on one leg, the abductors on the weight-bearing side contract so that the pelvis rises on the opposite side. A positive Trendelenburg test occurs when there is any *inefficiency of hip abduction*: The pelvis droops towards the unsupported side.

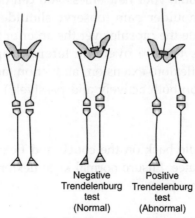

Negative   Positive
Trendelenburg   Trendelenburg
test   test
(Normal)   (Abnormal)

Figure 8.1: Trendelenburg test

Inefficiency of hip abduction occurs as a result of the following: *disturbance in the pivotal mechanism* (dislocation or sublaxation of the hip, shortening of the femoral neck) and *weakness of the hip abductors* (gluteus medius and minimus) (myopathy, usually bilateral, and neuropathy – L5 lesion, usually unilateral).

Arms

During the general inspection, you should inspect for abnormalities such as a swelling or deformity, and look for any skin changes which may be associated with arthritis, for example, digital vasculitis in SLE, or evidence of peripheral infarcts from Raynaud's phenomenon.

Ask the patient to show you his/her hands, palms down, and then turn them over – this is an assessment of the radioulnar joint, which is a common site for rheumatoid arthritis. Remember to keep the elbows tucked in, or patients can use their shoulders to perform this movement.

Ask the patient to make a tight fist with each hand; this is a position of function of the hands, and you can also assess power grip.

Ask the patient to place the tip of each finger onto the tip of the thumb in turn; this permits an assessment of the dexterity and fine finger movements of the hand which is limited in rheumatoid arthritis.

Squeeze across from the second to the fifth metacarpals; this is an assessment of joint tenderness. Tenderness across the metacarpophalangeal joints is a sign of rheumatoid arthritis.

Next, ask the patient to put his/her hands behind the head, pressing the shoulders right back; this is an assessment of abduction and external rotation of the shoulder with flexion of the elbow. It is a measurement of shoulder and elbow movement as well of function; it is not possible to put on a tie or comb your hair unless you can do this manoeuvre.

Look for any shoulder pain (observe shoulders for asymmetry and swelling; palpate the capsule over the anterior humeral head and the supraspinatus tendon over the lateral upper humerus for tenderness; assess flexion, extension, abduction, adduction, internal and external rotation both actively and passively).

Legs

Ask the patient to lie back on the couch and flex the hip and knee while holding the knee. Ensure normal knee flexion, feel for crepitus, and also test hip flexion.

Then passively and internally rotate the hip with the knee and hip still flexed; this is a measurement of knee movement and internal rotation of the hip.

Look for any hip pain (look for flexion deformity of the hip; assess flexion at the hip with the knee flexed to relax the hamstrings; assess internal and external rotation in flexion).

Look for any knee pain (look at the quadriceps muscle, wasted in significant knee disease; look for selling and perform the bulge test; flex and extend the knee to its fullest extent in either direction).

Ask the patient to flex, extent, invert, and evert the ankle in order to assess tibiotalar (affected by osteoarthritis) and subtalar (affected by inflammatory arthritis) movements.

Squeeze the metatarsals, again looking for rheumatoid arthritis, in the same way as looking over the metacarpals.

Spine

Observe the curvature of the cervical and thoracic spine in the posterior and lateral plane.

Ask the patient to stand up and put his/her ear to each shoulder in turn; this is an assessment of lateral fusion of the neck, which is lost with either osteoarthritis or rheumatoid arthritis affecting the neck.

Put two fingers over adjacent spinous processes in the lumbar region, and then ask the patient to bend over and touch his/her toes; your fingers should move apart. This is a modification of a Scrober's test which is designed to pick up a lack of movement associated with ankylosing spondylitis.

Ensure the pelvis is symmetrical/no abnormal rotation.

Look for low back pain (assess the curvature of the spine, palpate the erector spinae muscles to assess spasm, perform a Modified Schrober's test, ask the patient to lean over to each side in turn, ask the patient to lean over backards to assess extension, passively flex the hip keeping the knee extended and then passively dorsiflex the ankle – this is the sacral stretch test, and is positive if the patient complains of any sensory disturbance below the knee; the counterpart to this is the femoral stretch test by passively flexing the knee and extending the hip – a positive test is irritation over the front of the thigh).

MONOARTHRITIS

Table 8.3: Types of monoarthritis

Infective/trauma	Septic arthritis Gonococcal or meningococcal infection Rheumatic fever Viral infections
Seronegative arthropathies	Reiter's disease Reactive arthropathy Ankylosing spondylitis Psoriatic arthropathy Enteropathic arthropathy
Metabolic	Gout Pseudogout (associated with hyperparathyroidism, hyperuricaemia and gout, haemochromatosis, acromegaly, diabetes mellitus, renal failure, Wilson's disease, ochronosis)
Haematological	Haemophilia Sickle cell anaemia
Other	Osteoarthritis Rheumatoid disease

When discussing your management, always mention the importance of aspiration of the joint and culture of the fluid for bacterial infection/microscopy for crystals.

POLYARTHRITIS

- Rheumatoid arthritis
- Osteoarthritis
- Gout/pseudogout
- SLE
- Polyarteritis nodsa
- Rheumatic fever
- Ankylosing spondylitis
- Reiter's disease/reactive arthritis
- Psoriasis
- Still's disease
- Sarcoidosis
- Infective endocarditis
- *Others:* Systemic sclerosis, Whipple's disease, Behcet's disease, alkaptonuria.

  Tests: Rheumatoid factor, ANA, HLA typing.

CHARCOT'S JOINT

Painless deformity and destruction of a joint with new bone formation following repeated minor trauma secondary to loss of pain and sensation. The most important causes are tabes dorsalis: hip and knee, *Diabetes:* Ankle, syringomyelia: Elbow and shoulder. *Treatment:* Bisphosphonates can help.

PSORIATIC ARTHROPATHY

Psoriatic arthropathy affects up to 10% of patients with psoriasis and may proceed or follow skin disease by months or even years. There are in theory five types although overlapping pictures are common. *Types of psoriasis:* Pustular psoriasis, guttate psoriasis, flexural psoriasis, erythrodermic psoriasis.

- Asymmetrical distal interphalangeal joint arthropathy. This is relatively uncommon but the form most strongly associated with psoriasis. Affected digits often show nail changes such as pitting. This is an oligo- or monoarthritis.
- Rheumatoid like hands. This is the commonest arthropathy and is seronegative. Exclude rheumatoid nodules at the elbows and look for psoriatic changes. Predominantly affects DIP joints.
- Asymmetric large joint mono- or oligo-arthropathy. Tell the examiners you would ask about large joint pain or swelling.
- Spondyloarthropathy or sacroiliitis. Tell the examiners you would ask about low back pain. Appears like anykylosing spondylitis.
- *Arthritis mutilans:* A very uncommon, severely destructive form.

Tests: Skin biopsy, skin scrapings and nail clippings to rule out tinea, X-ray of the affected joints "pencil-in-cup" deformity, RA factor.

Treatment: Emollients, coal tar, short acting dithranol, talcacitol, steroids used topically, narrow band UVB phototherapy, retinoic acid derivatives, methotrexate in severe refractory disease/severe erythrodermic form/arthropathy, NSAIDs for arthropathy, and scalp psoriasis.

Sulphalazine and methotrexate are becoming established as treatment for psoriatic arthropathy. Ciclosporin may have a place in refractory disease.

RHEUMATOID DISEASE

An Extremely Common Case

Symmetrical, deforming arthropathy.

Signs

1. *Joints:* Typically a distal, symmetrical, small joint polyarthritis involving the proximal interphalangeal joint and metacarpophalangeal joints of the hand, wrist, metatarsophalangeal joints, ankles, knees and cervical spine.

2. *Upper limbs:* Soft tissue swelling around affected joints, spindle-shaped appearance of the fingers, trigger fingers due to tenosynovitis of the long finger tendons, compression of the Median nerve, Tinel's sign and Phalen's sign. Volar sublaxation of the metatarsocarpophalangeal joints, ulnar deviation and sublaxation of the fingers. Swan neck deformity. Boutonniere (button-hole) deformity and Z deformity of the thumb. Piano-key sign. Distal ulna migrates dorsally which can be depressed by pressure like a piano key. Subcutaneous nodules are commonly found on the extensor surface of the forearm of the elbow. Wasting of small muscles of the hand, use restricted by weakness, deformity and pain. Palmar erythema. Elbow and shoulder disease.

3. *Lower limbs:* Synovitis of the metatarosphalangeal joints resulting in larger shoe size. Valgus deformity of the hindfoot is normal and valgus deformity of the knee at a later stage.

4. *Extra-articular manifestations:* Rheumatoid nodules (subcutaneous and intracutaneous nodules), anaemia (moderate anaemia invariably), lung involvement (pleurisy, nodules and pulmonary fibrosis), cardiac (pericardial effusion), vasculitis (aortic valve more than mitral valve), Eye (Sjogren's syndrome, Episcleritis, Scleritis), peripheral nerve involvement (entrapment neuropathy), muscle (reflex inhibition and wasting resulting from severe joint pain), liver (hepatosplenomegaly), Felty's syndrome (splenomegaly + RA + leucopenia).

Assess disease activity: Red, swollen, hot, painful hands imply active disease.

Assess function: Power grip "squeeze my fingers", precision grip "pick up a coin", key grip "pretend to use this key", remember the wheelchair, walking aids and splints.

Extra points: Exclude psoriatic arthropathy (main differential), nail changes, *Psoriasis:* Elbows, behind ears, scalp, and around the umbilicus.

Surgical scars: Carpal tunnel release (wrist), joint replacement (especially thumb), tendon transfer (dorsum of the hand); steroid side effects; C-spine stabilization scars; systemic manifestations.

Causes of anaemia in rheumatoid disease: Anaemia of chronic disease, GI bleeding due to NSAIDs, bone marrow suppression (gold, indomethacin, methotrexate, penicillamine, sulphalasine), megaloblastic anaemia, Felty's syndrome.

Systemic manifestations: Pulmonary (pleural effusions, fibrosing alveolitis, obliterative bronchiolitis, Caplan's nodules), eyes (secondary Sjogren's, scleritis), neurological (carpal tunnel syndrome, atlanto-axial sublaxation, peripheral neuropathy), haematological (Felty's syndrome, all types of anaemia), pericarditis.

Investigations: Elevated inflammatory markers, radiological changes (soft tissue swelling, loss of joint space, articular erosions, periarticular osteoporosis), positive rheumatoid factor in 80%. The presence of nodules clinically means that the disease is seropositive.

Management: Medications: First-line. NSAIDs, oral, daily. COX-2 (e.g. celecoxib, rofecoxib, meloxicam) inhibitors had been recommended by NICE for those people with rheumatoid arthritis or osteoarthritis who are at high risk of developing serious gastrointestinal problems, but have been discontinued due to adverse effects.

Second line: Disease modifying drugs. Gold salts. D-penicillamine, antimalarials (hydroxychloroquine) and sulphalazine.

Third line: Cytotoxic drugs and corticosteroids. Steroids are still commonly used, as background therapy or large oral pulses. They are also used as intra-articular injections into inflamed joints. I/m injection as flare-up. Azathioprine, cyclophosphamide, chlormabucil and methotrexate, anti-tumour necrosis factors (e.g. infliximab/etanercept). Some trials show dramatic improvement in symptoms and apparent halting of disease progression. Early treatment is critical. Methotrexate is a medication where alcohol consumption should ideally not exceed eight units per week.

Surgery: Soft tissue procedures, repair of ruptured tendons, tendon transfers, decompression and transfer of nerves, synovectomy, arthrodesis, joint replacement arthrodesis.

Life-style modification: Splinting of affected joints, gentle massage, local heat or cold application, regular exercise.

Explanation and education (patient, carer)

Dietary advice (weight reduction, fish oil, fish supplements, primrose oil).

Side effects of NSAIDs: Renal, neurological (uncommon), dermatological (rare, erythema multiforme), haematological (aplastic anaemia), hepatitis, systemic anaphylactoid reactions.

OSTEOARTHRITIS

Elderly patient ± walking stick.

Asymmetrical distal interphalangeal joint deformity with Heberden's nodes (and sometimes Bouchard's nodes at the proximal interphalangeal joint).

Disuse atrophy of hand muscles.

Crepitation, reduced movement and function.

Carpal tunnel syndrome, reduced movement and function.

Extra points: Carpal tunnel syndrome or scars.

Other joint involvement and joint replacement scars.

Prevalence: 20% (common)

Radiographic features: Loss of joint space, osteophytes, peri-articular sclerosis and cysts.

Investigations: In the hand none essential, if there is involvement of the hip, knee – X-ray.

Complications: Pain, deformity, ankylosis, entrapment of nerves, cervical spondylosis.

Treatment: Simple analgesia, weight reduction (if OA affects weight bearing joint), physiotherapy and occupational therapy, joint replacement, exercise for hip, knees, surgery for major joints.

ANKYLOSING SPONDYLITIS

Common symptom: Difficulty in bending down to tie shoelaces.

Key signs: Males more often than females, pain worse on waking, eased with exercise; progression loss of spinal movements, kyphosis later on, reduced thoracic expansion. Stooped question-mark posture, buttock atrophy, protuberant abdomen due to diaphragmatic breathing, reduced chest expansion (< 5 cm increase in girth), increased occiput-wall distance (> 5 cm), Schober's Test (two points marked 15 cm apart on the dorsal spine expand by less than 5 cm on maximum forward flexion).

Features

Iritis 30% (acute, deep aching pain, redness, photophobia, miosis, sluggish papillary reflex).

Aortitis 4% (Collapsing pulse and early diastolic murmur of aortic incompetence).
- Anterior uveitis.
- Aortic regurgitation (4%) "I would like to listen to the aortic valve".
- Apical fibrosis – rare (apical inspiratory crackles; probably secondary to diminished apical ventilation).
- Cardiac conduction defects – 10% (usually atrio-ventricular nodal block; other cardiac abnormalities may occur).
- Neurological (atlantoaxial dislocation).
- Secondary amyloidosis.
- Anaemia of chronic disease.
- IgA nephropathy.

Spinal fracture, cauda equina syndrome, pulmonary mycetoma secondary to apical fibrosis and cavitation are potential complications, as are those related to therapy, i.e. use of NSAIDs may result in GI haemorrhage, and previous use of deep X-ray treatment led to increased episodes of leukaemia and renal obstructive problems.

Tests: ESR, plasma viscosity, CRP (elevated), FBC (a mild normochromic, normocytic anaemia in an untreated patient), X-ray of the sacroiliac joints, lumbar, thoracic and cervical spine. The radiological findings are characteristic, although their specificity depends on the stage of the disease. Radiologically there is bilateral sacroiliac joint involvement, with blurring the cortical margins of the subchondral bone, followed by erosion and sclerosis. End-stage involvement is that of ankylosis and obliteration of the joints. Vertebral involvement starts in the lumbar region, with erosisons and sclerosis producing a squaring of the vertebral bodies. Subsequent involvement of the annulus fibrosis leads to syndesmophye formation and eventual ankylosis of the spine.

90% association with HLA B27.

Management: Physiotherapy (exercise is of paramount importance, attendance to posture throughout the day and night is essential, hydrotherapy and physiotherapy are needed as an initial introduction to a lifelong exercise programme), NSAIDs (needed by around 80% of patients), anti-tumour necrosis factor medications now licensed for this indication.

GOUT

Typically an asymmetrical polyarthropathy.

Key signs: Acute gout would be unusual in the exam, look for gouty tophi of helix of ear and elbow, remember to look at the ears for tophi. Asymmetrical swelling of the small joints of the hand and feet. Joint deformity.

Cause: Urate excess. Secondary hyperuricaemia may occur in drugs – diuretics (thiazides), ethambutol, nicotinic acid; myeloproliferative and lymphoproliferative disease (e.g. PRV, CML); chronic renal failure; alcoholism; obesity.

Differential diagnosis: Septic arthritis, pseudogout, rheumatoid arthritis.

Investigation: Aspirate acute joints and look for crystals, negative birefringent crystals for gout and pyrophosphate for pseudogout; serum urate is normal or raised. FBC, U&E, serum uric acid, urinary urate excretion.

Radology: Characteristic periarticular erosions without surrounding osteoporosis; soft-tissue swelling.

Management: Weight reduction, alcohol and protein intake reduced, stop drugs that make it worse–low dose aspirin/thiazides, increase hydration, high fluid intake, NSAIDs for acute episodes; intra-articular injection of a corticosteroid may be used if necessary. NSAIDs should be avoided in patients with renal insufficiency–colcichines if not tolerated, and allopurinol. Long-term treatment is recommended if there are recurrent attacks, evidence of tophi or gouty arthritis, there is associated renal disease, the patient is young with a high serum uric acid, and normal levels of serum uric acid cannot be achieved by lifestyle modification.

Non-pharmacological management of gout.

Chronic tophaceous gout: Asymmetrical swelling of the small joints of the hands and feet (commonly first MTP), gouty tophi around the joints, ear and tendons. Reduced movement and function.

Associaions: Urate stones (nephrectomy scars).

Cause: Drug card (diuretics), lymphadenopathy (lymphoproliferative disorder), chronic renal failure (fistulae).

DIABETIC FOOT

Ulcer, callous formation, concavity of the transverse arch lost, feet cold, foot pulses not palpable, loss of hair. Factors which may contribute to the production of diabetic foot lesions: Injury, neuropathy, trivial injury is not noticed; consequent formation of callosities at repeatedly traumatized pressure points; small vessel disease; large vessel disease producing ischaemia and gangrene of the foot; increased susceptibility to infection.

ENDOCRINE

Pituitary

ACROMEGALY

This 52-year-old man has had tingling in his hands. What is the endocrine diagnosis?

An Extremely Common Cause

Important clinical signs: Prominent supraorbital ridges, prognathism (protrusion of lower jaw), soft tissue enlargement of the nose and ears, macroglossia with thick lips, thick skin with hypertrichosis, spade-like hand, broad toes, acanthosis nigricans. Broad nose. *Sweaty skin:* Interdentular spaces are increased. *Cranial nerve involvement in acromegaly:* Bitemporal hemianopia, optic atrophy–affection of the optic nerve, external ophthalmoplegia and deafness; *Metabolic features:* Diabetes and hypertension. Coarsening of features. Voice may be husky. *Other features:* Heart failure, hirsuite, hypopituitary, kyphosis, lactation, myopathy (proximal), multinodular goitre in 10-20%. Paraesthesia may be due to carpal tunnel syndrome or a peripheral neuropathy secondary to diabetes mellitus.

Ask the patient if any member of he family has noticed any change in facial appearance, whether there has been any recent changes in the size of clothes, gloves or shoes, whether her/she suffers from headaches, whether there has been any sweating, and whether there has been any problems with sweating.

The scar of previous neurosurgery is often difficult to detect, and sometimes observed only on the gum line. Carpal tunnel scars can also be difficult to observe.

Measures of severity: (a) Blood pressure, (b) Diabetes, (c) Bitemporal hemianopia, (d) Carpal tunnel syndrome, (e) Obstructive sleep apnoea (f) Colorectal cancer risk. Acromegaly develops insidiously and newly diagnosed patients often have symptoms for years.

Signs of activity: Tight rings of hands, sweaty, headaches.

Aetiology: 99% of cases are due to a pituitary growth-hormone-secreting. adenoma; 5% of patients have MEN-1 syndrome; very rarely, ectopic GHRH secreted from neuroendocrine carcinoid tumour.

Investigations include CXR (cardiomegaly), ECG (ischaemia), blood pressure, baseline prolactin, testosterone, LH and thyroxine levels, plain skull X-ray to demonstrate enlargement of pituitary fossa and thickening of skull vault, visual field test (formal Goldman perimetry), fasting glucose, lipid profile, colonoscopy, sleep studies. The diagnosis is confirmed by a failure of serum growth hormone to suppress below 2 mU/L in a prolonged 75 g oral glucose tolerance test and by an elevated IGF-1. When the diagnosis is confirmed, further dynamic tests may be needed to determine the overall function of the anterior pituitary (e.g. insulin tolerance test, thyroid releasing hormone and LHRH test). Consider MRI or CT of the pituitary fossa. Other features: ECG, skin thickness, visual fields and acuity.

Management: Most patients proceed to transphenoidal surgery (transcranial if significant suprasellar extension), by an experienced pituitary surgeon to remove the adenoma. Cure rates of 40-90% have been achieved. Surgery is invariably complicated by early but transient diabetes inspidius. Larger adenomas are difficult to excise. Dopamine agonists are generally not very effective at reducing GH secretion and do not reduce tumour size. Somatostatin analogues such as ocreotide can be very effective at inhibiting GH secretion, but do not cause significant tumour shrinkage. A newly developed growth-hormone receptor antagonist 'Pegvisomant' is more efficacious, normalising IGF-1 in > 90% of patients. External pituitary radiotherapy alone takes several years to achieve GH reduction and often ultimately reduced hypopituitarism and is usually for failed surgery. Radiotherapy is given routinely post incomplete surgery to prevent tumour recurrence and to reduce GH secretion. The greatest decrease in growth hormone concentration occurs during the first 2-year. Measures to reduce vascular risk factors are paramount from the outset.

MEN (multiple endocrine neoplasia) I: Inherited tumours (parathyroid hyperplasia, pituitary tumours, pancreatic tumours). Causes of macroglossia: Acromegaly, amyloidosis, hypothyroidism, Down's syndrome.

Carpal tunnel syndrome: Thenar wasting, weakness of opposition, abduction and flexion of the thumb, and weakness of the index finger and middle finger lumbicals. Sensation is impaired over the palmar aspect of the lateral side of the hand, thumb, index finger, middle finger, and lateral radial border of the ring finger. The palm is spared as the palmar branch of the nerve lies superior to the retinaculum. Percussing over the medial nerve may reproduce the tingling (Tinel's sign). Flexing the wrist for 1 minute may do the same (Phalen's sign). *Causes:* Often idiopathic, occupational trauma, signs of rheumatoid arthritis, gout, pregnancy, osteoarthritis, amyloid, and sometimes there is a family history of carpal tunnel syndrome. *Management:* Rest, splinting, diuretics and local hydrocortisone injection may help temporarily while an underlying cause is relieved. Division of the flexor retinaculum will rapidly relieve symptoms. Sensory function will return over 6-12 months and muscle power, if impaired, may return almost to normal.

GALACTORRHOEA

Prolactin release from the anterior pituitary is normally inhibited by dopamine-derived from the hypothalamus.
Causes of hyperprolactinaemia are:
- Physiological (stress, sleep, coitus, pregnancy/lactation)
- Drugs (dopamine receptor antagonists such as metoclopromaide)
- Hypothalamic or pituitary stalk disease (granulomas or meningiomas causing disconnection hyperprolactinaemia)
- Macroadenomas (e.g. acromegaly) which may secrete prolactin
- Prolactinomas
- Polycystic ovarian syndrome
- Hypothyroidism
- Idiopathic
- Post seizure.
  Men may present with hypogonadism causing erectile dysfunction.

KLINEFELTER'S SYNDROME

This man has a testosterone patch. Why?
Revise the features of this condition. Remember that the patient with the classical form will be tall and have eunuchoidal proportions (span more than 5 cm greater than height; sole to symphysis pubis greater than symphysis pubis to crown); patients are also generally tall. The testes are small and firm. Gynaecomastia is usually present.

Axillary and facial hair will be sparse. The patient may have obesity and varicose veins. Men are not fertile being azoospermic due to a lack of germ cells within the testes which tend to be hyalinized.

HYPOPITUITARISM

Key signs of hypopituitarism: Cases unlikely to be in the exame but complaing of tiredness and postural hypotension; signs include pallor, fine facial skin, breast atrophy in females and other signs of hypogonadism, reflecting that FSH and LH are hormones lost early. Tell the examiners that your further assessment would include:

- Decreased axillary/pubic hair.
- History of brain surgery or obstetric problems.
- Blood pressure measurement for postural hypotension.
- Visual field assessment for bitemporal hemianopia.
- Examination of the testes for hypogonadism in males.
- Eliciting a history of amenorrhoea in females.

Causes of hypopituitarism are pituitary tumours, infiltration by granulomatous disease, pituitary infarction. Diagnosis of hypopituitarism is by combined anterior pituitary function testing, which may include LHRH, TRH, insulin stress tests with measurement of cortisol, growth hormone, LSH, TH, and prolactin.

Investigations: I would like to know the patient's previous history. T_4/TSH. LH/FSH and testosterone for men. Short synachten test. Arginine growth hormone releasing test.

Management: Hydrocortisone first, thyroxine, sex hormone, growth hormone for younger patients.

ADRENOCORTICAL OVERACTIVITY (e.g. abnormalities of body weight distribution, presence of striae, hypertension, or associated features of Cushing's syndrome or adrenal virilism).

Hyperaldosteronism may be secondary to hyperreinaemia or primary, in which rennin levels are suppressed.

Causes of primary hyperaldosteronism include adrenal adenoma/Conn's syndrome, bilateral adrenal hyperplasia, and carcinoma. Effects include hypokalaemic alkalosis with hypertension, especially diastolic hypertension. Sodium is retained and extracellular fluid volume decreases. But there is insufficient water retention for oedema. Investigations for primary hyperaldosteronism may reveal a low rennin level and a low ambulant or erect renin-aldosterone ratio (screening test). Endocrine causes of hypertension are: Cushing's syndrome, Conn's syndrome, acromegaly, phaeochromocytoma, Liddle's syndrome, glucocorticoid remediable hypertension, and apparent mineralocorticoid excess.

Hirsutism is excessive hair growth, particularly over the face and limbs, in androgen-dependent areas (male pattern). There may be acne. There may be other signs of virilisation. The diagnosis of PCOS rests on a combination of symptoms, clinical findings and biochemical abnormalities. In addition to hirsutism, common associations are acne, obesity, male pattern hair thinning, subfertility and oligomenorrhoea or secondary amenorrhoea. Always consider the possibility of a virilising adrenal tumour causing Cushing's syndrome. Check for glycosuria. Virilization refers to male pattern hair loss and other physical changes including voice change, breast atrophy and clitoromegaly. Hirsuitism may be constitutional, or it may be due to adrenal or ovarian disorders, such as androgen excreting tumours in either of these organs. It may be caused by congenital adrenal hyperplasia. It may be caused by drugs.

CUSHING'S SYNDROME

This 42-year-old lady on the wards at present experienced some weight gain and regularly has a bone scan. What is the endocrine diagnosis?

Signs of corticosteroid excess. The examiners expect: Centripetal fat distribution, truncal obesity, acne, proximal muscle wasting/weakness ("lemon on a stick" appearance), cataracts, ankle oedema, supraclavicular fat pads/moon face, thoracocervical fat pads or 'buffalo lump', protein wasting, skin: thin, striae, wound healing, easy bruising, hirsutism, oedema.

Most patients are on long-term corticosteroids for a chronic inflammatory disease such as COPD, asthma or inflammatory bowel disease or a retinal transplant. Rarely, pseudo-Cushing's syndrome may result from obesity, depression or sometimes alcohol excess. *Investigations:* Many will be iatrogenic in the exam, "Before undertaking further tests, I would like to check that the patient is not taking steroids for another medical problem".

Consider hypertension, glucose intolerance/diabetes mellitus. *Signs of decompensation:* Osteoporosis/wedge fractures, immunosuppression, recurrent infections.

Cause: E.g. asthma, signs of RA (requiring steroids)

Diagnosis: 24-hour urinary cortisol (increased in Cushing's and adrenal tumours). Overnight dexamethosone suppression test. Low-dose suppression test (all cases apart from pseudo-Cushing's, i.e. alcohol/depression and normal should fail to suppress). ACTH is easily detectable in Cushing's disease, and suppressed in adrenal adenoma (secretes cortisol leading to hirsutism and virilization). Ectopic ACTH does not suppress and is high. Circadian rhythm of cortisol secretion is normally lost in Cushing's although can be lost in stress, illness and venepuncture.

Imaging is unsatisfactory as pituitary adenomas may be only a few mm wide. Incidentalomas are common. CT/MRI modalities.

Treatments: Cushing's disease: Transsphenoidal hypophysectomy is the treatment of choice for proven pituitary disease, complications being CSF rhinorrhoea, diabetes insipidus, hypopituitarism, visual field disturbance, recurrent disease; radiotherapy; drugs such as metyrapone; bilateral adrenalectomy if primary evacuation is not possible (which may be complicated by Nelson's syndrome where ACTH levels rise and cause melanin-induced hyperpigmentation). Iatrogenic: discontinue drug. An adrenal tumour requires surgical removal. Ectopic ACTH – surgical if possible, or medical treatment, e.g. metyrapone, aminoglutethimide, ketoconazole.

POLYCYSTIC OVARIAN SYNDROME

This 42-year-old lady, on clomiphene, was concerned about her weight gain. What is the endocrine diagnosis?

The pathophysiology of PCOS is incompletely understood. It is a condition of androgen excess, characterized biochemically by: Raised testosterone and androstenedione levels, a raised LH:FSH ratio with an abnormality in the usual pulsatile secretion of gonadotrophin releasing hormones, normal or elevated oestradiol levels, mild hyperprolactinaemia, low sex hormone binding globulin levels, low HDL cholesterol.

Congenital adrenal hyperplasia are a group of disorders, all autosomal recessively inherited, the commonest being 21-hydroxylase deficiency. There can be a spectrum of clinical manifestations from mild, late onset signs resembling PCOS in females, to ambiguous sexual differentiation at birth. The enzyme defect results in a deficiency of glucocorticoids or mineralocorticoids leading to hyperstimulation of the adrenal gland which can only respond by producing excess hormones from unaffected pathways–testosterone precursors and testosterone.

PRIMARY HYPOADRENALISM (e.g. weight loss, associated with disturbance of pigmentation such as buccal pigmentation).

There is hyperpigmentation, especially of skin creases (palms, elbows), lips and mouth, and surgical scars. There may be signs of other autoimmune disease such as vitiligo, and sparse axillary (and pubic) hair. There is postural hypotension. Ask about nausea and vomiting, and weakness, fatigue and weight loss. Mention that tachycardia would be a critical sign. Wish to know the results of serum electrolytes (tendency to hypokalaemic, hyperchloraemic metabolic acidosis with hyponatraemia, but results may be normal).

A short Synachten test would be the next step (teratosactrin 250 um IM), to determine whether or not administered synthetic ACTH can stimulate an appropriate rise in cortisol levels to greater than 500 nmol/L. The diagnosis can then be confirmed by measurement of plasma ACTH which is greatly raised. Causes of hypoadrenalism include Addison's disease, TB, HIV, amyloid, metastatic, fungal infiltration (histoplasmosis), adrenoleucodystrophy, Waterhouse-Friederechsen syndrome.

Management: Steroid warning card, patients should be taught how to give a IM injection in case of vomiting or coma, hydrocortisone, warn patient about intercurrent illnesses, Medicalert bracelet, Fludrocortisone only if high renin electrolyte problems or continuing postural hypotension.

HYPOGONADISM

What is the endocrine diagnosis?

Testosterone deficiency is becoming increasingly recognised, and is not uncommon. It may be as a result of a specific hypogonadal disorder or age-related decline. It can present in many ways, most commonly as:

Sexual dysfunction, reduced muscle mass, reduced bone mass with an increased risk of osteoporosis, reduced facial, body or pubic hair, small testes, tiredness, depression or non-specific cognitive changes such as poor concentration.

It may be hypergonadotrophic or hypogonadotrophic:

1. Hypergonadotrophic hypogonadism refers to primary testicular failure, often with elevated FSH and LH levels. Acquired causes includes mumps, trauma, torsion, surgery, radiotherapy, drugs (spironolactone, chemotherapy, marijuana) and myotonic dystrophy. Congenital disorders include Klinefelter's syndrome (XXY, tall stature, small testes, azoospermia, raised gonadotrophins, gynaecomastia) and 5a reductase deficiency (androgen resistance).

2. Hypogonadotrophic hypogonadism is gonadic failure secondary to hypothalamic/pituitary disease, usually with low or normal FSH and LH levels.

GOITRE/NECK LUMPS

Examine this lady's neck.

This is most likely to be a 'thyroid case'.

Key signs: Swelling in the neck, scar (horizontal skin crease incision is most common following thyroid surgery), look for regularity/ nodularity/ movement on swallowing, ask the patient to stick her tongue out (checking for a thyroglossal cyst), work out whether the thyroid is diffusely enlarged or nodular, look for other evidence of thyroid problems but most cases but will be well treated in the exam, look at eyes, some examiners will want you to percuss over the sternum to check for mediastinal extension.

Table 8.4: Signs in Grave's disease and hyperthyroidism

	Specific to Grave's	*Hyperthyroidism*
Eye signs	• Proptosis • Chemosis • Exposure keratitis • Ophthalmoplegia	• Lid retraction • Lid lag
Peripheral signs	• Thyroid acropachy • Pretibial myxoedema	• Agitation • Sweating • Tremor • Palmar erythema • Sinus tachycardia/AF • Brisk reflexes

Check for thyroid status in the hands: Increased sweating (hyperthyroidism), thyroid acropachy (pseudoclubbing of Graves' disease), pulse (tachycardia or atrial fibrillation in hyperthyroidism, bradycardia in hypothyroidism), fine tremor (best demonstrated by placing a sheet of paper on the outstretched hands with the palms facing downwards). Check also for loss of hair on the upper third on the eyebrows (hypothyroidism).

Grave's disease patients may be hyperthyroid, euthyroid or hypothyroid depending on their stage of treatment.

Eyes

Features to look for are:
• Lid retraction–raised upper eyelid but the whiteness of the sclera is not visible around the iris (Dalyrimple's sign).

- Lid lag.
- Proptosis.
- Exophthalmosis.
- Chemosis (the venous and lymphatic drainage is disturbed by the protrusion of the eye and the appearance is oedematous and wrinkled).

Types of goitre include diffuse multinodular, toxic goitre, neoplastic goitre and autoimmune.

Optic nerve compression: Loss of colour vision initially then develops to a central scotoma and reduced visual acuity. Papilloedema may occur.

Investigation: Thyroid function tests (TSH and T3/T4), thyroid antibodies (positive in Hashimoto's disease), u/s thyroid (solid versus cystic), FNAC, bloods (calcium is raised in medullary Ca of the thyroid), radio-isotope scanning (increased uptake of ^{131}I in Graves', reduced in thyroiditis). *Treatment:* β-blocker, e.g. propanolol, carbimazole or propylthiouracid (both thionamides). Block and replace with thyroxine. Titrate dose and monitor endogenous thyroxine. Stop at 18 months and assess for return of thyrotoxicosis. 1/3 of patients will remain euthyroid. The dose of carbimazole should be titrated according to thyroid function tests. The risks of carbimazole are rash (1:200) and agranulocytosis (1:2000); the patient should attend for a blood count if they experience a sore throat within the first three months on medication. If thyrotoxicosis returns, the options are a repeat course of a thionamide, radioiodine (hypothyroidism common) and subtotal thyroidectomy.

Severe ophthalmopathy may require high-dose steroids, orbital irradiation or surgical decompression to prevent visual loss.

Both radioactive iodine therapy and surgical thyroidecomy are extremely effective and usually result in permanent cure. Patients will require lifelong thyroxine replacement. Radioiodine is considered to be the treatment of choice. Treatment with radioiodine may worsen Graves thyroid eye disease. The exact mechanism by which it does this may be related to the release of antigens by the damaged thyroid gland in response to the radioiodine. Currently, it is thought that radioiodine should not be used in patients with active and/or severe thyroid eye disease, and in patients with mild eye disease, radioiodine may be used together with oral corticosteroids (BMJ 1999; 319: 68-9).

Contraindications to radioiodine therapy are breastfeeding and pregnancy, situations in which it is clear that the safety of other persons cannot be guaranteed, allergy to iodine, and patients who are incontinent who are unwilling to have a urinary catheter. Risks include early hyperthyroidism, late hypothyroidism and late hyperparathyroidism. Thyroid surgery is expensive and inconvenient, but offers a definitive cure and leaves a scar. In Graves' disease, the indications for surgery include: A large goitre, the patient's preference, drug non-complance, patients who refuse radiation therapy, patients wishing to become pregnant within 4 years, and disease relapse when radioiodine is not available.

Method of Examination

Observe

- Is the jugular venous pressure elevated?
- Are there any scars?
- Are there any enlarged lymph glands visible?
- Is there an obvious goitre?

If there is an obvious goitre:
- Arrange the patient comfortably in a chair;
- Give the patient a glass of water, there is usually one conveniently nearby. Inspect and palpate the gland from the front;
- Stand behind the patient and palpate the gland, one lobe at a time. The patient should be asked to swallow some water, at appropriate intervals.

You should be assessing:
- Size
- Texture
- Mobility
- Tenderness.

Palpate the cervical lymph glands:
- Check for tracheal displacement.
- Percuss for retrosternal extension
- If there is a thyroidectomy scar, test for Chvostek's sign.
- Auscultate over the gland for bruits.

Now perform simple tests of thyroid function:
- Observe for myxoedematous facies.
- Feel pulse (check rate, rhythm and volume).
- Feel palms (sweaty). Look for palmar erythema.
- Ask patient to hold hands outstretched. Look for postural tremor.
- Inspect for acropachy.

- Test supinator jerks (observe relaxation phase).
- listening over the thyroid for a systolic bruit (this hypervascular thyroid is almost pathognomic of Graves; disease) (look for other eye signs above).
- *Observe shins:* Pretibial myxoedema.

Features of Hypothyroidism

Slow pulse, dry skin, cool peripheries, "peaches and cream" complexion, periorbital oedema, thinning hair, goitre or thyroidectomy scar, slow relaxing ankle jerk, pericardial effusion, congestive cardiac failure, carpal tunnel syndrome (Phalen's, Tinel's test), proximal myopathy (stand from sitting) and ataxia. *Causes:* Autoimmune (Hashimoto's thyroiditis) and atrophic hypothyroidism, iatrogenic (post thyroidectomy, amiodarone, lithium, antithyroid drugs), iodine deficiency, dyshormonogenesis. *Tests:* Thyroid function tests, autoantibodies, cholesterol, 24-hour urinary collection for cortisol, pericardial effusion and ischaemia on ECG, pericardial effusion and CCF on chest X-ray. *Management:* Thyroxine titrated to TSH suppression and clinical response.

DYSTHYROID EYE DISEASE

This 42-year-old lady has double vision. What is the underlying endocrine diagnosis?

Investigations: Thyroid function, ultrasound to see if it is cystic, scan–old spots may be malignant, adenomas are usually hot, FNA if there are concerns about malignancy.

Management: Check that the airway is secure – at least tell the examiner that this would be a thought, management is then of the underlying problem – thyroxine/radioiodine, etc. as appropriate to case.

PAROTID ENLARGEMENT

This 66-year-old man with a previous alcohol dependence syndrome has noticed some changes in the appearance in his face. What are the possibilities here?

Ask the patient whether the parotids are painful and the mouth dry.

Ask about dry eyes or the use of artificial tears.

Consider history of sarcoidosis, lymphoma or leukaemia.

Examination demonstrates bilateral parotid enlargement.

Causes: Sarcoidosis, Sjogren's syndrome or keratoconjuncivitis sicca, lymphoma, leukaemia.

Schirmer's test: Filter paper is hooked over the lower eyelid.

Manage patients with artificial tears (e.g. hypromellose) and artificial saliva for dry mouth.

TURNER'S SYNDROME

This 42-year-old lady has had fertility problems. What is the underlying diagnosis?

Turner's syndrome (45XO, XO, XX mosaicism) causes primary amenorrhoea, short stature and delayed puberty. There may be webbed beck, shield-like chest (broad chest with widely spaced nipples and poorly developed breasts), short 4th metacarpals, high-arched palate, numerous naevi, secondary sexual characteristics are under-developed, and widely spaced nipples. Sometimes there is a horseshoe kidney or aortic coarctation. Other features are lymphoedema, hypertelorism, epicanthal fold, strabismus, ptosis, intestinal telengectasia, premature osteoporosis, premature ageing in appearance, higher incidence of diabetes mellitus and Hashimoto's thyroiditis. Examine the cardiological system for coarctation of the aorta and pulmonary stenosis. Oestrogen levels are low with raised FSH and LH levels: Turner's syndrome (gonadal dysgenesis) is the most common cause of primary ovarian failure. Congenital renal abnormalities (horse-shoe kidneys and double ureters) may be present in some cases. Differential diagnosis for short stature: familial, achondroplasia (small limbs, relatively normal trunk, large head bulging), Turner's syndrome, Noonan's syndrome.

GYNAECOMASTIA

Examine this man's chest (observation only), and discuss with the examiners.

Make sure that there is gynaecomastia not excessive breast tissue in an obese person, confirmed on palpation by the presence of increased glandular tissue. Note for height (Klinefelter's syndrome), acromegalic features, thyrotoxic features, Addisonian features, signs of cirrhosis, heart failure (spironolactone), atrial fibrillation (digoxin), clubbing and cachexia (carcinoma of the lung), absence of body hair (hypogonadism, oestrogen therapy), or an evidence of an endocrine disorder. Palpate for a testicular tumour.

Causes of Gynaecomastia

Physiological: Pubertal (very common, often unilateral–due to transient dominance of circulating oestradiol over testosterone).

Senile (normal rise in oestrogens and fall in androgens with age).

Pathological

- Cirrhosis of the liver.
- Thyrotoxicosis.
- Carcinoma of the lung and liver.
- Klinefelter's syndrome (47XXY, small testes, mental deficiency, incomplete virilization, raised LH and FSH, azoospermia, cryptochordism, personality disorders, diabetes, chronic obstructive airways disease: Span > height, sparse body hair, timid behaviour).
- Pituitary disease (acromegaly, hypopituitarism, visual field defect).
- Isolated gonadotrophin deficiency (e.g. Kallman's syndrome).
- Testicular tumours (due to HCG secretion, oestrogen secretion).
- Testicular failure.
- Addison's disease.
- Adrenal carcinoma.
- Testicular femininization.
- Drug-induced.
- Rare (X-linked androgen-insensitivity; also may cause fasciculations in the tongue).

Investigations: FBC, ESR, U&Es (renal failure), LFTs (liver failure), TFTs (thyroid disorders), CXR (primary tumour), mammography, chromosome analysis (Klinefelter's syndrome), HCG and AFP (testicular tumour), prolactin (prolactinoma), CT head (pituitary tumour).

PAGET'S DISEASE

Simply look at this man's face, arms and legs, and discuss with the examiners.

There is enlargement of the skull. Bowing of tibia. Warm. Bony enlargement. Patient may be kyphotic (vertebral involvement may lead to loss of height and kyphosis from disc degeneration and verebral collapse). Occurs in 3% of population over 70. Bone pain, headaches, tinnitus and vertigo. Deafness (conductive) – look for hearing aid. Cardiac failure (high-output), entrapment neuropathies; optic atrophy and angioid streaks.

Symptoms: Usually asymptomatic, bone pain and tenderness (2%).

Investigations: Grossly elevated serum alkaline phosphatase, urinary hydroxyproline elevated.

Calcium and phosphate usually normal.

High serum uric acid and high ESR.

Radiology: "moth-eaten" appearance on plain films (*osteoporosis circumscripta*).

Bone scans (increased uptake).

Other complications: Urolithiasis, sarcoma.

Causes of bowing tibia: Paget's disease, rickets, apparent bowing, congenital syphilis, yaws.

OSTEOMALACIA

This 42-year-old lady who is an Indian lady with coeliac disease has been under follow-up following initiation of a gluten-free diet. Look at her legs and discuss what may be the diagnosis.
- Legs are bilaterally and symmetrically curved.
- Short-stature.
- Deformity long-standing.
- Diagnosis of old rickets.
- Main causes of rickets/osteomalacia:
- Decreased availability of vitamin D–insufficient sunlight exposure, low dietary intake

Malabsorption: Billroth type II gastrectomy, celiac disease, jejunoileal bypass, regional enteritis, pancreatic insufficiency, biliary cirrhosis.

Abnormal metabolism: Chronic renal failure, liver disease, X-linked hypophosphataemia, RTAs, anticonvulsants, vitamin-D resistant rickets

Miscellaneous: Aluminium toxicity, hypophosphataemia, nephritic syndrome.

EYES

You are likely for this bit to be taken away into a separate darkened room, if you are asked to examine any eyes.

Look at this patient's eyes and discuss the diagnosis with the examiners.

Examination of fundi

It is helpful to have your own ophthalmoscope with which you are familiar.

Most people find ophthalmoscopy difficult because they become lost and disorientated within the eye. It you take the time to position yourself and the patient correctly, you should find it easier to navigate your way around the fundus.

Introduce yourself.

Observe any external signs, e.g. nystagmus may be present in a patient with demyelinating eye disease providing a clue to the presence of optic atrophy.

Instruct the patient to fix his eyes at a point behind you, which is chosen for height so that you are comfortably able to look into their eye.

Ask for the room to be darkened to facilitate your examination.

Use your right eye to examine the patient's right eye and vice versa. When examining the right eye, hold the ophthalmoscope in your right hand and vice versa, placing your index finger on the rotating disc to allow you to alter the power as necessary.

Before looking at the posterior segment start from 50 cm away, and look at the red reflex. This provides information about the clarity of the media in front of the retina, such as the presence of cataracts or vitreous haemorrhage, which will be of some diagnostic help if the retina is difficult to visualize.

Move closer to the eye and look at the cornea, anterior chamber, lens and vitreous in turn. Opacities in any of these media will appear as black spots against the red reflex.

The optic disc (blind spot) is located 20 degrees of the visual angle medial/nasal to the macula (centre of fixation). It also lies just below the horizontal.

Look into the eye from about 20 degrees lateral/temporal to the line of fixation and from just below the horizontal meridian. The optic disc should come into view immediately and you need to adjust the power of the ophthalmoscope to obtain a sharper image. Check for cupping, colour (pallor/neovascularisation/haemorrhages) and contour (swelling/drusen).

If the patient's eyes have not been dilated for the examination, the abnormality is usually located at the optic disc.

Next follow each of the four major vascular arcades looking for abnormalities such as arterio-venous crossings, vessel calibre and tortuosity.

Examine the peripheral retina in the four quadrants by asking the patient to look in the direction of each quadrant. Look for the presence of pigmentary abnormalities, exudates, haemorrhages and new vessels.

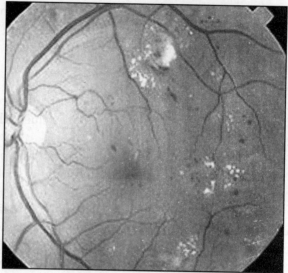

Figure 8.2: Diabetic retinopathy
(*For colour version, see Plate 1*)

Examine the macula by asking the patient to look at the light of the ophthalmoscope. The macula in health is darker than the surrounding retina in colour and free of vessels at its centre. It is located 1 – 2 disc diameters lateral and a little below the temporal margin of the optic disc. The central depression, the fovea, should be identified. Abnormalities in this region will affect visual acuity. Look for exudates, haemorrhages or drusen.

CATARACT/RUBEOSIS

Causes: Diabetes, old age, trauma, metabolic (Cushing's syndrome. Willson's disease, galactosaemia), congenital disorders such as dystrophia myotonica, Turner's syndrome, congenital infections such as rubella or cytomegalovirus, dermatological disorders such as atopic dermatitis/ichthyosis, chronic anterior uveitis, hypoparahyroidism, radiation, myotonic dystrophy, retinitis pigmentosa, steroid therapy, chlorpromazine, chloroquine.

DIABETIC RETINOPATHY

This 58-year-old woman has had insulin-dependent diabetes mellitus (IDDM) for the past 12-years. Examine her fundi to establish whether or not she has retinopathy and discuss her further management in the light of your findings (Figure 8.2).

An Extremely Common Cause

Signs

Early background retinopathy (mild non-proliferative diabetic retinopathy) microaneurysms, sparse scattered haemorrhages, few hard exudates. Routine 13-week referral time to eye-clinic, annual follow-up.

Moderate non-proliferative diabetic retinopathy: Hard exudatives. 6 weeks referral. Focal laser treatment. 3 months follow-up.

Maculopathy: Clinically significant macular oedema (CSME), ischaemic maculopathy (untreatable), CSME, which appears as retinal thickening, is difficult to appreciate without the aid of binocular vision. Warning signs include hard exudates (circinate if in the form of rings), which indicate oedema and multiple haemorrhages indicating the presence of ischaemia.

Severe non-proliferative: >20 intra-retinal haemorrhages in each of the 4 quadrants, venous beading in 2+ quadrants, intraretinal abnormalities in 1+ quadrant. 6 weeks referral time and 3 week month follow-up.

Proliferative retinopathy: One or more of the following: Neovascularization of the retina, optic nerve or iris; vitreous haemorrhage; pre-retinal haemorrhage ± retinal detachment ± fibrous tissue adherent to vitreous face of the retina. 2 weeks referral time and 2 month follow-up.

Investigations

- Ordinary eye exam–May not detect non-advanced cases.
- Dilated eye exam.
- Eye test (vision test)–Only detects very advanced cases of retinopathy
- Dye test (fluorescein angiogram)–This is a special eye test that shows retinal circulation.
- Amsler grid–A special test that helps you identify what parts of your visual field are damaged.
- Slit lamp examination–Often does as part of a dilated eye exam. This test examines the front or back of the eye.
- Colour fundus photography examination (dilated). A form of photography of the retina.
- Eye ultrasound test (ultrasonography). A rarely used test that is mainly used when there is a vitreous haemorrhage or cataract that makes a visual dilated eye checkup not possible.

Non-mydiatric camera. A new form of retinal examination for retinopathy that does not require pupil dilation.

Management

Accelerated deterioration occurs in poor diabetic control, hypertension and pregnancy.

Control blood sugars (lower blood sugar HBA1c <7.5% is associated with less retinopathy), quit smoking, control blood pressure (BP < 140/80 improves micro- and macrovascular complication rates), laser eye surgery, laser photocoagulation, scatter photocoagulation or panretinal photocoagulation which usually avoids the macular region (prevents the ischaemic retinal cells secreting angiogenesis factors causing neovascularization), focal photocoagulation: A focussed attack on certain retinal areas.

(Indications: Maculopathy, proliferative and pre-proliferative diabetic retinopathy).

DCCT trial was a 6½ year study into the effects of tight glucose control on microvascular complications in type I diabetes patients. Patients maintained on intensive insulin regimen showed 54% reduction in retinopathy.

Table 8.5: Summary table of referral speed for diabetic retinopathy in the UK, at time of publication

Immediately (1 day)	Urgently (1 week)	Soon (4 weeks)
Sudden loss of vision Retinal detachment	New vessel formation Preretinal and/or vitreous haemorrhage Rubeosis iridis	Unexplained drop in visual acuity Hard exudates within 1 disc diameter of the fovea Macular oedema Unexplained retinal findings Pre-proliferative or more advanced (severe) retinopathy.

PAPILLOEDEMA

Features: Bilateral, disk hyperaemia, indistinct margins, absence of spontaneous venous pulsation, dilated veins, splinter haemorrhages, cotton wool spots, hard exudates, optic atrophy (late stage). *Causes:* Intra-cranial space-occupying lesion, tumour, abscess, haematoma, benign intracranial hypertension; meningitis; hypercapnoea; sinus thrombosis. Optic disc swelling causes include ischaemic optic neuropathy, accelerated (malignant) hypertension, pseudopapilloedema; central retinal vein thrombosis. cavernous hypoparathyroidism; severe anaemia; Guillain-Barré syndrome, Paget's disease, Hurler's syndrome, poisoining with vitamin A, tetracyclines, ocular toxoplasmosis, cereberal anoxia, aqueduct stenosus.

OLD CHOROIDORETINITIS

Scars of old choroidoretinitis appear as well-defined white patches (where the retina is atrophic) with pigmented edges (due to proliferation of the retinal pigment epithelium). The blood vessels can be seen to pass over the lesions undisturbed. Differential diagnosis of the pigmented retina include normal racial variant, malignant melanoma, retinitis pigmentosa, scans of panretinal photocoagulation. Causes of choroidoretinitis include cytomegalovirus, congenital toxoplasmosis, toxocara, AIDS, sarcoidosis, Behcet's disease, TB, syphilis.

DYSTHYROID EYE DISEASE

Key signs: Exopthalmos, look from above in the plane of the forehead; look for opthalmoplegia; if allowed check for other signs of hyperthyroidism; visual acuity.

Investigations: Those for thyroid function, visual acuity, MRI of orbit.

Management: If affecting vision, surgical help is critical. Control hyperthyroidism but this will not necessarily help eyes. Long-term supervision – eye drops/lid surgery/etc. to protect cornea.

OCULAR PALSY AND NYSTAGMUS (SEE NEUROLOGY)

Key signs: III ptosis, large pupil, eye down and out, IV diplopia on looking down and in, VI horizontal diplopia on looking out.

Investigations: Are for underlying cause, III–diabetes, temporal arteritis, posterior communicating artery aneurysm and tumours which are more likely to enlarge the pupil and therefore less common in the exam, IV- trauma history, VI alone Wernicke's, false localizing sign with raised intracranial pressure, pontine stroke (unlikely in the exam).

OPTIC ATROPHY

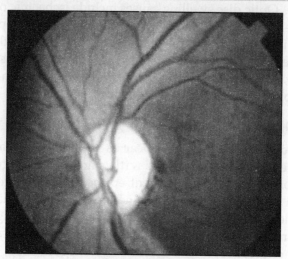

Figure 8.3: Optic atrophy
(For colour version, see Plate 1)

Degeneration of the nerve fibre bundles of the optic nerve and their replacement by glial cells leads to the pale appearance of the optic disc. Certain characteristics can give a clue as to the cause. In optic nerve disease (primary optic atrophy), the edges of the disc will be well defined in contrast to chronic papilloedema where the edge is indistinct or blurred. In glaucoma, the blood vessels will appear to dip at the edge of a cupped optic disc. Consider also retinitis pigmentosa, central retinal artery occlusion, Foster-Kennedy syndrome (papilloedema in one eye and optic atrophy in the other).

End of bed: Cerebellar signs (Fredreich's ataxia, multiple sclerosis), large bossed skull (Paget's), Argyll-Robertson pupil.

To confirm findings, look for a central scotoma, abnormalities of colour perception, and a relative afferent papillary defect.

Key signs: Reduced visual acuity often severe, pale discs, may be signs of specific problem such as pigmentation with retinitis pigmentosa.

Common Causes

- Multiple sclerosis: May be young, ask to examine the central visual field and the cerebellar system.
- Compression of optic nerve by tumour or aneurysm (pituitary or meningioma).

- Glaucoma (older patient).
- Ischaemic optic atrophy (abrupt onset of visual loss in an elderly patient); examine the pulse and listen for carotid bruits; giant cell arteritis or idiopathic acute anterior ION.
- Leber's optic atrophy.
- Retinal artery occlusion.
- Toxic ambylopia (lead, methyl alcohol, arsenic, insecticides, quinine).
- Nutritional amblyopia (tobacco, vitamin B_{12} deficiency and hyperglycaemia in diabetics).
- Tabes dorsalis.
- Paget's disease.
- Trauma (birth hypoxia).
- Infections (meningitis, encephalitis, neurosyphilis).
  Secondary optic atrophy – secondary to chronic papilloedema
  Consecutive optic atrophy – caused by extensive retinal disease such as retinitis pigmentosa and chorioretinitis.

Investigations: History including family history, underlying conditions such as a demyelinating disease or tumours.

Management: Remember practical issues, aids for poor sight, registration so that patients receive appropriate benefits, is there any underlying problem to treat, if not support only.

RETINAL VEIN OCCLUSION

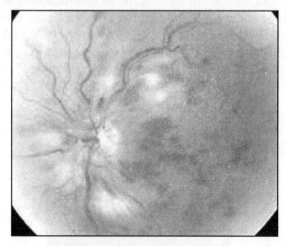

Figure 8.4: Retinal vein occlusion
(For colour version, see Plate 2)

Veins are tortuous and engorged. Haemorrhages are scattered +++ riotously over the whole retina, irregular and superficial, like bundles of straw along the veins. Multiple cotton wool spots. Optic disc swelling in the acute stage. Disc collateral vessels, retinal exudates, aterial and venous sheathing in chronic stages.

Look for diabetic or hypertensive changes.

Rubeosis iridis causes secondary glaucoma (CRVO), visual loss or field defect.

Risk factors: There may be hypertension, hyperlipidaemia or diabetes mellitus, or there may be an underlying hyperviscosity syndrome, especially Waldenstrom's macroglobulinaemia, retinal periphlebitis (sarcoidosis, Behcet's disease), collagen vascular disorders. *Young adults:* OCP is risk factor. 20% can lose sight in the eye due to acute secondary glaucoma.

Management: Refer to an ophtlamologist within 2-3 weeks. Principles of management lie in the prevention of neovascularisation and macular oedema. Flourescein angiography will define the degree of ischaemia and hence the risk of neovascularisation. Retinal ischaemia or macular oedema are treated by panretinal photocoagulation which may decrease the risk of subsequent neovascular glaucoma.

RETINAL ARTERY OCCLUSION

Features include: Reduced visual acuity, a RAPD, the retinal artery shows cattle-tracking, cotton wool spots, cherry red spot at the fovea (this is the intact choroidal circulation which is visible where the retina is at its thinnest and stands out against the ischaemic milky white macula, it may disappear after 2 weeks); in chronic cases there is retinal atrophy, arteriolar swallowing and optic atrophy. Visual field defect, sectoral retinal ischaemia and changes, embolism may be visible.

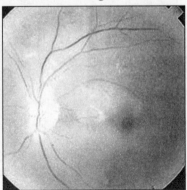

Figure 8.5 : Retinal artery occlusion
(For colour version, see Plate 2)

Cherry red spot differential diagnosis: Sphingolipidoses (deposition of GM2 gangliosidase with the retinal ganglion cells gives the retina a pale colour), quinine toxicity, traumatic retinal oedema.

Extra points: Cause–AF (irregular pulse) or carotid stenosis (bruit).

Effect: Optic atrophy and blind (white stick).

Causes: Emboli from the heart, three types of emboli (cholesterol, platelet-fibrin emboli associated with large vessel arteriosclerosis and calcific emboli from cardiac valves), vaso-obliterative disorders, excessively high intraocular pressure.

This is an ophthalmic emergency. An ophthalmologist must see the patient within 48 hours of the onset of symptoms.

GLAUCOMA

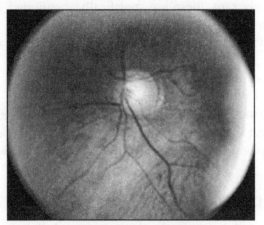

Figure 8.6: Glaucoma
(For colour version, see Plate 3)

There is unilateral visual field defect.

This could be due to a space-occupying lesion compressing the lateral part of the optic chiasma or it could be due to simple glaucoma.

The visual fields are grossly constricted and the patient only has central vision.

Differential diagnosis: Retinitis pigmentosa, advanced chronic glaucoma or diffuse choroidoretinitis. In the early stages, a sickle-shaped extension of the blind spot may be demonstrated and some impairment of the nasal field may be seen on the Bjerrum screen. The problem is when to start treatment in a patient with chronic open angle glaucoma.

In general, patients who have a raised intraocular pressure of 24 mmHg, family history of disease, and those in the 7th decade have miotics (e.g. pilocarpine) aimed at reducing the intraocular pressure, hence slowing the progression of visual failure.

There are three cardinal features of POAG:

- Raised IOP > 21–22 mmHg (> 30 mmHg warrants urgent referral to an ophthalmologist).
- A cupped optic disc with an increased cup: disc ratio.
- Visual field loss.

The pathophsiological changes in POAG have been traditionally been attributed to raised IOP causing damage to the optic nerve head. Increasingly, however, vascular and toxic damage to the optic nerve fibres are thought to contribute.

ANGIOID STREAKS

Whilst relatively rare, these are specifically mentioned in the MRCP Clinical Guidelines.

Dark brown streaks with serrated edges, radiating out from the optic disc.

Deep to the retinal veins.

Darker and wider than retinal vessels.

Systemic associations are found in 50% of patients. Pseudoxanthoma elasticum, Paget's disease, Sickle cell anaemia, Ehler-Danlos syndrome, thrombocytopaenic purpura, Marfan's syndrome, acromegaly, lead poisoning.

MYELINATED OPTIC DISC

A benign congenital abnormality known as medullated or myelinated nerve fibres. Myelination begins in fetal life at the lateral geniculate body reaching the optic disc at birth. In 1% of the population myelination does not stop at the lamina cribrosa but extends onto the nerve fibres surrounding the optic disc.

Features the optic disc contains a white irregular streaky patch. The myelination may extend from the disc and terminate peripherally in a feather-like pattern. It usually obscures the retinal vessels. Look for other clinical findings associated with myelinated optic disc: Enlargement of the blind spot, variable visual loss depending on the extent of myelination, ambylopia (reduced visual acuity in the affected eye), myopia.

HYPERTENSIVE RETINOPATHY

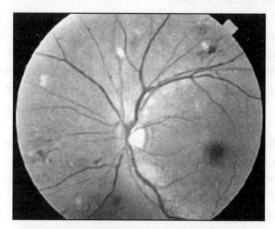

Figure 8.7: Hypertensive retinopathy
(For colour version, see Plate 3)

Keith-Wagner-Barker classification based on the severity and duration of hypertension:

Grade I   Generalized arteriolar attenuation
Grade II   Severe grade I changes, AV nipping, varying vessel calibre
Grade III   Haemorrhages, exudates, cotton wool spots
Grade IV   Accelerated malignant, optic disc swelling, hypertension

Causes: 90% essential, 10% renal/endocrine/eclampsia/coarctation of the aorta.

RETINITIS PIGMENTOSA

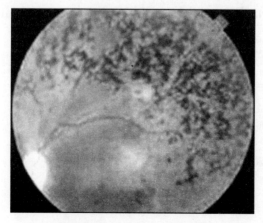

Figure 8.8: Retinitis pigmentosa
(For colour version, see Plate 3)

- Retinal pigmentary changes in a bone-spicule pattern.
- Attenuated retinal vessels.
- Pale optic disc.

The pigment conceals the course of retinal vessels. This is in contrast to choroidoretinitis where the vessels can be traced over the areas of hyperpigmentation. Also look for associated findings of optic drusen, optic disc cupping and cataracts. Look for peripheral constriction of visual fields. You should enquire about a history of night blindness and take a family history.

RP is a slow degenerative disorder of the rod photoreceptors with the cones affected late in the disease. Most are registered blind at 40-years, with central visual loss in the seventh decade. No treatment.

Patterns of inheritance: Autosomal recessive 51%

Autosomal dominant 26%

X-linked recessive 23%

Secondary RP: Phytanic acid storage disorders (Refsum's disease): Eliminate phtates present in dairy products and green vegetables. Look for icthyosis.

Kearynes-Sayre disorder. Look for deafness, ophthalmoplegia and permanent pacemaker.

Abetalipoproteinaemia (Bassen-Kornweig syndrome)

Fredreich's Ataxia

Laurence-Moon-Bardet-Biedle syndrome (polydactyly)

Usher's syndrome

Cockayne's syndrome

Mucopolysaccharidoses (Hurler's syndrome, Hunter's syndrome)

Pseudo-RP: Trauma, posterior ocular inflammation, drug toxicity, following central retinal artery occlusion.

Management: Essential to exclude and treat associated systemic disease.

Index